Cardiopulmonary Medicine from
Imperial College Press

Echocardiography in Congenital Heart Disease Made Simple

Siew Yen Ho
Imperial College & Royal Brompton Hospital, UK

Michael L. Rigby
Royal Brompton Hospital, UK

Robert H. Anderson
Institute of Child Health, UK

Cardiopulmonary Medicine from
Imperial College Press

Echocardiography in Congenital Heart Disease Made Simple

ICP Imperial College Press

Published by

Imperial College Press
57 Shelton Street
Covent Garden
London WC2H 9HE

Distributed by

World Scientific Publishing Co. Pte. Ltd.
5 Toh Tuck Link, Singapore 596224
USA office: 27 Warren Street, Suite 401-402, Hackensack, NJ 07601
UK office: 57 Shelton Street, Covent Garden, London WC2H 9HE

Library of Congress Cataloging-in-Publication Data
Ho, Siew Yen.
Echocardiography in congenital heart disease made simple / by Siew Yen Ho, Michael L. Rigby, Robert H. Anderson.
p. ; cm.
Includes index.
ISBN 1-86094-124-9 (alk. paper)
1. Congenital heart disease--Ultrasonic imaging. I. Rigby, Michael L. II. Anderson, Robert Henry. III. Title.
[DNLM: 1. Echocardiography--Handbooks. 2. Heart Defects, Congenital--diagnosis--Handbooks. WG 39 H678e 2005]
RC687.H6 2005
616.1'20437543--dc22

2004065845

British Library Cataloguing-in-Publication Data
A catalogue record for this book is available from the British Library.

Typeset by Stallion Press
Email: enquiries@stallionpress.com

Printed by FuIsland Offset Printing (S) Pte Ltd, Singapore

Contents

Preface

Echocardiography has probably become the most commonly used diagnostic tool in congenital heart disease, with many a senior physician now lamenting the fact that their younger colleagues resort to the 'echo' machine before they even place the stethoscope on the patient's chest. This textbook aims to facilitate understanding of cardiac malformations as seen in cross-sectional views, notwithstanding that some echocardiographic machines come equipped with software for three-dimensional reconstruction. The variation of structural malformations is legion and daunting to the beginner. With a systematic approach, and describing what we see, instead of speculating on what went wrong during development, congenital heart defects need not be complicated.

This slim volume is the culmination of many years of our short courses on Echo-Anatomic Correlates at the Royal Brompton Hospital. Indeed it is produced in response to continual requests from many of our students. Without their enthusiasm and overwhelming interest in learning about congenital heart defects, this textbook would not have come to fruition. One of us, SYH, would not have found the extra energy to complete this task had it not been for the gentle reminders from many of a series of commissioning editors at Imperial College Press. The patience of Lenore Betts, the current editor, has paid off.

We are indebted to our clinical colleagues at the Royal Brompton for the images taken from patients under their care and to Manjit Josen and Jo Wolfendon who performed many of the echocardiograms.

We are extremely grateful to the patients and their relatives for consenting to tissues and organs being used for education and research. We hope that this book provides ample evidence of the immense contribution that such donations make to diagnosis and treatment of current and future patients.

We also express our thanks to the Cardiac Morphology team at the Royal Brompton for their support. Specifically, Karen McCarthy and Tony Philip helped in the initial phase of collating some of the images and Carina Lim printed final copies. Joy Quek, Senior Editor at World Scientific Publishing Co. managed the project.

SYH prepared all the illustrations and all mistakes and omissions are her sole responsibility.

S. Y. Ho
(SYH)
M. L. Rigby
(MLR)
R. H. Anderson
(RHA)

Abbreviations

AAo	Ascending aorta
AD	Arterial duct
Ao	Aorta
ASD	Atrial septal defect
ASL	Antero-superior leaflet
CS	Coronary sinus
DAo	Descending aorta
HV	Hepatic vein
IBL	Inferior bridging leaflet
ICV	Inferior caval vein
IND.V	Indeterminate ventricle
LA	Left atrium
LAA	Left atrial appendage
LSc	Left subclavian artery
LV	Left ventricle
MV	Mitral valve
OS	Outlet septum
PT	Pulmonary trunk
PV	Pulmonary vein
RA	Right atrium
RAA	Right atrial appendage
RV	Right ventricle
RVOT	Right ventricular outflow tract
S	Septum
SBL	Superior bridging leaflet
SMT	Septomarginal trabeculation
T	Truncal valve
TV	Tricuspid valve
VSD	Ventricular septal defect

1

The Normal Heart

Introduction

Our purpose in this short volume is to show how echocardiographers can demonstrate nowadays the morphological details of congenitally malformed hearts with as much accuracy as the morphologist who holds the heart in his (or her) hands. Recognition of the abnormal, of course, depends on a thorough knowledge of the normal. This is nowhere more true than in the analysis of congenitally malformed hearts. Cardiac structures can often be thought to be abnormal simply because they occupy an unexpected location; yet, in strict anatomical terms, they can still be considered as 'normal'. In this opening chapter, therefore, we will demonstrate the features of the various components of the normal heart, comparing the anatomical features with cross-sectional echocardiographic images. This pattern, of comparing anatomy in autopsied hearts with cross-sectional echocardiographic images, will be followed throughout the remainder of this book.

The Cardiac Chambers and Arterial Trunks

The echocardiographer dealing with acquired heart disease, and the pathologist, usually describe the heart in terms of 'right' and 'left' sided chambers. In reality, the 'right' chambers are more anteriorly positioned within the body (Fig. 1.1), but the convention of using 'right' and 'left' is unlikely to disappear. At any event, in the normal heart, it is difficult to argue with the use of these terms. Problems arise in congenitally malformed hearts, however, since the chambers that would normally be described as 'right' may occupy a left-sided position, and vice versa. The continuing

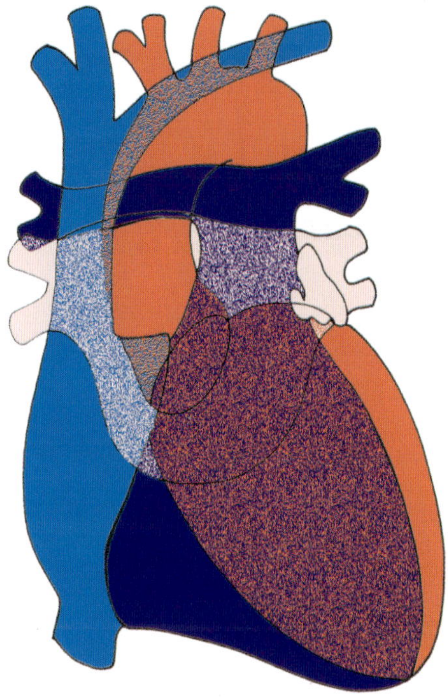

Figure 1.1 There is considerable overlap between the right heart chambers (blue) and left heart chambers (red) when the cardiac silhouette is viewed from the front.

use of 'right' and 'left', when the chambers being described do not occupy these locations, is confusing, but difficult to avoid. The difficulty is overcome in congenitally malformed hearts by adding the description 'morphologically' to 'right' and 'left'. This is not necessary when describing the normal heart. An important feature of the normal heart, nonetheless, and particularly important to the echocardiographer, is that its long axis is not parallel to the long axis of the body (Fig. 1.2). This means that the ventricles are inferior and to the left of the atriums, rather than sitting beneath them as in the St Valentine's heart. The relationships of the 'right' and 'left' structures of the normal heart are further complicated by the marked twisting of the ventricular outflow tracts. The aorta, even though emerging from the left ventricle (and, therefore, a 'left' component of the heart) has its valve in the right-sided position relative to the pulmonary valve (Fig. 1.3). Indeed, it is the appreciation of this central 'keystone' location of the aortic valve which leads to the proper interpretation of echocardiographic images.

The Morphologically Right Atrium

The right atrium, anatomically, is divided into the venous component, the vestibule, the septum, and the appendage (Fig. 1.4). The venous component receives

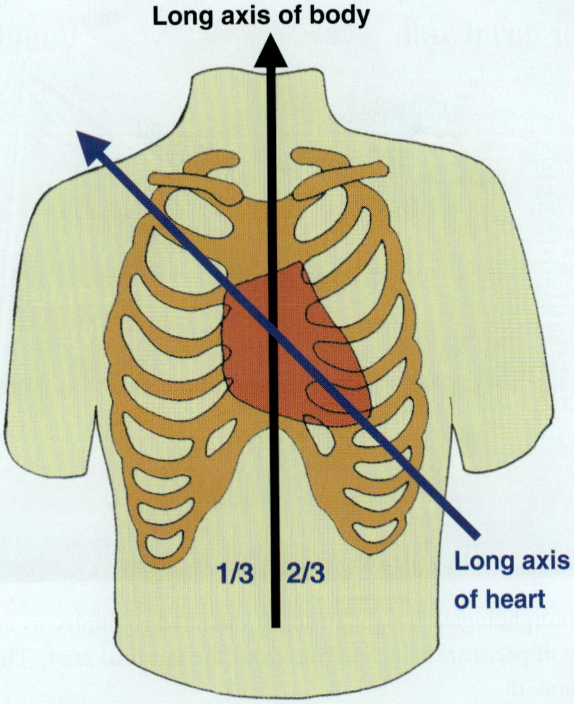

Figure 1.2 The long axis of the heart is at an angle to the long axis of the body. Two-thirds of the cardiac mass is to the left of the midline. The sternum, rib cage and lungs obscure much of the heart when viewed from the front.

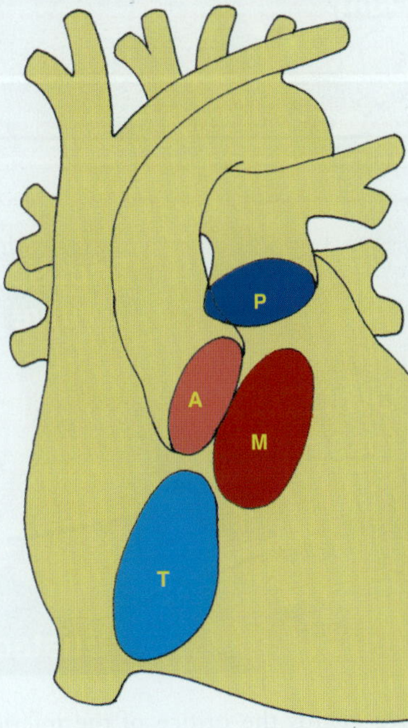

Figure 1.3 The pulmonary (P) and tricuspid (T) valves are well separated from one another. The valves of the left heart, the aortic (A) and mitral (M), are adjacent to one another.

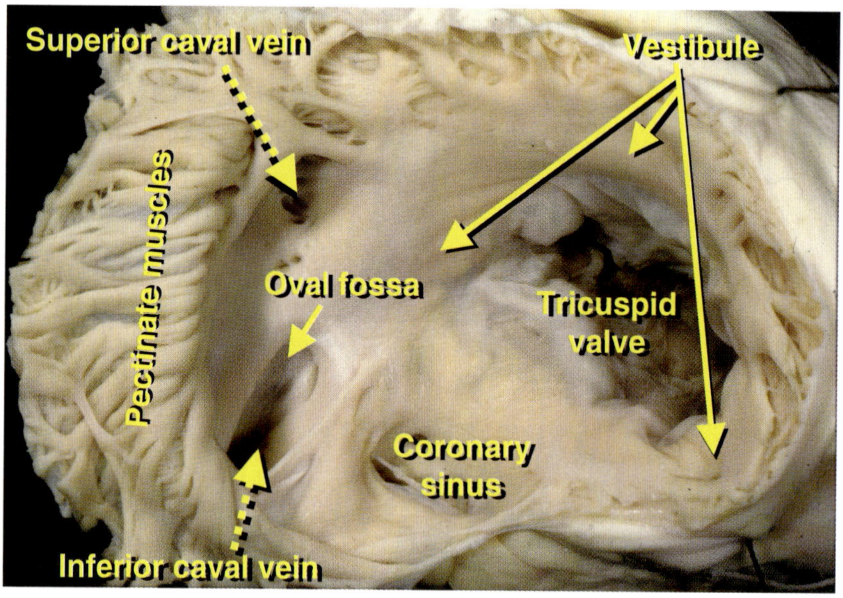

Figure 1.4 The morphologically right atrium is dissected to display its endocardial aspect. An extensive array of pectinate muscles arises from the terminal crest. The vestibule to the tricuspid valve is smooth.

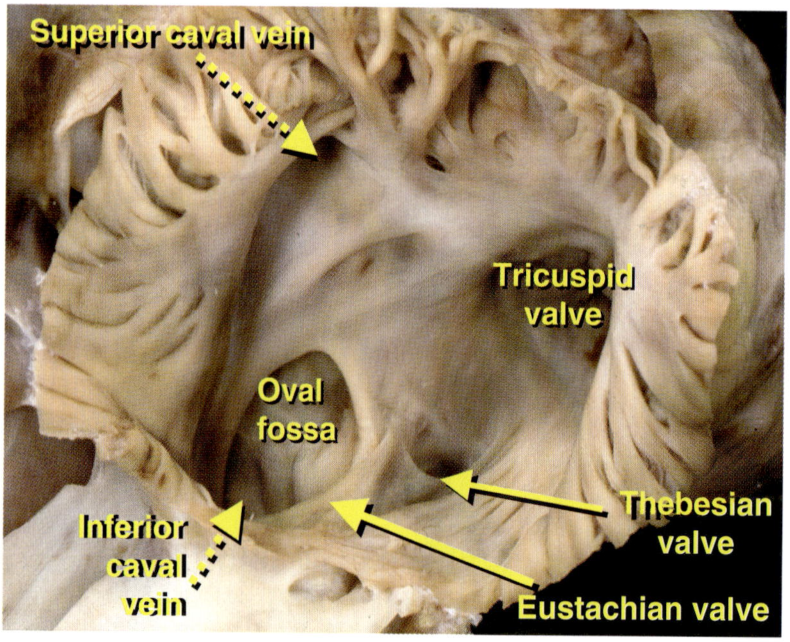

Figure 1.5 The Eustachian valve guards the orifice of the inferior caval vein while the Thebesian valve guards the coronary sinus.

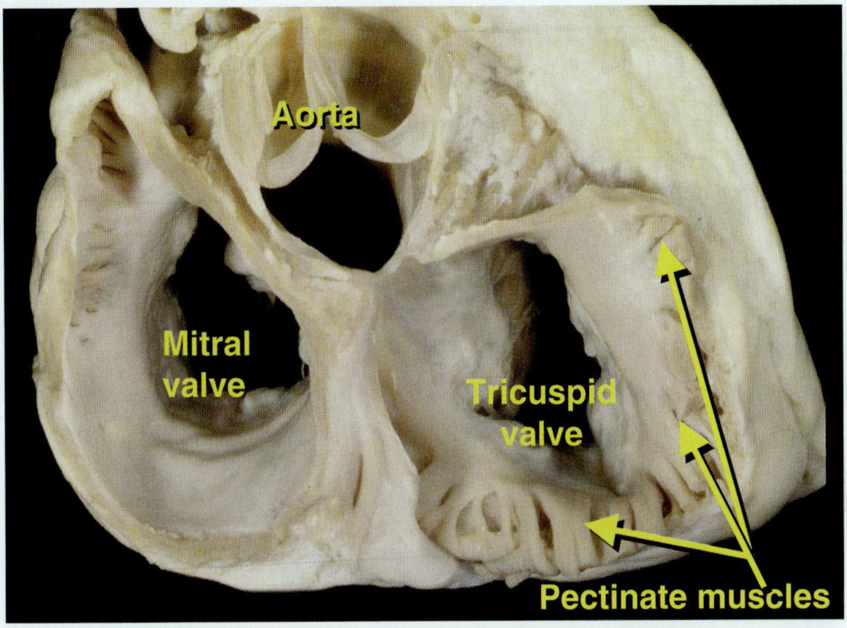

Figure 1.6 This dissection of the base of the normal heart shows the array of pectinate muscles that is characteristic of the morphologically right atrium. In contrast, the pectinate muscles are confined to the atrial appendage on the left side, leaving a smooth left atrial wall.

the superior and inferior caval veins together with, at the junction with the septal component, the coronary sinus. The terminal crest (crista terminalis) divides the venous component from the appendage, and pectinate muscles branch from the crest at right angles to run into the appendage. Fibro-muscular webs attach to the crest in the regions of the openings of the inferior caval vein and the coronary sinus. These are the so-called venous valves, the Eustachian valve in relation to the inferior caval vein, and the Thebesian valve at the coronary sinus (Fig. 1.5). There is a fibrous structure which runs from the union of these valves into the septum between the coronary sinus and the oval fossa as the tendon of Todaro. The most characteristic anatomic feature of the morphologically right atrium is the extension of the pectinate muscles around the atrioventricular junction (Fig. 1.6). The junction between the appendage and venous component is particularly wide. The septal surface is made up of the floor and inferior rim of the oval fossa, the superior rim of the fossa, the so-called 'septum secundum', being an infolding of the atrial wall between the superior caval vein and the right pulmonary veins (Fig. 1.7). The coronary sinus opens into the right atrium having extended through the left inferior atrioventricular groove. We used to think that the atrial surface of the triangle of Koch was also a septal structure. We now know that a fibro-adipose tissue plane separates this wall from the crest of the ventricular septum. The vestibule of the morphologically right atrium is smooth-walled, and supports the attachments of the leaflets of the tricuspid valve.

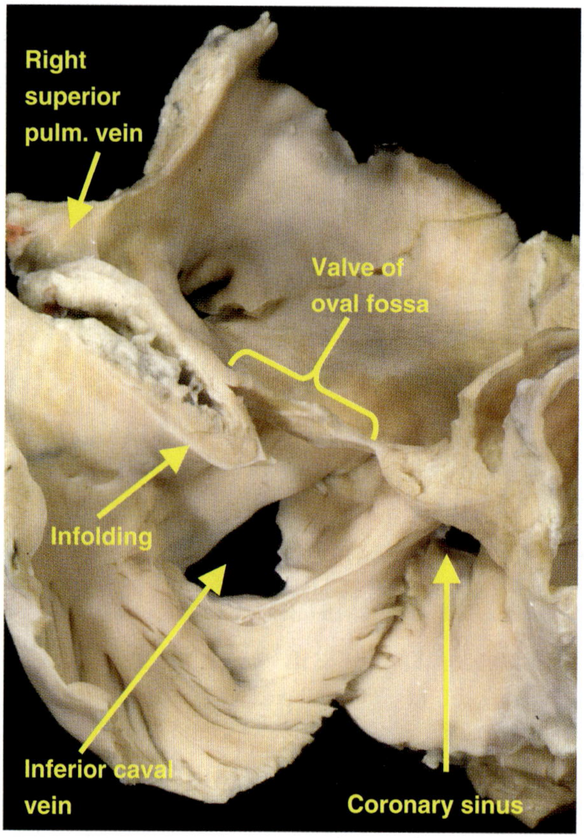

Figure 1.7 This longitudinal section through the heart profiles the atrial septum which is marked by the oval fossa. The atrial septum is not as extensive as suggested by the right atrial view as displayed in Fig. 1.4. The infolding of the right atrial wall ('septum secundum') forms the muscular rim around the oval fossa.

The Morphologically Left Atrium

The left atrium, like its morphologically right counterpart, has a venous component, a septal surface, a vestibule and an appendage. Unlike its partner, it also possesses an extensive body (Fig. 1.8). The venous component, with smooth walls, receives the four pulmonary veins. The septal surface is roughened on its left atrial aspect, and is the flap valve of the oval fossa. The flap valve overlaps the infolded atrial walls (the 'septum secundum') superiorly. Even if the flap valve is not fused with the rim of the oval fossa, there will be no shunting across the septum as long as the pressure in the left atrium exceeds that in the right. Indeed, probe patent foramens are found in up to one-third of the normal population. The vestibule of the left atrium supports the leaflets of the mitral valve and is smooth. The body of the atrium is best appreciated in the setting of the totally anomalous pulmonary venous connection, giving volume to the chamber in the absence of the venous component.

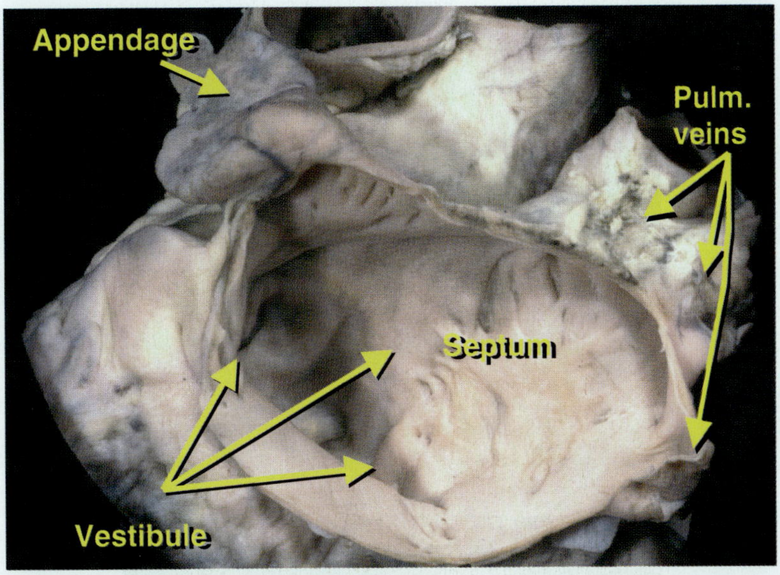

Figure 1.8 The endocardial aspect of the left atrium is displayed to show its relatively smooth wall compared to the right atrium. The flap valve of the oval fossa is the septal area.

The pectinate muscles are much less obvious within the left atrium, being confined within the appendage, which itself has a narrow, tubular junction with the rest of the chamber (Fig. 1.9). Only occasionally do pectinate muscles spill into the body of the atrium. Unlike the situation in the right atrium, they never extend around the atrioventricular junction. The appendage also differs markedly from the normal right appendage in terms of its shape, but this is variable in malformed hearts. It is the morphology of the junctions between the venous components, the appendages and the vestibules which is the most reliable marker for the morphologist to differentiate between the morphologically right and left atriums. It has yet to be established if this distinction can consistently be made echocardiographically, but the shape of the appendages can certainly be distinguished in normal hearts.

The Morphologically Right Ventricle

The right ventricle possesses inlet, apical trabecular and outlet components. The pathway between them swings from inferiorly and rightwards to superiorly and leftwards within the ventricular mass (Fig. 1.10). The inlet component surrounds and supports the leaflets and tension apparatus of the tricuspid valve. The leaflets occupy septal, antero-superior and inferior (or mural) locations within the atrioventricular junction (Fig. 1.11). The most characteristic feature of the tricuspid valve, particularly for the echocardiographer, is the presence of tendinous cords attaching its septal leaflet to the ventricular septum (Fig. 1.12). Another useful marker is the moderator

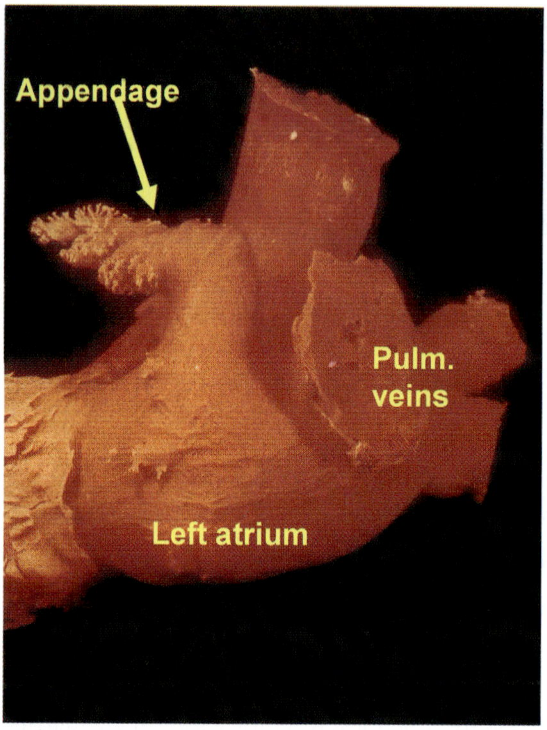

Figure 1.9 This endocast of the left atrium shows the rough region (pectinate muscles) confined to the appendage.

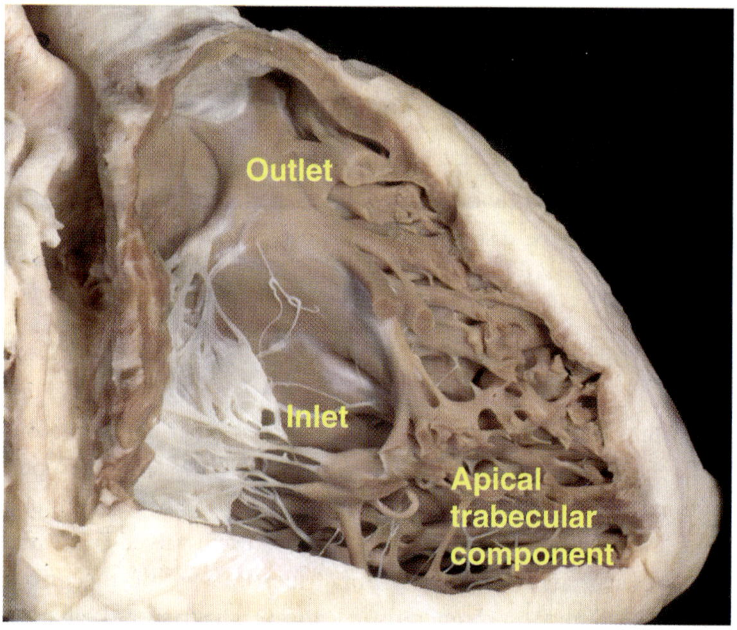

Figure 1.10 The cavity of the right ventricle is displayed by removing its anterior wall. Note the coarse trabeculations in the apical component.

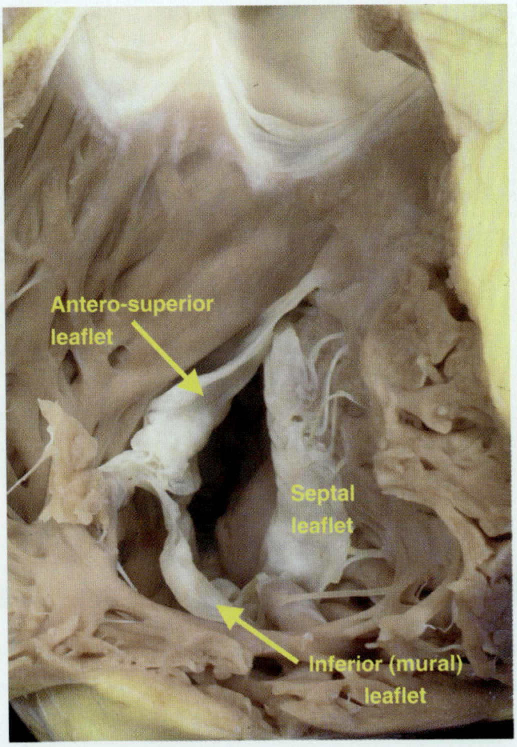

Figure 1.11 The orifice of the tricuspid valve is viewed from the apex of the right ventricle. The three leaflets are displayed.

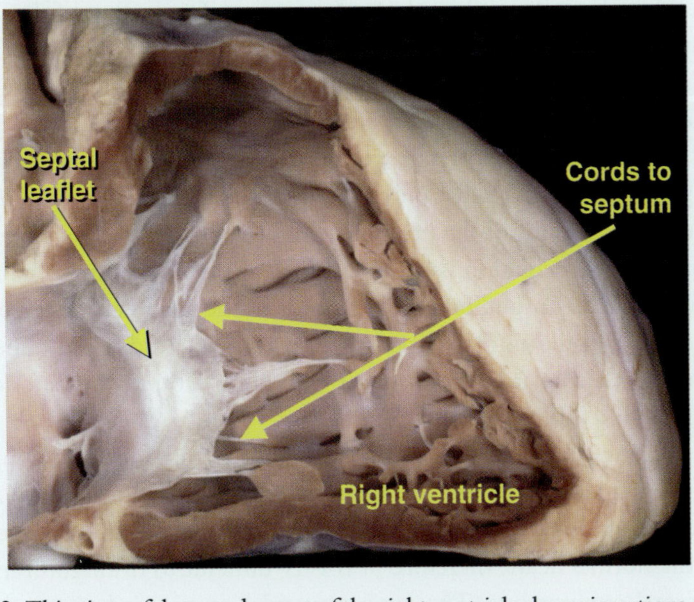

Figure 1.12 This view of the septal aspect of the right ventricle shows insertions of tendinous cords from the septal leaflet to the septum.

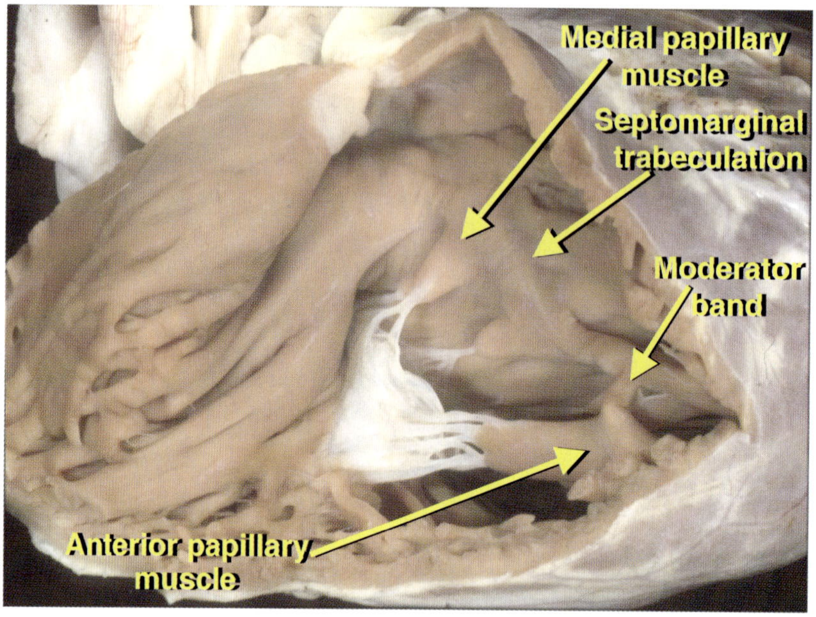

Figure 1.13 The parietal wall is reflected to show the cavity of the right ventricle. The moderator band extends from the septum across the ventricular chamber.

band, usually a broad muscular strap that crosses the ventricular cavity (Fig. 1.13). The apical trabecular component of the right ventricle has characteristically coarse trabeculations (Fig. 1.10). This is the best morphological criterion for ventricular identification in those chambers that lack an inlet and do not possess a tricuspid valve, but cannot always be used by the echocardiographer. The leaflets of the pulmonary valve are supported completely by the muscular infundibulum. It is important to note that much of the 'septal' surface of the infundibulum is, in reality, a free-standing muscular sleeve, which is separated from the aorta by extracardiac space (Fig. 1.14). Previously, we had argued incorrectly that this component of the infundibulum was an outlet septal structure. In reality, only a small part of the infundibulum, namely that inserted between the limbs of the prominent right ventricular muscle bundle called the septomarginal trabeculation, is truly a muscular outlet septum. The rest of the posterior margin of the infundibulum, which forms the supraventricular crest (crista supraventricularis), is the infolded roof of the ventricle. Additional trabeculations, the septoparietal trabeculations, are found extending around the anterior parietal margin of the infundibulum (Fig. 1.15).

The ventricular septum itself has muscular and membranous components, the latter being very small. Because of the central 'keystone' location of the aorta, part of the muscular septum separates the inlet of the right ventricle from the outlet of the left. In the normal heart, therefore, it is very difficult to distinguish inlet, apical and outlet septal components. The entire muscular septum is best considered as a continuous entity.

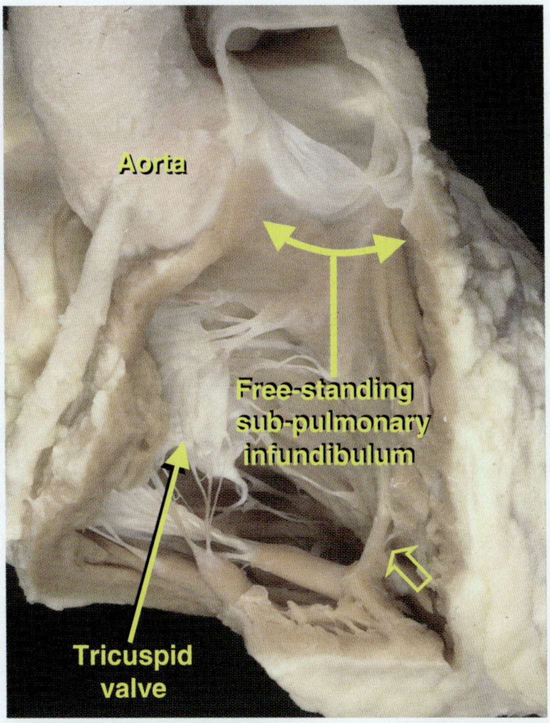

Figure 1.14 The pulmonary valve is supported by a cone of right ventricular myocardium — the sub-pulmonary infundibulum. The aortic root is exposed in this dissection by removing the parietal part of the ventriculo-infundibular fold. The open arrow denotes the moderator band.

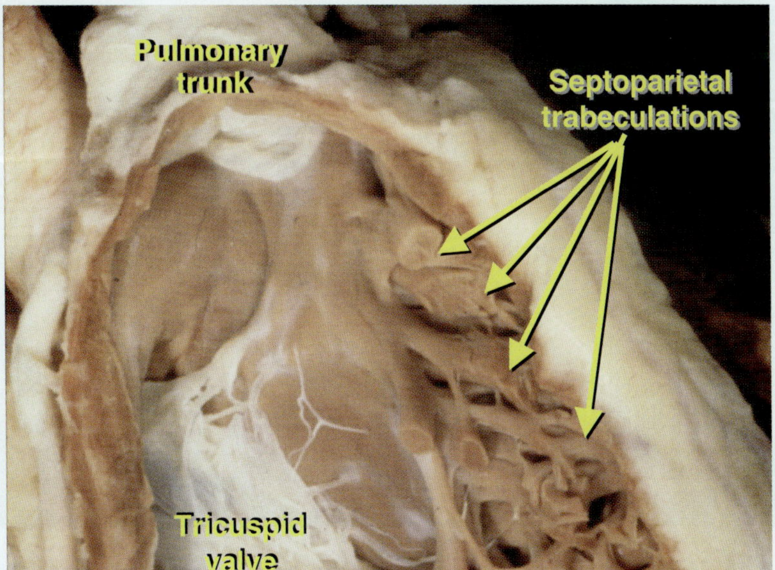

Figure 1.15 Several septoparietal trabeculations have been cut across in this dissection that displays the right ventricular outflow tract.

The Morphologically Left Ventricle

Like its morphologically right counterpart, the left ventricle has inlet, apical trabecular and outlet components (Fig. 1.16). The inlet component contains and surrounds the mitral valve, which has aortic and mural leaflets, so named because of their relationship with the leaflets of the aortic valve and the parietal atrioventricular junction, respectively (Fig. 1.17). The zone of apposition between the two leaflets has antero-lateral and postero-medial ends, the so-called commissures, each supported by one of the paired left ventricular papillary muscles. The most characteristic echocardiographic feature of the mitral valve is that it has no cordal attachments to the ventricular septum (Fig. 1.18). The apical part of the ventricle has fine criss-crossing trabeculations, and the septal surface is smooth. The leaflets of the aortic valve are supported in semilunar fashion but, unlike the pulmonary valve, the leaflets are attached in part to fibrous structures, specifically the leaflets of the mitral valve and the membranous septum, and in part to the muscular walls of the ventricle.

The Aorta

The aorta springs from the centrepoint of the base of the heart and curves upwards to the aortic arch, where it gives rise to the brachiocephalic arteries. The three sinuses

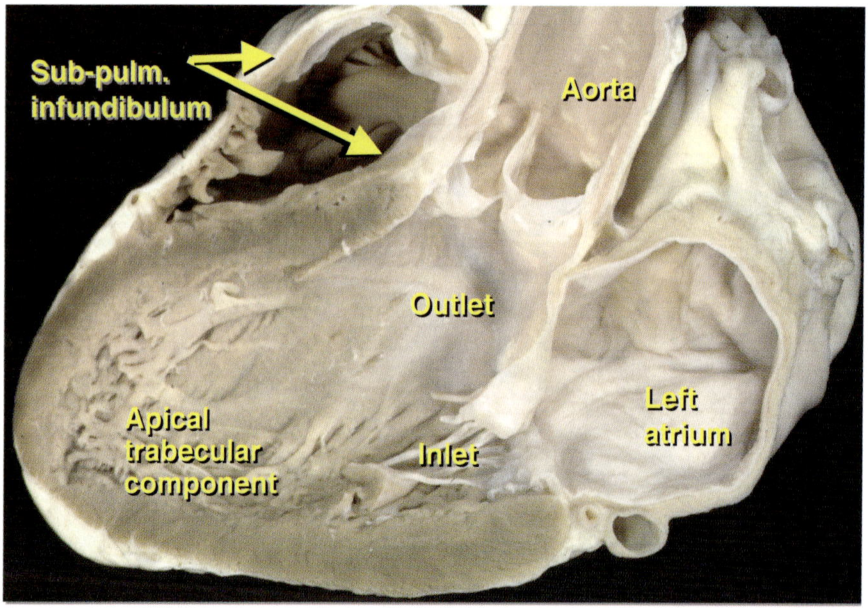

Figure 1.16 This section through the long axis of the heart simulates the echocardiographic section obtainable through the parasternal window. The three components of the left ventricle are shown. The criss-crossing muscular bundles in the apical component are finer than that in the right ventricle (compare with Fig. 1.10).

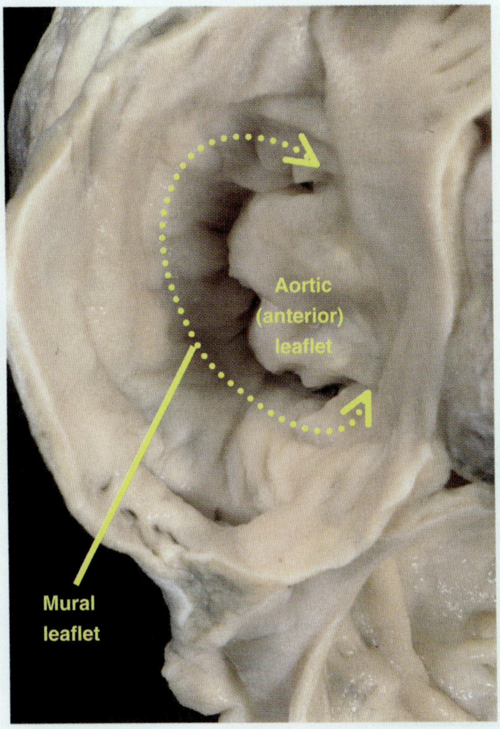

Figure 1.17 This view of the mitral valve from the left atrium shows the arrangement of its leaflets. The mural leaflet occupies nearly two-thirds of the valvar perimeter.

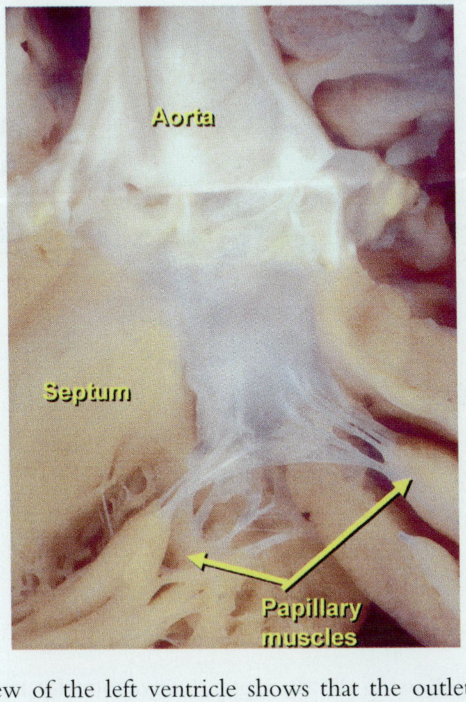

Figure 1.18 This view of the left ventricle shows that the outlet to the aortic valve is wedged between the ventricular septum and the aortic ('anterior') leaflet of the mitral valve. The mitral valve is supported by two groups of papillary muscles.

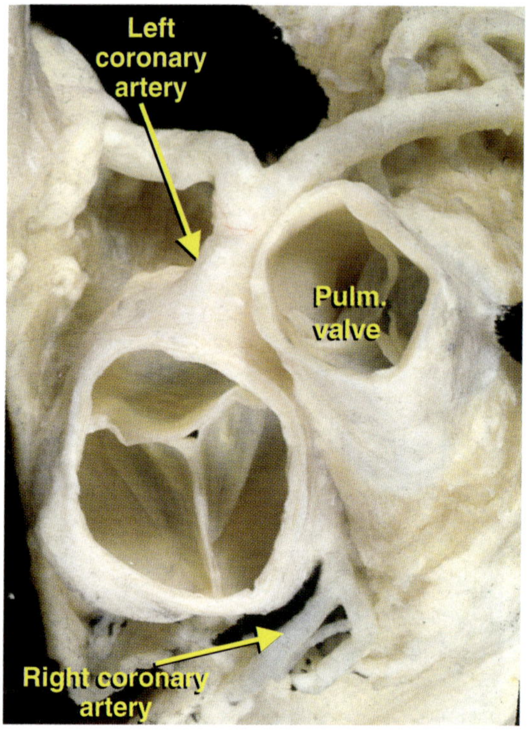

Figure 1.19 This dissection shows the aortic valve and the pulmonary valve. The coronary arteries arise from the aortic sinuses that are adjacent to the pulmonary valve. The non-facing sinus is also non-coronary.

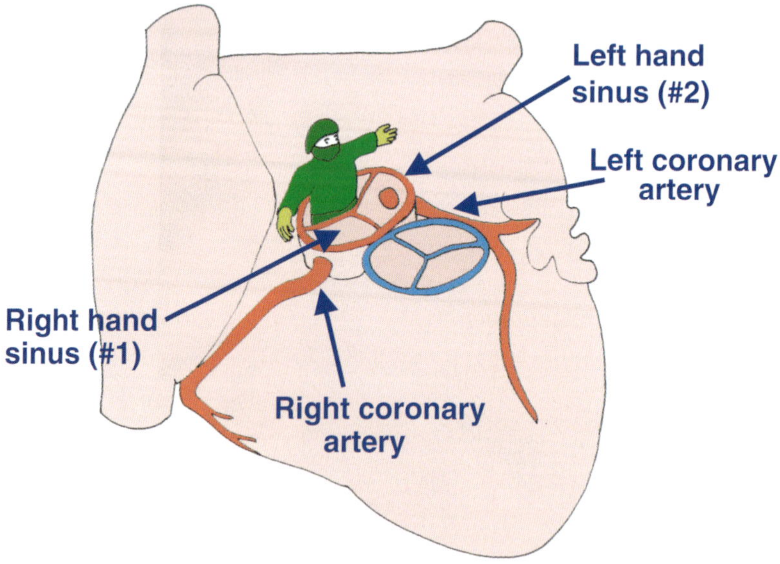

Figure 1.20 Diagram showing the descriptive convention for naming the aortic sinuses by positioning oneself at the non-facing sinus of the aortic valve. The Leiden convention designates the facing sinuses as #1 and #2.

of Valsalva support the leaflets of the aortic valve. Two of these sinuses give rise to coronary arteries. Almost without exception, these sinuses are the ones adjacent to, or 'facing', the pulmonary trunk (Fig. 1.19). Because of this relationship, the sinuses can be called the coronary aortic sinuses. They can then be distinguished as right hand and left hand facing sinuses as seen from the vantage point of the observer positioned at the non-facing sinus and looking towards the pulmonary trunk (Fig. 1.20).

The Pulmonary Trunk

The pulmonary trunk runs from the pulmonary infundibulum, where its sinuses support the leaflets of the pulmonary valve, to its bifurcation into the right and left pulmonary arteries (Fig. 1.21). Two of the sinuses of the pulmonary trunk are always adjacent to the aorta, the facing sinuses, while the third sinus is non-facing. The facing sinuses can again be considered right-handed and left-handed structures from the vantage point of the observer standing at the non-facing sinus and looking towards the aorta. In the foetal circulation, the arterial duct ('ductus arteriosus') extends from the pulmonary trunk into the descending aorta. The isthmus of the

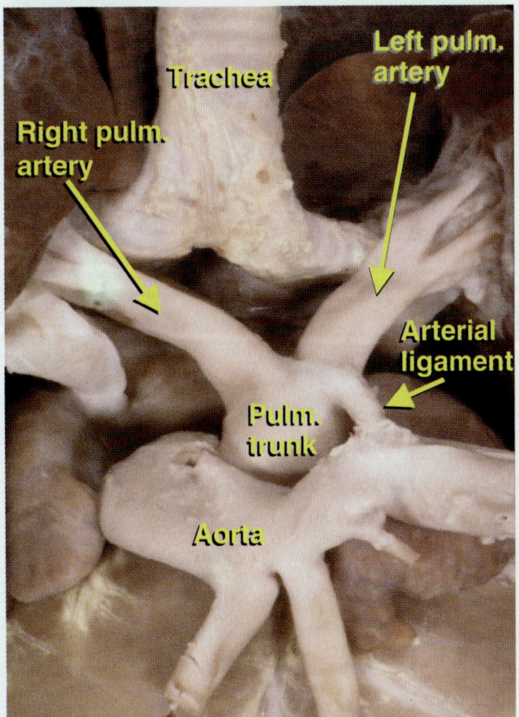

Figure 1.21 A specimen viewed from the front with the aortic arch pulled forward to show the pulmonary trunk and its bifurcation.

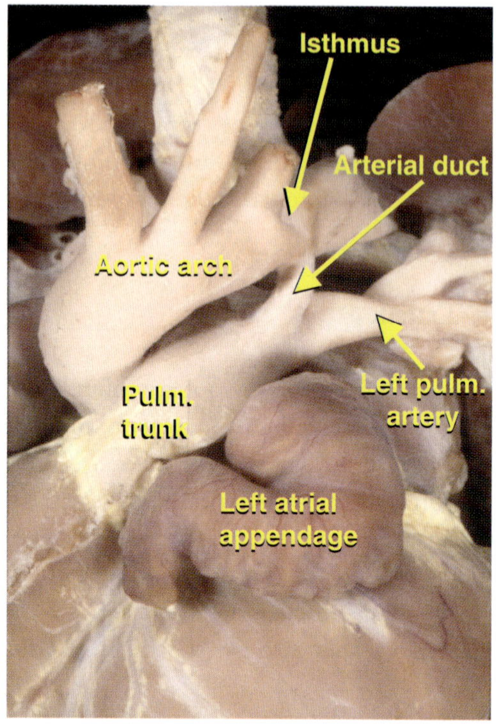

Figure 1.22 The normal aortic arch passes to the left of the trachea. The isthmus of the arch lies between the left subclavian artery and the arterial duct.

aorta is the segment between the site of take-off of the left subclavian artery and the aortic insertion of the duct (Fig. 1.22). Subsequent to birth, the duct closes and is converted to the arterial ligament.

The Cardiac Crux

In cross-sectional anatomy, the crux is an important landmark. The morphologist refers to the crux as the area on the diaphragmatic surface of the heart where the plane of the normal septal structures crosses the inferior atrioventricular groove. The echocardiographer cannot see this point on the epicardial surface. Instead, he/she can identify the echocardiographic crux at the inferior atrioventricular junction. This is the area of the atrioventricular muscular sandwich that we previously described incorrectly as the muscular atrioventricular septum (see Chapter 5). It is the off-set attachments of the leaflets of the tricuspid and mitral valves that produce the cruciate appearance on the echocardiographic image.

2

The Normal Cross-sectional Echocardiographic Study

With cross-sectional echocardiography, the clinician has the technique to demonstrate cardiac anatomy in patients in similar detail as the morphologist with the heart in his/her hands. Complemented with colour flow and quantitative Doppler measurements, an echocardiographic examination by an experienced operator can provide adequate information on the pathophysiology of the cardiac defect. Because echocardiographic images are cross-sectional views, interpretation of the cardiac structures requires a thorough knowledge of the relationships between the cardiac chambers, the great arteries and the veins. We have discussed these relationships, and the morphological characteristics of each chamber, in the previous chapter. In this chapter, we review the anatomy of the normal heart as displayed by cross-sectional echocardiography. With modern ultrasonic equipment, facilities are available for displaying the images in as close to anatomical orientation as possible. The practice of orientating the image with the apex of the heart at the top of the screen is to be deprecated.

There are two portals for imaging the heart with the ultrasonic beam. The most convenient, and non-invasive, is to place the transducer on the walls of the chest or abdomen, called the transthoracic approach. The other portal, via the mouth to provide the transoesophageal and transgastric approaches, is used in cases where transthoracic images are inadequate, and in monitoring interventional procedures.

Transthoracic Echocardiography

Since the bony structures of the sternum and rib cage, together with the lungs, cover most of the heart, imaging from the body surface is limited to a

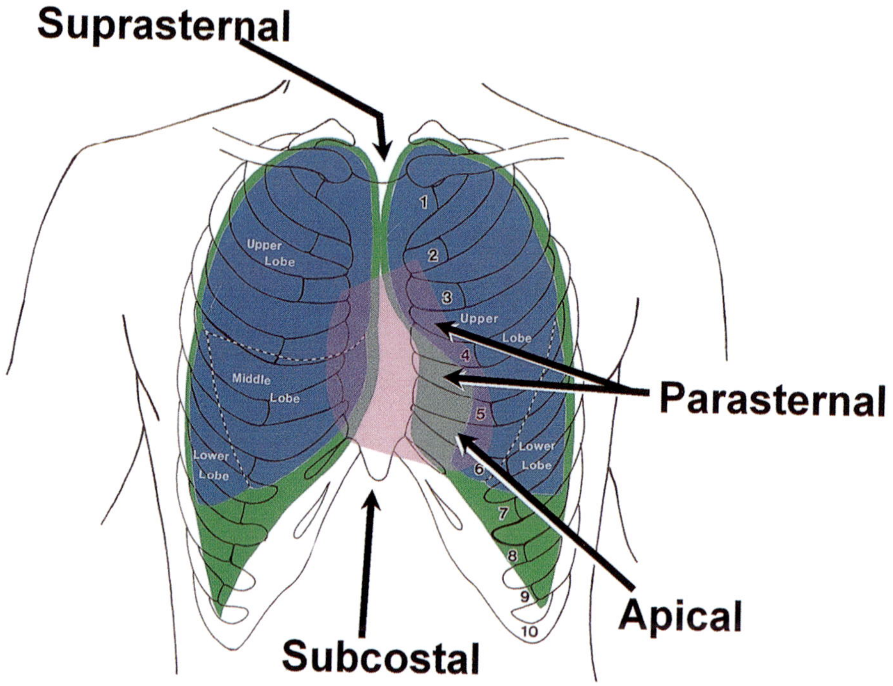

Figure 2.1 The transthoracic approach is restricted to 'echocardiographic windows'.

few echocardiographic windows. Unobstructed views can be obtained from the cardiac apex, from the intercostal spaces (parasternal window), from beneath the rib cage (the subcostal approach), from the suprasternal notch and from the supraclavicular regions (Fig. 2.1). From each of these windows, it is possible to obtain a myriad of cross-sectional planes. Interpretation of cross-sectional anatomy, however, can be simplified by describing the heart, whatever its position, in terms of three orthogonal planes. Since the long axis of the heart rarely coincides with the long axis of the body, the orthogonal planes of the body, namely the sagittal, coronal and short axis planes, do not correspond to the orthogonal planes of the heart (Fig. 2.2). For the heart itself there are again two series of long axis planes and one of short axis planes. From each window, the ultrasonic beam can obtain two basic series of planes, together with intermediate cuts towards the third plane. The basic planes should be used as reference points, and not as ends in themselves. The more views the echocardiographer can use, the greater will be the morphological detail.

The two long axis index planes through the heart are at right angles to the short axis planes. In normal hearts, the inlet portion of the right ventricle is almost at right angles to its outlet portion. Long axis planes through the inlets of both ventricles are conventionally termed four-chamber views. Those at right angles to the four-chamber cuts produce views in the 'two-chamber plane'. The index section also displays the right ventricular outlet, in addition to the left atrium and left ventricle. The 'two-chamber plane' is also one of the standard planes obtained from

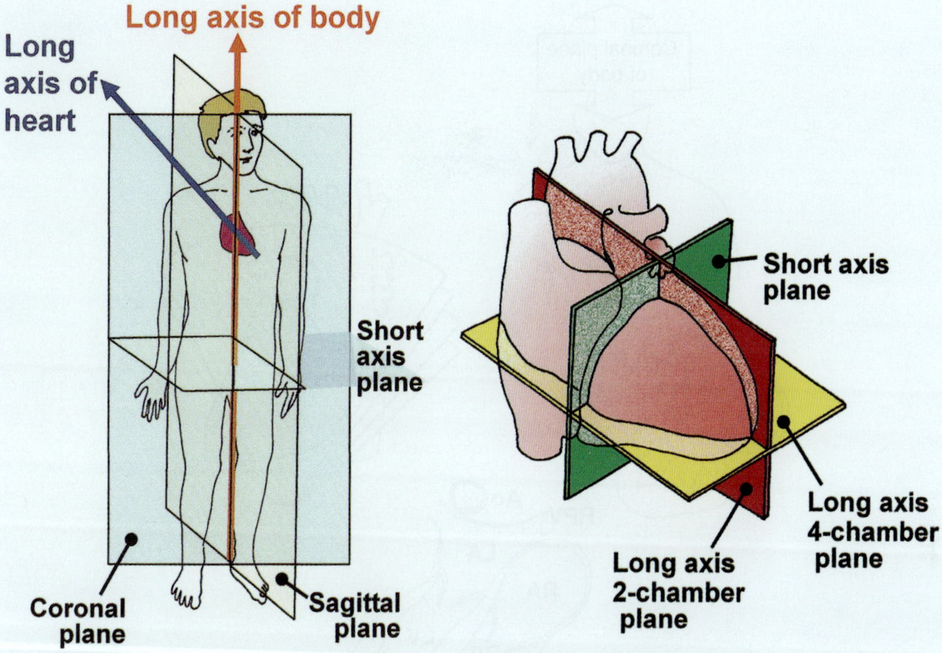

Figure 2.2 The long axis of the heart is at an angle to that of the body. The orthogonal planes of the heart do not correspond to those of the body.

the parasternal window, together with a series of short axis planes. When scanning from the subcostal and suprasternal windows, it is no longer possible to image a normally positioned heart along its own axes. Instead, the heart is cut in paracoronal and parasagittal planes. From a subcostal position, such cuts produce sections that are similar to, but differ in some aspects from, 'four chamber' and short axis planes. The suprasternal window is usually best for long axis views of the aortic arch and the great veins.

To obtain a complete picture of cardiac structures, many views and series of planes must be used. Despite the description of echocardiagraphic findings in terms of 'cuts', it is advisable to obtain continuous scans from one view to another in order to build up in one's mind a three-dimensional picture.

Subcostal Planes

In infants and children, the subcostal window is often the first port of access. The best images are achieved by placing the transducer in the epigastrium below the liver rather than above it. With the transducer directed to the left of the midline, posterior sections in the paracoronal plane will demonstrate the atrial septum and the superior right and left pulmonary veins (Fig. 2.3). On occasion, this plane can replicate a heart with absence of the right atrioventricular connection, even when two normal

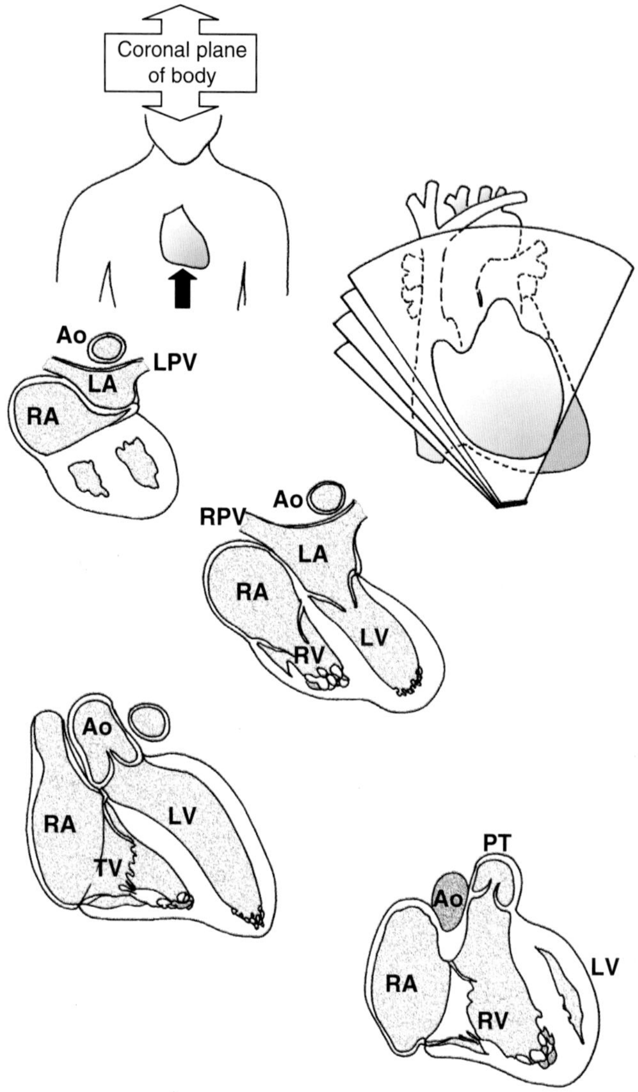

Figure 2.3 The subcostal approach produces a series of sections that approximate to the coronal plane of the body. Ao = aorta; LA = left atrium; LPV = left pulmonary vein; LV = left ventricle; PT = pulmonary trunk; RA = right atrium; RPV = right pulmonary vein; RV = right ventricle.

atrioventricular valves are present. In this series, the hepatic veins can also be traced into the inferior caval vein, and the inferior caval vein then followed to the right atrium. As the transducer is tilted anteriorly, the beam cuts the superior caval vein. Clockwise rotation of the transducer will then image a series of short axis sections of the left ventricle (Fig. 2.4). In this view, the right ventricular outflow tract, together with the pulmonary valve and proximal pulmonary trunk, are seen. Anticlockwise rotation will show the left atrium and its connection to the left ventricle. By tilting

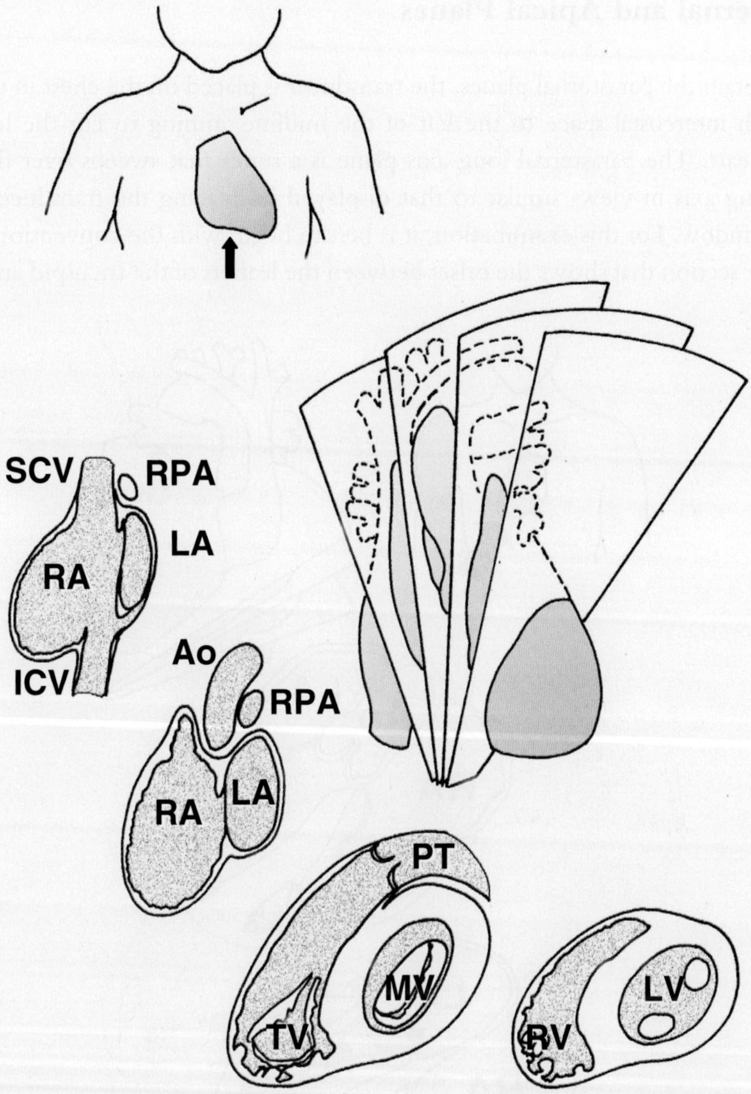

Figure 2.4 This series of short axis sections through the heart from the subcostal approach approximates to the sagittal plane of the body. ICV = inferior caval vein; MV = mitral valve; RPA = right pulmonary artery; SCV = superior caval vein. Other abbreviations as in Fig. 2.3.

the transducer from this position towards the right shoulder, the right oblique section will be displayed. This is one of the most important views in defining abnormalities of the right ventricular outflow tract. Tilting anteriorly in the midline will then demonstrate the left ventricular outflow tract, the aortic valve, the ascending aorta and the proximal aortic arch.

Parasternal and Apical Planes

To obtain the parasternal planes, the transducer is placed on the chest in the third or fourth intercostal space to the left of the midline, aiming to cut the long axis of the heart. The parasternal long axis plane is a series that sweeps over the heart in its long axis in views similar to that displayed by placing the transducer in the apical window. For this examination, it is best to begin with the conventional four-chamber section that shows the offset between the leaflets of the tricuspid and mitral

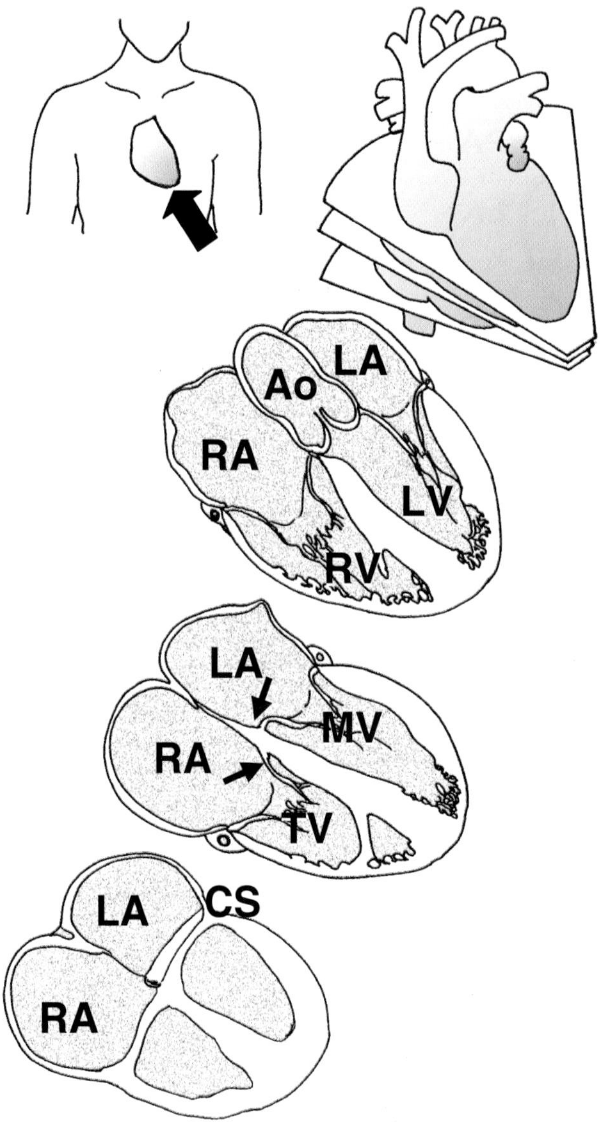

Figure 2.5 The apical approach produces a series of four-chamber sections through the long axis of the heart. Arrows indicate offset between tricuspid and mitral valves. CS = coronary sinus. Other abbreviations as in Figs. 2.3 and 2.4.

valves (Fig. 2.5). Clockwise rotation of the transducer will produce, in turn, long axis sections of the left and right ventricle, followed by the left ventricular short axis view (Figs. 2.6 and 2.7). The short axis view can be used to demonstrate the papillary muscles and the mitral valve and for defining the septal attachments of the tricuspid valve (Fig. 2.7). With slight superior angulation, the morphology of the aortic valve, and the origins of the coronary arteries, can be seen. From the four-chamber cuts, anterior and rightward tilting of the transducer produces the so-called five-chamber view, showing the central position of the aorta (Fig. 2.5). The left ventricular outflow

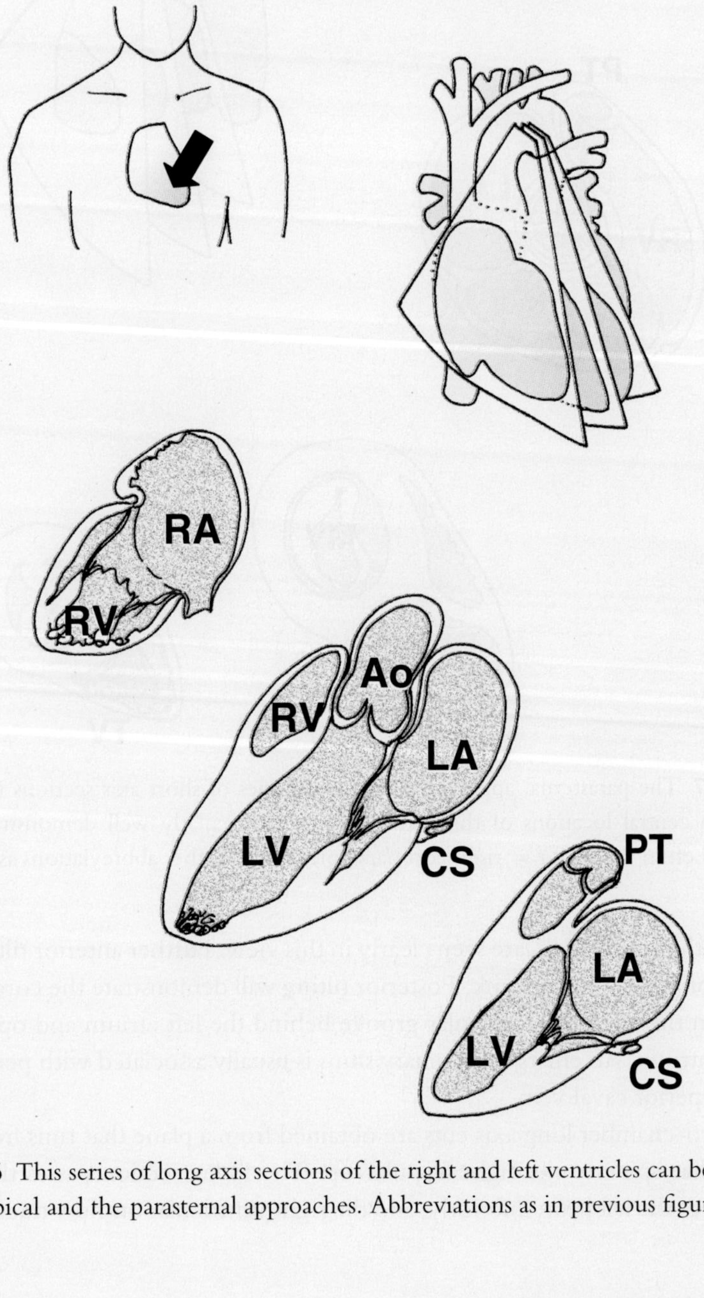

Figure 2.6 This series of long axis sections of the right and left ventricles can be produced from the apical and the parasternal approaches. Abbreviations as in previous figures.

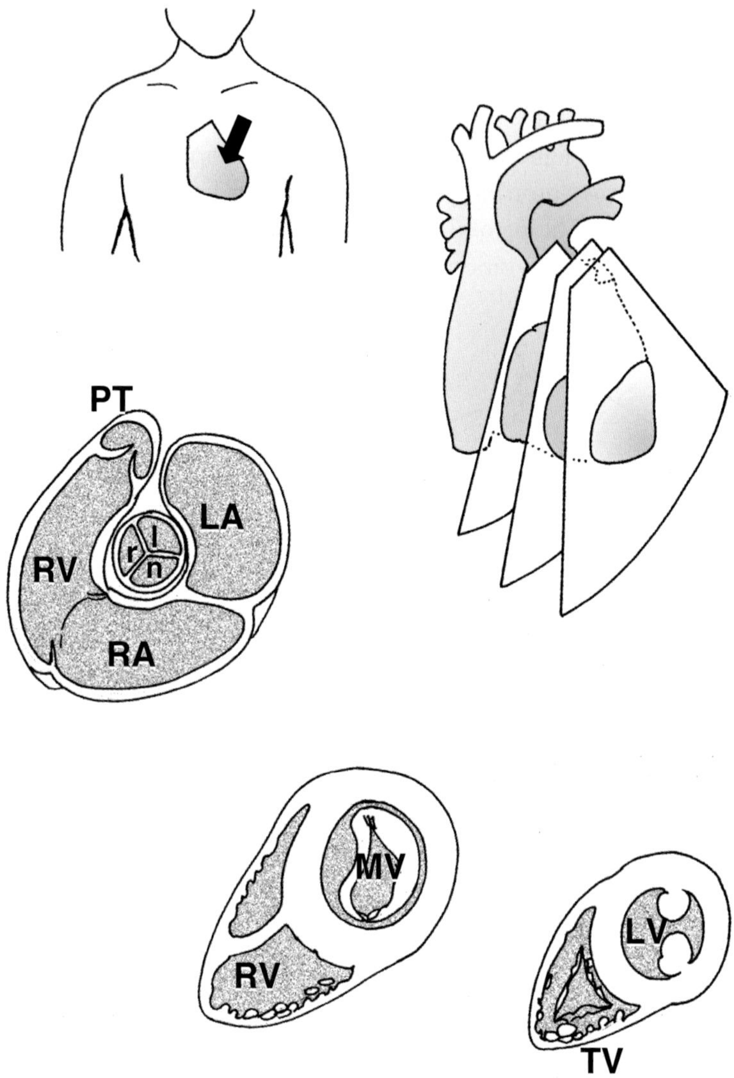

Figure 2.7 The parasternal approach produces a series of short axis sections through the heart. The central locations of the aortic root are particularly well demonstrated in this view. l = Left; n = non-; r = right coronary aortic sinus. Other abbreviations as in previous figures.

tract, and the aortic valve, are seen clearly in this view. Further anterior tilting reveals the pulmonary valve and trunk. Posterior tilting will demonstrate the coronary sinus running in the left atrioventricular groove behind the left atrium and opening into the right atrium. An enlarged coronary sinus is usually associated with persistence of the left superior caval vein.

The two-chamber long axis cuts are obtained from a plane that runs from the left anterior iliac spine to the right scapular tip. The index section passes through the chambers of the left heart inferiorly, and the right ventricular outflow tract superiorly

(Fig. 2.6). The mitral valve, the left ventricular outflow tract and the ascending aorta are also seen clearly in this view. High on the precordium, the left parasternal long axis sections are best for showing the left and right ventricular outflow tracts. When the pulmonary trunk is seen in long axis, the arterial duct, if present, will be detected. Sweeping slightly to the right, the juxtaductal region of the aorta can be seen, important in the context of aortic coarctation.

Suprasternal Planes

The suprasternal notch provides a window for the ultrasonic beam to define, by angulation and rotation of the transducer, paracoronal or parasagittal cuts relative to the bodily planes. The standard paracoronal section will demonstrate, from superior to inferior, the brachiocephalic vein, the aortic arch, the right pulmonary artery and the left atrium (Fig. 2.8). The four pulmonary veins entering the left atrium posteriorly produces the so-called 'crab sign'. Failure to demonstrate normal pulmonary venous connections should alert the echocardiographer to the possibility of partially or totally anomalous pulmonary venous connections. The right superior caval vein is seen to the right. A more anterior section will show the ascending aorta running parallel to the right superior caval vein. Extreme anterior angulaton will display the ascending aorta, together with parts of the left ventricular outflow tract.

Anticlockwise rotation of the transducer produces two index parasagittal sections (Fig. 2.8). One section shows the aortic arch, while the other section shows the left pulmonary artery crossing the descending aorta. Better views of the aorta are sometimes obtained with the transducer to the right of the suprasternal notch, or in a high parasternal position. The thoracic aorta can be cut in its entirety from the aortic valve through the ascending aorta, into the aortic arch with the head and neck vessels, and onwards to the aortic isthmus and the descending aorta. In this view, the right pulmonary artery is cut in cross section, and lies in the hollow under the aortic arch.

Transoesophageal and Transgastric Echocardiography

This mode of investigation is increasingly used to complement conventional transthoracic echocardiography when investigating patients with congenital heart disease. It is especially useful for documenting the adequacy of surgical repair in the early post-operative period, and is indispensable in the monitoring of interventional cardiac catheterisation. It should also be considered in adolescents and adults with an inadequate thoracic window. The procedure should be carried out only by a trained operator. In this section we describe the series of views that can be obtained by directing the ultrasonic beam from within the oesophagus and the stomach.

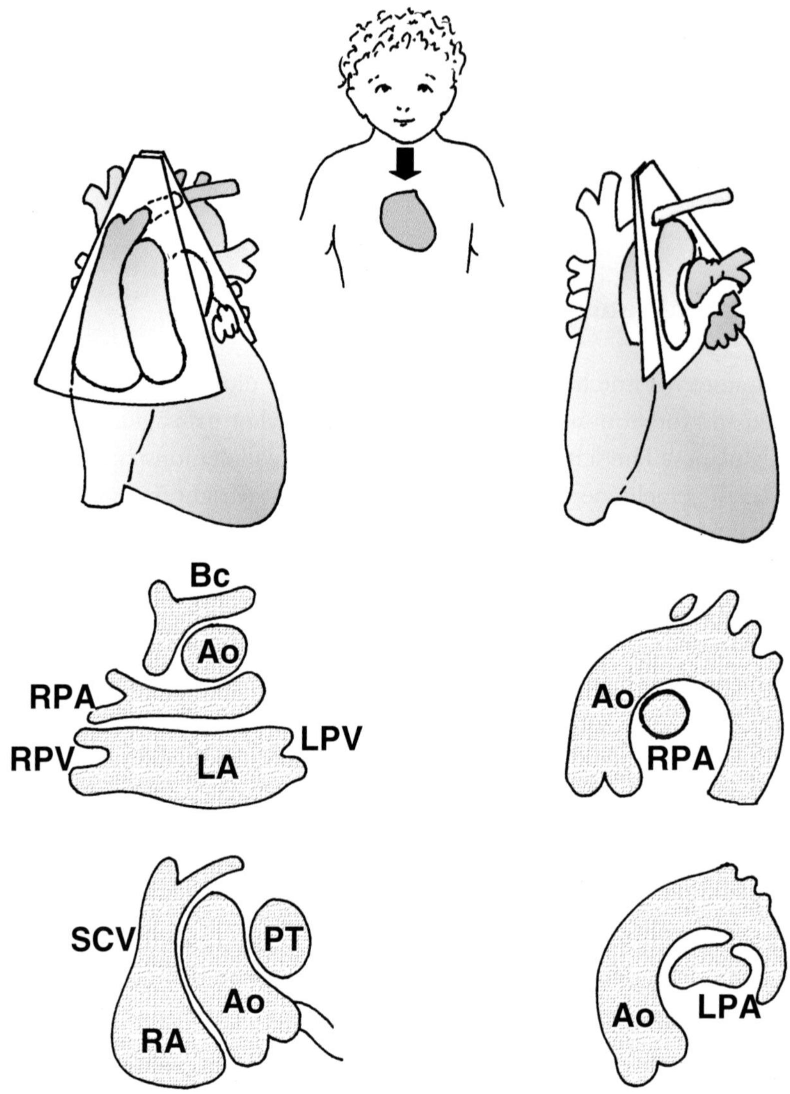

Figure 2.8 The paracoronal and parasagittal planes obtainable from the suprasternal window demonstrate the great veins and great arteries. Bc = brachiocephalic vein; LPA = left pulmonary artery. Other abbreviations as in previous figures.

Transoesophageal Basal Short Axis Plane

These sections are the first to appear as the transducer is advanced into the oesophagus (Fig. 2.9). They show the junction of the superior caval vein with the right atrium, together with the entrances of the pulmonary veins into the left atrium. The distinctive shapes of the right and left atrial appendages are evident. It is also possible, with care, to demonstrate the extent of the pectinate muscles. By varying the extent

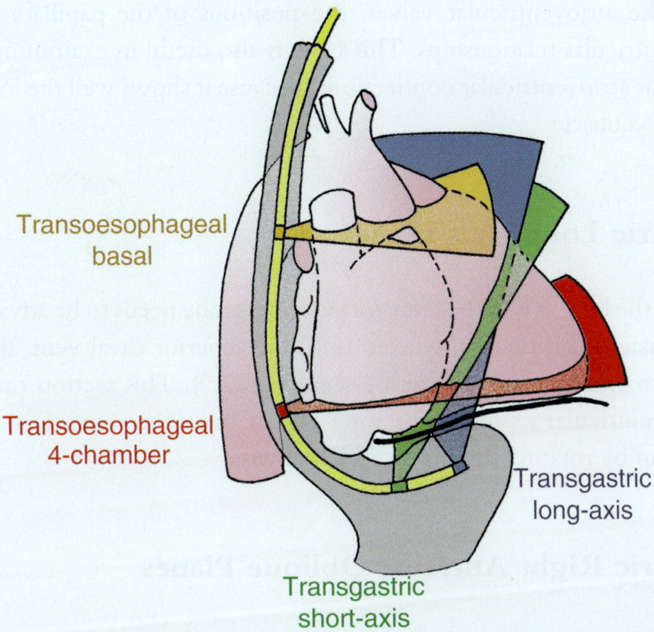

Figure 2.9 The transoesophageal and transgastric approaches allow views that complement conventional transthoracic approaches.

of clockwise or anticlockwise rotation, and flexion and antiflexion of the transducer, basal sections will also display the atrial septum, the proximal coronary arteries, the pulmonary valve and proximal pulmonary trunk, and the right pulmonary artery.

Transoesophageal Four-chamber Planes

From the basal short axis view at the level of the aortic root, retroflexion of the transducer will cut through the left ventricular outflow tract, showing the aortic valve in its long axis. This section is similar to that obtained transthoracically by tilting anteriorly in the four-chamber view (Fig. 2.9). With further retroflexion of the transducer, a conventional four-chamber view will be seen, showing the normal offsetting of the leaflets of the atrioventricular valves at the crux of the heart. This plane can reveal anatomical and functional abnormalities of the mitral and tricuspid valves and their tension apparatus. The coronary sinus running in the left atrioventricular groove will often be seen in the inferior cuts.

Transgastric Short Axis Planes

When the probe is advanced into the stomach, and anteflexed to image the heart from the fundus, the first cuts are through the short axis (Fig. 2.9). These allow analysis of the atrioventricular valves, the positions of the papillary muscles and show the ventricular relationships. This view is also useful in examining hearts with univentricular atrioventricular connections, because it shows well the location of the rudimentary ventricle.

Transgastric Long Axis Planes

To obtain the long axis of the left ventricle, the probe needs to be advanced further into the stomach. It is then anteflexed until the superior caval vein, the ascending aorta, and proximal aortic arch can be seen (Fig. 2.9). This section can be used to display the ventricular septum. The long axis of the right ventricle is displayed in similar fashion by rotating the probe anticlockwise.

Transgastric Right Anterior Oblique Planes

These sections are very similar to the right anterior oblique view obtained with the conventional subcostal approach. They show the tricuspid valve and inlet of the right ventricle, its apical component and outflow tract, together with the pulmonary trunk and its bifurcation.

Transgastric Four-chamber Planes

This is similar to that obtained from the conventional subcostal window. The liver is imaged to show the hepatic veins, and the inferior caval vein is traced to the right atrium. This plane gives good views of the postero-superior part of the atrial septum, together with the superior pulmonary veins. It is useful for imaging the occlusion device used in transcatheter closure of atrial septal defects.

Longitudinal Planes

Using the transoesophageal and the transgastric approaches, it is also possible to obtain sections along the bodily long axis. Longitudinal planes can be used to image the caval veins, the ascending aorta and right coronary artery, the right ventricular outflow tract, the long axis of the left ventricle and the ventricular septum. Because the septum is sectioned obliquely, it appears thickened.

3

Basic Principles of Diagnosis

The essence of simple and straightforward diagnosis of complex congenital cardiac malformations is sequential segmental analysis. All hearts, normal or abnormal, are built from three segments — the atriums, the ventricular mass and the arterial trunks (Fig. 3.1). Congenital abnormalities can be present in one or more of these segments. There may also be abnormalities of the great veins entering, or the arteries leaving, the heart. The basic structure must be described first. Then all associated malformations must be identified. In many abnormal hearts, the associated malformations will be the only abnormality, but it is important in all cases to establish whether the basic structure is normal.

Usual Findings

Each of the three segments of the normal heart possesses a right and a left side. One of the major features of hearts which are congenitally malformed is that these structures are not always in their expected locations. As already explained, we use the terms 'morphologically right' and 'morphologically left' when describing abnormally located chambers. Descriptions will then make sense even when the structures are not at their expected location. To determine whether cardiac chambers are normal, we must look at the features of their most constant components, making use of the principle that has become known as the morphological method. For the atriums, the most constant component is the atrial appendage. The differences between the morphologically right and left atrial appendages always allow us to determine which is which when we are able to view the heart directly. The morphologically right appendage has the shape of a broad triangle, whereas the left appendage is tubular

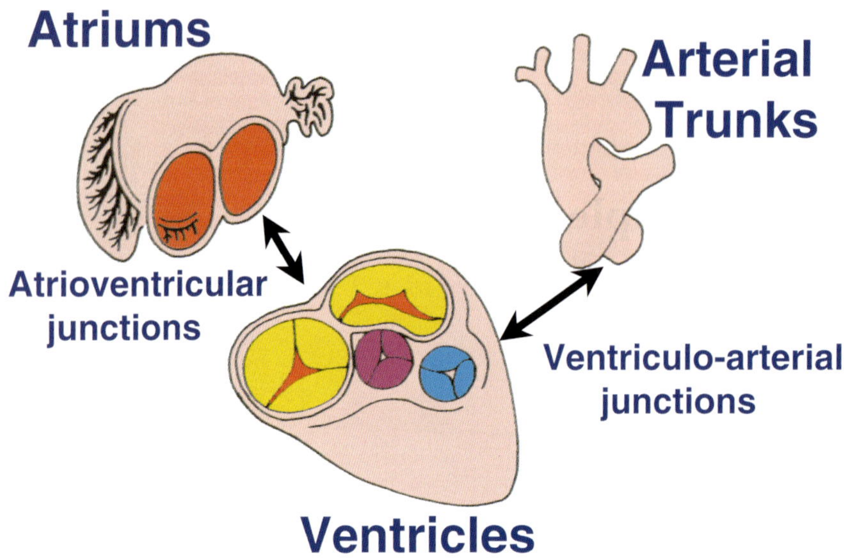

Figure 3.1 The heart is analysed in terms of three segments: atriums, ventricles and great arteries. The segments are connected, or not connected, across the atrioventricular and ventriculo-arterial junctions.

and hooked. Even more distinctive is the junction between the appendage and the smooth walled venous component of the atrium. This is wide, and marked by an extensive crest with pectinate muscles, in the morphologically right appendage. It is narrow with no crest and few pectinate muscles, in the left. It is the extent of the pectinate muscles, nonetheless, which is most distinctive. They extend to the crux in atriums with a morphologically right appendage. The infero-posterior vestibule is smooth in atriums with a morphologically left appendage (Fig. 3.2). These features are more difficult to distinguish echocardiographically, but the shape is distinctive when viewed from the transoesophageal window (Fig. 3.3).

The second segment of the heart, the ventricular mass, almost always contains two ventricles (Fig. 3.4), although very rarely there may be a solitary ventricle of indeterminate morphology (Fig. 3.5). When two ventricles are present, they are always of right and left morphology. The distinction between the two is best determined from the structure of their apical trabecular components. Coarse trabeculations are the characteristic feature of the morphologically right ventricle (Fig. 3.6), whereas fine trabeculations characterise the morphologically left ventricle (Fig. 3.7). These are better seen in specimens than in echocardiographs. All ventricles may possess inlet and/or outlet components. Normal ventricles have one of each. In ventricles with only one inlet, the best guide to which one is the morphologically right ventricle is the presence of tendinous cords fixing the tricuspid valve to the septum. This feature is not found in the morphologically left ventricle (Fig. 3.8). It is an excellent sign for the echocardiographer (Fig. 3.9).

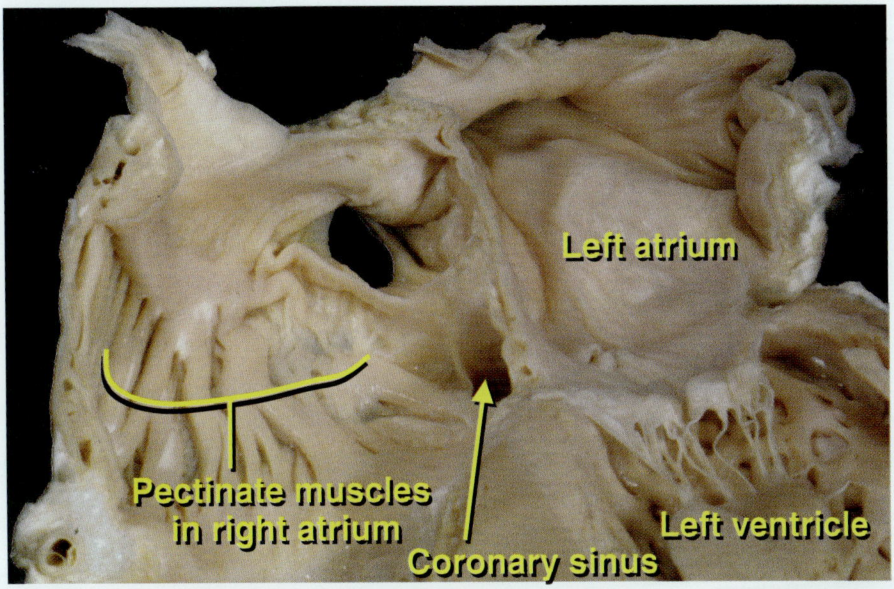

Figure 3.2 This view of the inferior parts of the atrial chambers in a simulated four-chamber section shows the extensive pectinate muscles giving the right atrium a rough appearance compared to the smoother wall of the left atrium.

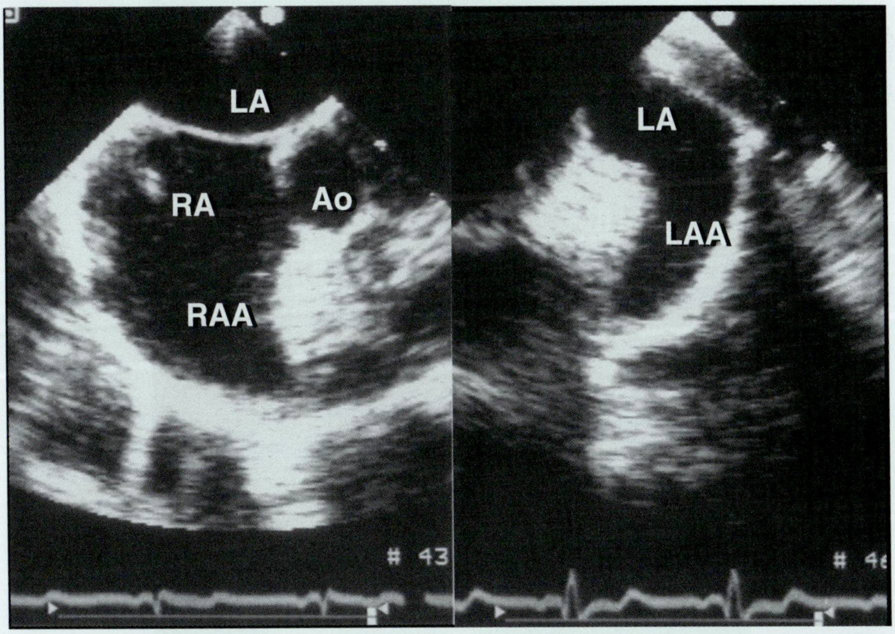

Figure 3.3 Transoesophageal echocardiograms showing the broad right atrial appendage and narrow left atrial appendage.

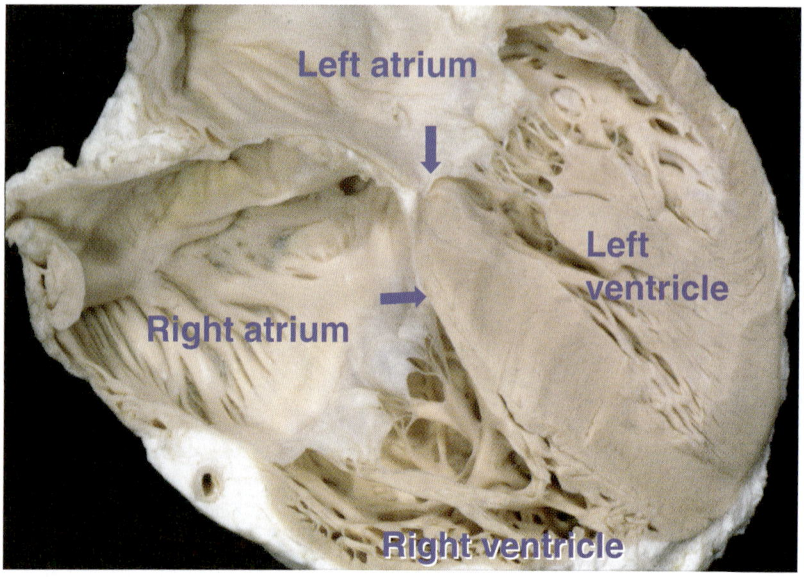

Figure 3.4 This four-chamber section shows each atrium connected to a ventricle. The attachment of the hinge of the tricuspid valve at the septum is nearer to the cardiac apex than the hinge of the mitral valve. This 'offset' arrangement between tricuspid and mitral valves allow ventricular morphology to be inferred.

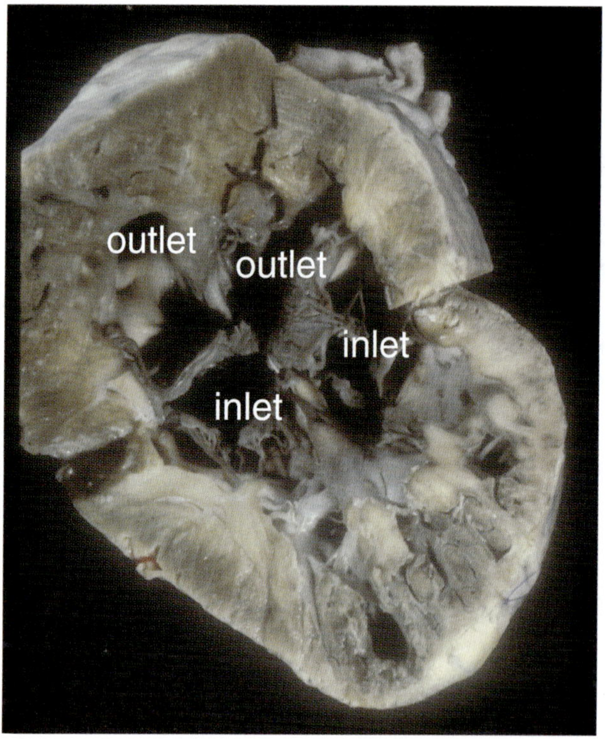

Figure 3.5 This heart has only one ventricular chamber. The trabecular pattern is coarser than that of a morphologically right ventricle.

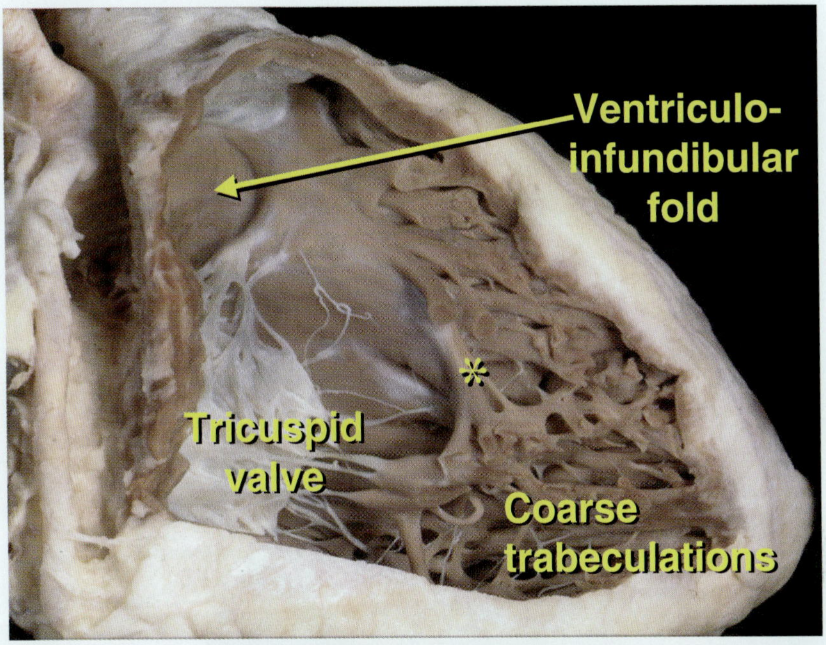

Figure 3.6 The right ventricle is displayed by removing its parietal wall. The normal ventricle has three components: inlet, outlet and apical trabecular. In the normal and morphologically right ventricle, the inlet portion receives the tricuspid valve while the outlet portion leads to the pulmonary valve. Characteristically, the apical portion contains coarse-looking muscle bundles or trabeculations. Note the moderator band (*) passing between the septum and the parietal wall.

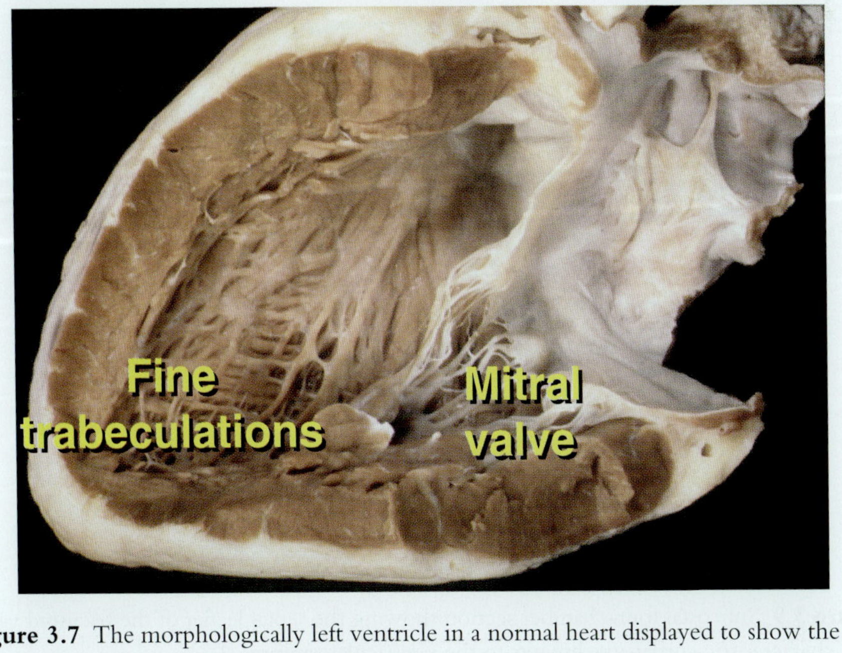

Figure 3.7 The morphologically left ventricle in a normal heart displayed to show the fine apical trabeculations and the smooth upper part of the septum leading to the aortic valve.

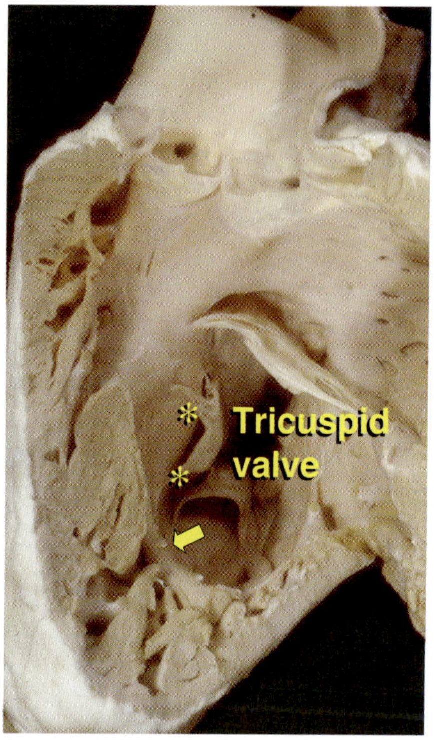

Figure 3.8 In this heart with congenitally corrected transposition, the morphologically right ventricle is located to the left of the morphologically left ventricle. Despite its location, its morphological features still allow indentification. Note the attachment of the septal leaflet to the septum (**) and the moderator band (arrow).

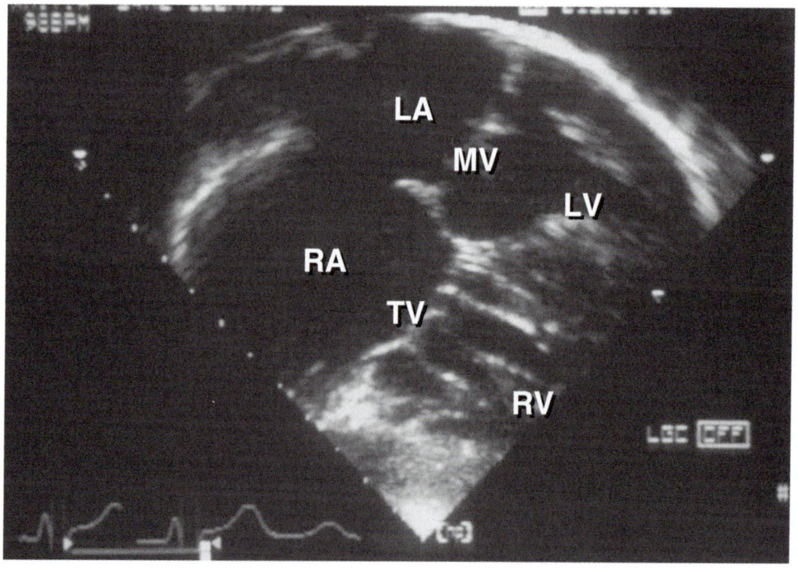

Figure 3.9 Subcostal four-chamber section showing the septal leaflet of the tricuspid valve with characteristic cordal attachments to the ventricular septum.

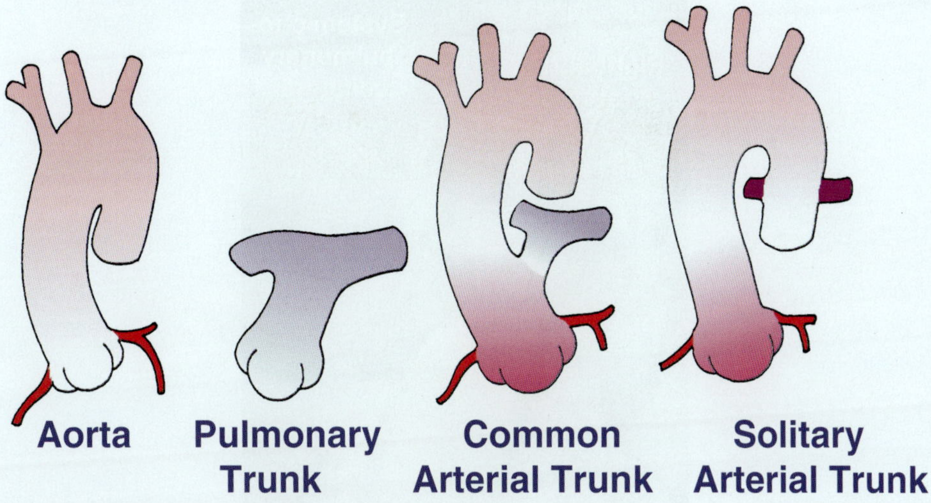

Figure 3.10 The branching patterns of the four variants of great arteries are distinctive although variabilities exist within each form.

The arterial trunks, making up the third segment of the heart, can always be identified on the basis of the pattern of branching of their arteries. In normal hearts, the aorta gives rise to systemic and coronary arteries, whereas the pulmonary trunk divides into right and left pulmonary arteries. These rules hold good for normal or abnormal trunks, but two other arrangements may be seen (Fig. 3.10). A common arterial trunk supplies directly all the coronary, systemic and pulmonary arteries. The second variant is found in hearts with no central intrapericardial pulmonary arteries. There is then a single great artery arising from the heart. In the absence of a pulmonary trunk, it is impossible to define accurately whether the solitary trunk is an aorta or potentially a common structure (Fig. 3.11). It is best described, therefore, as a solitary arterial trunk.

The morphological features of right sidedness and left sidedness are also seen in the rest of the thoracic and abdominal organs. With usual and mirror-imaged arrangements, there is usually harmony between the sidedness of different organs (Fig. 3.12). There are then important patterns, however, in which the abdominal organs are jumbled-up, giving the arrangement often called heterotaxia. Within the chest in such patients, the bronchial tree and atrial appendages can be identified as showing evidence of isomerism (Figs. 3.13 and 3.14).

Atrial Arrangement

The first step in sequential analysis is to determine the arrangement of the atriums, assessed according to the morphology of the appendages. There are four possible

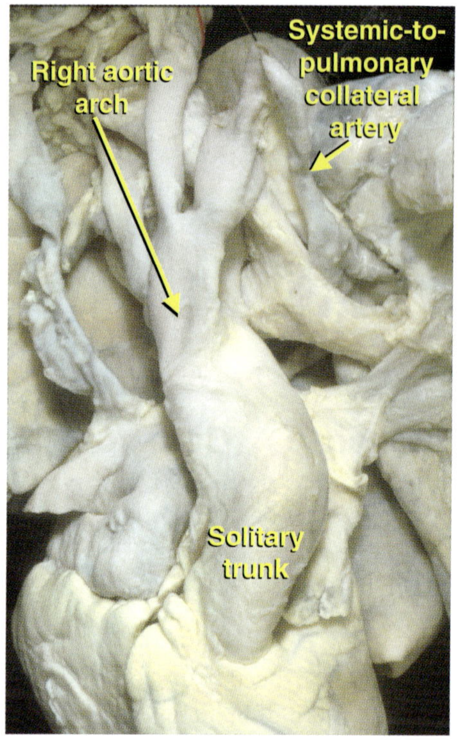

Figure 3.11 This example of a solitary arterial trunk shows the lungs supplied by collateral arteries in the absence of intrapericardial pulmonary arteries.

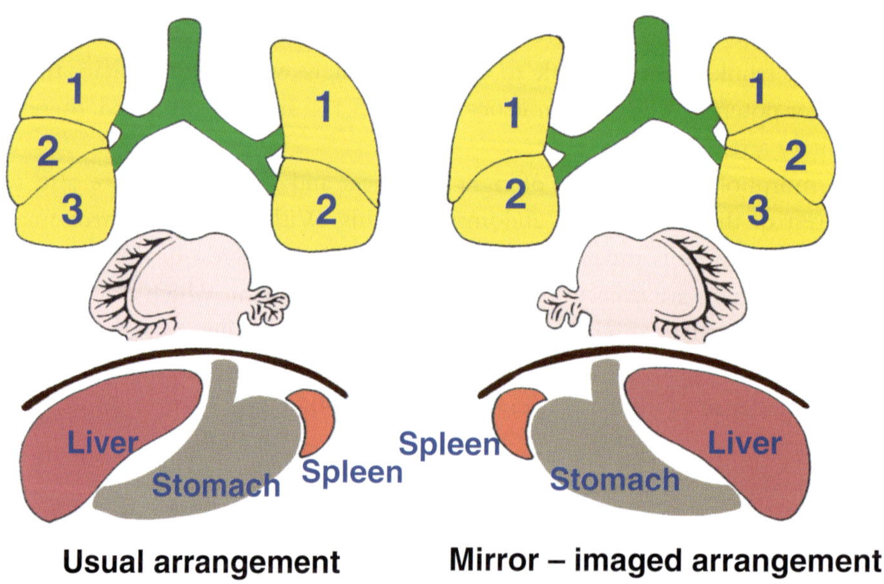

Figure 3.12 Schematic representation of usual and mirror-imaged arrangements of atrial appendages with their respective arrangement of thoracic and abdominal organs.

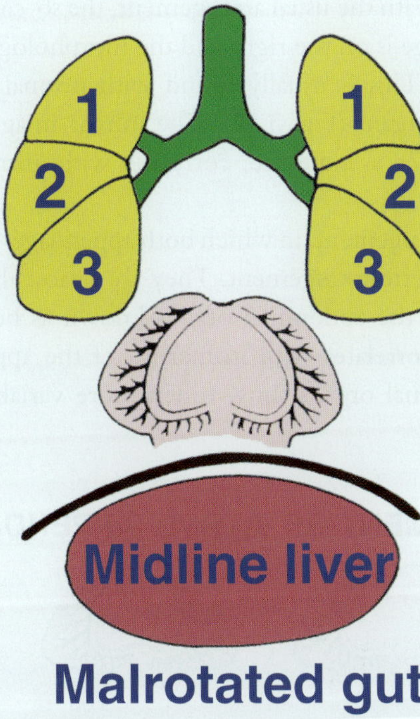

Figure 3.13 Diagram of isomeric arrangement of right atrial appendages and associated arrangement of thoracic and abdominal organs.

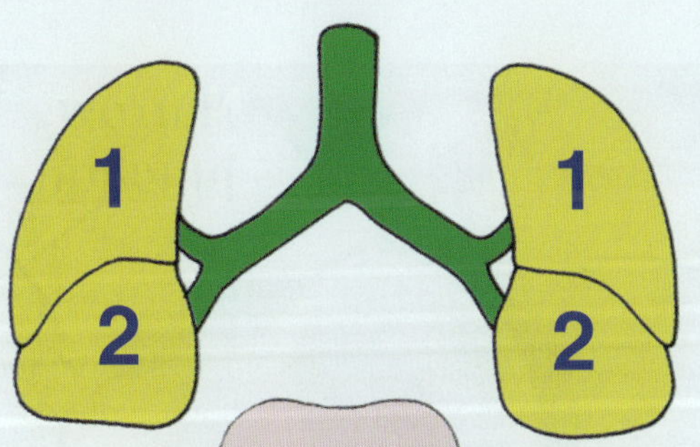

Figure 3.14 Diagram of isomeric arrangement of left atrial appendages and associated arrangement of thoracic and abdominal organs.

arrangements (Fig. 3.15). With the usual arrangement, the so-called solitus, the morphologically right appendage is on the right and the morphologically left appendage is on the left (Fig. 3.16). This is usually found with normal lateralisation of the other thoraco-abdominal organs (Fig. 3.12). The mirror-imaged arrangement, the so-called inversus (Fig. 3.17), as expected, correlates with mirror-imagery of other organs (Fig. 3.12).

The other patterns of arrangement, in which both appendages are of the same morphology, represent an isomeric arrangement. They are almost always associated with the jumbled-up pattern of the abdominal organs known as heterotaxy. Bronchial isomerism almost always correlates with isomerism of the appendages (Figs. 3.13 and 3.14), but the abdominal organs show much more variability. In most cases,

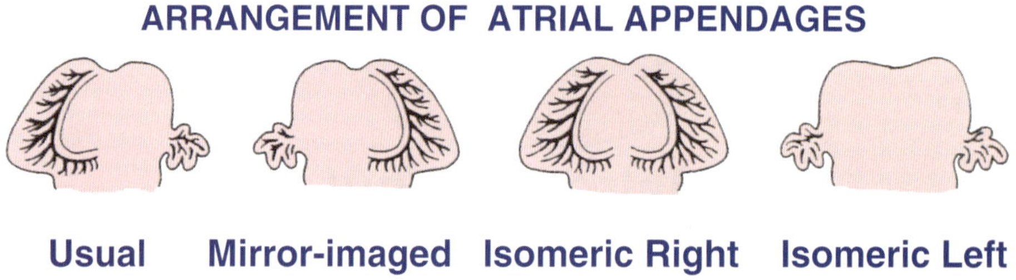

Figure 3.15 Schematic representation of the four possible arrangements of atrial appendages.

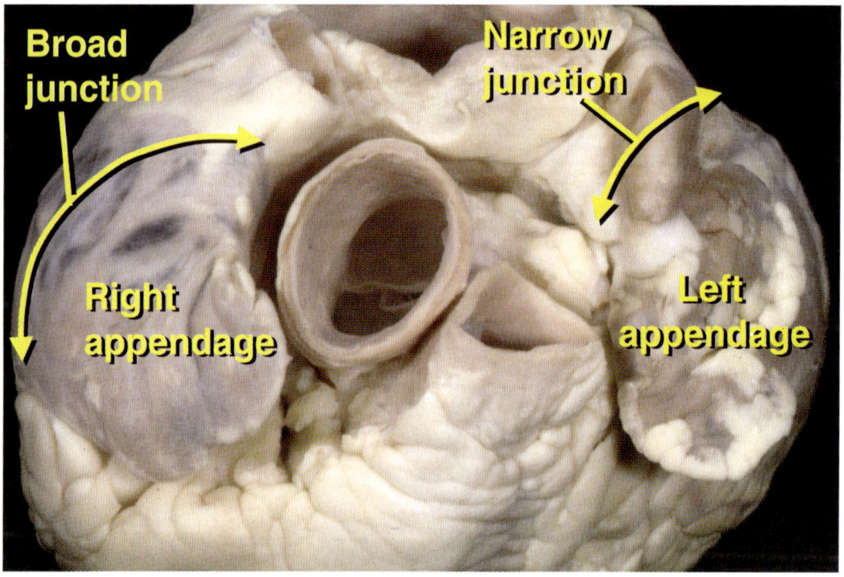

Figure 3.16 The morphologically right appendage is triangular in shape and has a broad junction with the atrium. In contrast, the morphologically left atrial appendage is finger-like and has a narrow junction with the atrium.

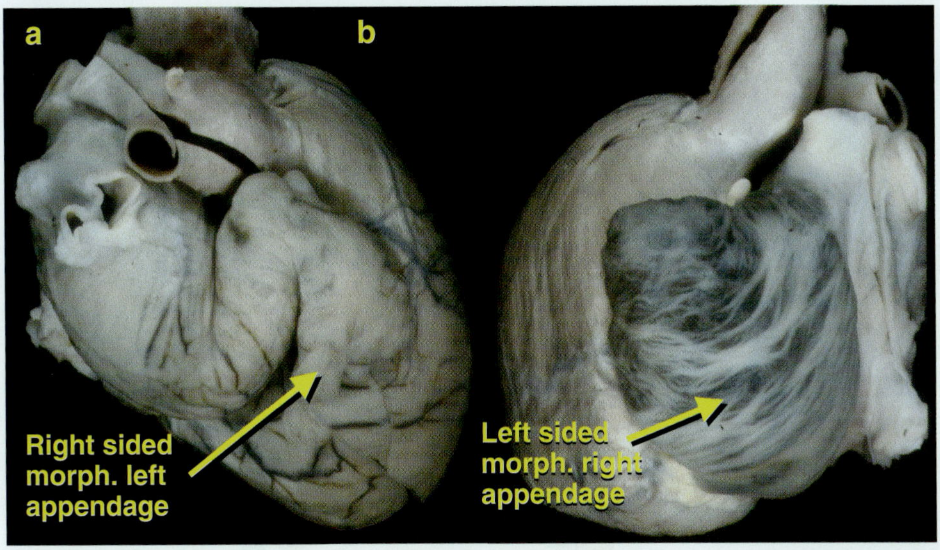

Figure 3.17 The arrangement of the atrial appendages in this heart is the mirror-image of the usual.

absence of the spleen accompanies right isomerism, while multiple spleens are found in patients with left isomerism.

Atrial arrangement is best determined clinically by direct recognition of the morphology of the appendages. This is not always possible echocardiographically. More usually, therefore, the diagnosis is made indirectly, either from the bronchial morphology seen on the x-ray, or from the location of the aorta and inferior caval vein as determined echocardiographically within the abdomen. The aorta can be recognised by its pulsations coincident with the cardiac apex, while the inferior caval vein expands with inspiration. When transverse sections through the abdomen show symmetrical positions of the aorta and the inferior caval vein anterior to the spine, lateralised atrial arrangement can be assumed provided the morphologically right atrium is found to the same side as the inferior caval vein. With the usual arrangement of the atrial appendages (solitus), the aorta will be to the left and the inferior caval vein to the right of the spine (Fig. 3.18). A left-sided caval vein with right-sided aorta will be characteristic of mirror-imagery (inversus). In infancy, the inferior caval vein may not always be demonstrated clearly in transverse sections. Long axis parasagittal sections are then useful to confirm the relative positions of the two vessels. Almost always, all the hepatic veins will drain to the inferior caval vein, entering just proximal to its junction with the right atrium. Isomeric arrangement of the right atrial appendages is almost always found with the aorta and inferior caval vein located on the same side of the spine, either to the right or to the left, with the vein slightly anterior (Fig. 3.18). Isomerism of the left atrial appendage can usually be distinguished from right isomerism because transverse sections show a midline aorta closely associated with an azygos vein (Fig. 3.18). It must then be remembered

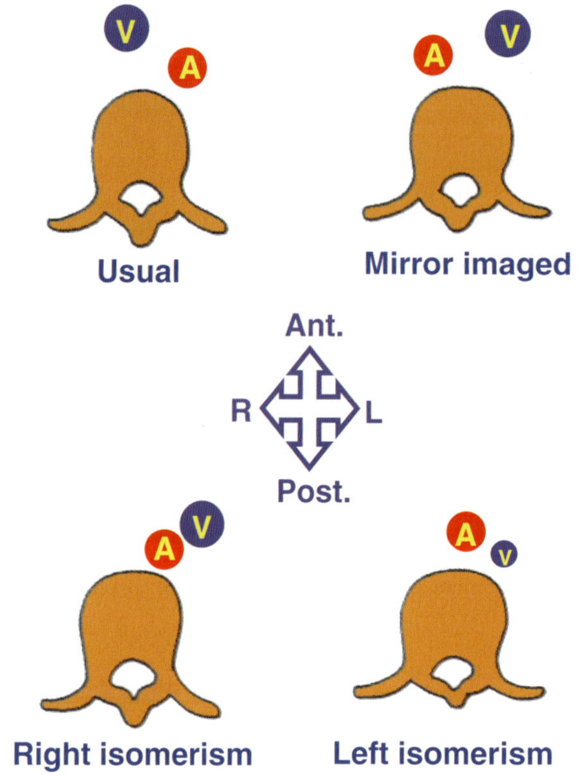

Figure 3.18 The arrangements of the aorta and inferior caval vein relative to the spine allow inferences to be made with regard to atrial arrangement.

that these are only inferential techniques, and that discrepencies may occur. This is unlikely to give problems in clinical management, since the cardiac anomalies themselves are also characteristic (see Chapter 4).

Variation at the Atrioventricular Junction

To describe the atrioventricular junction, it is first necessary to establish how the segments of the atrial myocardium are connected to the ventricular mass. The pattern of the atrioventricular valves should then be described. Subcostal, parasternal, and apical four-chamber sections are useful for analysing atrioventricular connections. There are three basic groups of atrioventricular connections. With biventricular connections, each atrium is connected to its own ventricle. With usual and mirror-imaged arrangement of the atriums, such biventricular connections can be concordant when the right atrium is connected to the right ventricle and the left atrium to the left ventricle. The connections are discordant when the right atrium is connected to the left ventricle and the left atrium to the right ventricle (Fig. 3.19).

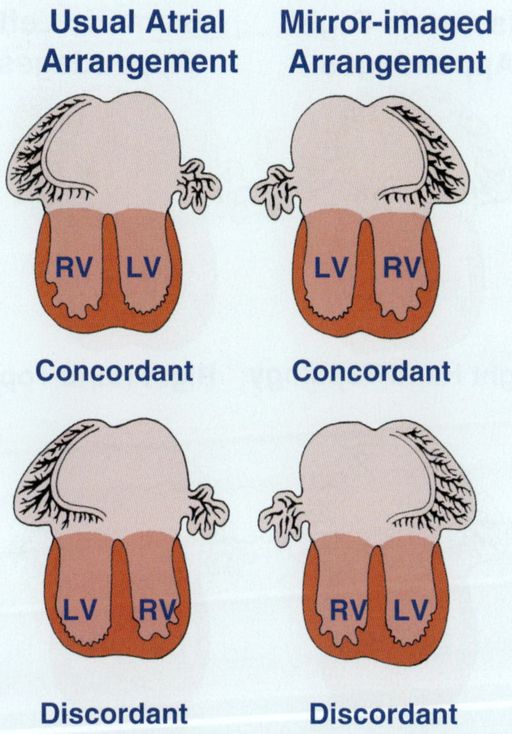

Figure 3.19 Diagram of biventricular atrioventricular connections in the setting of usual and mirror-imaged arrangements of atrial appendages.

When the atrial appendages are isomeric, biventricular connections cannot be subdivided in this way. Instead, they are biventricular and ambiguous (Fig. 3.20). In the setting of such ambiguous and biventricular atrioventricular connections, it is also essential to describe the three-dimensional structure, or topology, of the ventricular mass. There may be one of two patterns, right-hand or left-hand topology. The pattern can be determined by imagining a hand placed on the septal surface of the morphologically right ventricle (Fig. 3.21).

The second group of atrioventricular connections produce the univentricular arrangement. This is found in the setting of a double inlet ventricle, or when either the right-sided or left-sided atrioventricular connection is absent (Fig. 3.22). Univentricular atrioventricular connections can be found with the atriums connected to a dominant left ventricle, when the right ventricle will be rudimentary and incomplete; to a dominant right ventricle, found with a rudimentary and incomplete left ventricle; or to a solitary ventricle of indeterminate morphology. In hearts where one ventricle is dominant, the rudimentary ventricle can vary markedly in its position. Almost always, however, rudimentary right ventricles are found antero-superiorly, while rudimentary left ventricles occupy a postero-inferior position within the ventricular mass.

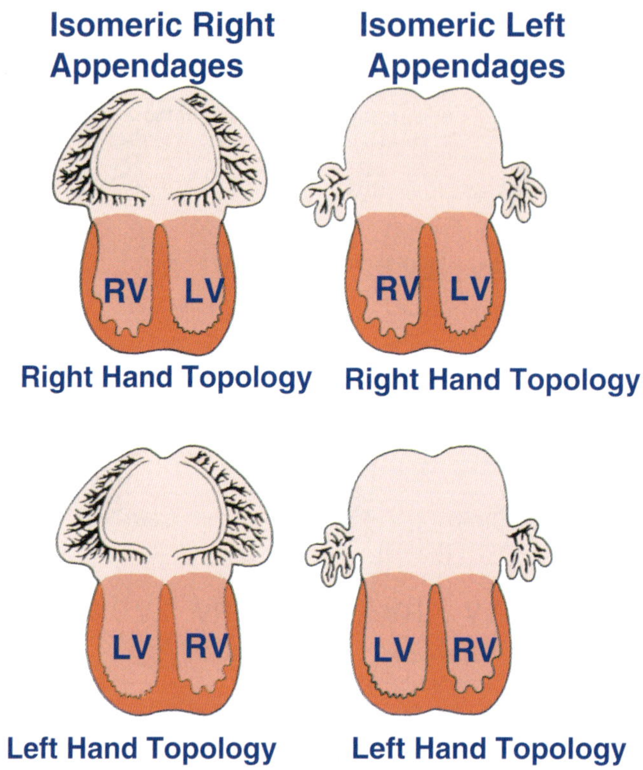

Figure 3.20 Diagram of biventricular and ambiguous atrioventricular connections in the setting of isomeric arrangements of the atrial appendages.

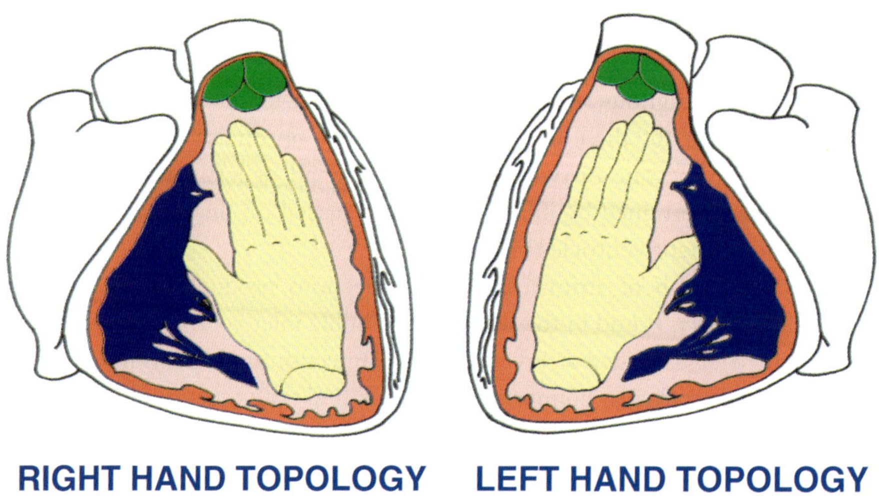

Figure 3.21 Ventricular topology is determined by placing the palm of one's hand, figuratively speaking, on the septal surface of the morphologically right ventricle in such a way that the wrist is in the apex, the thumb in the inlet and the fingers in the outlet.

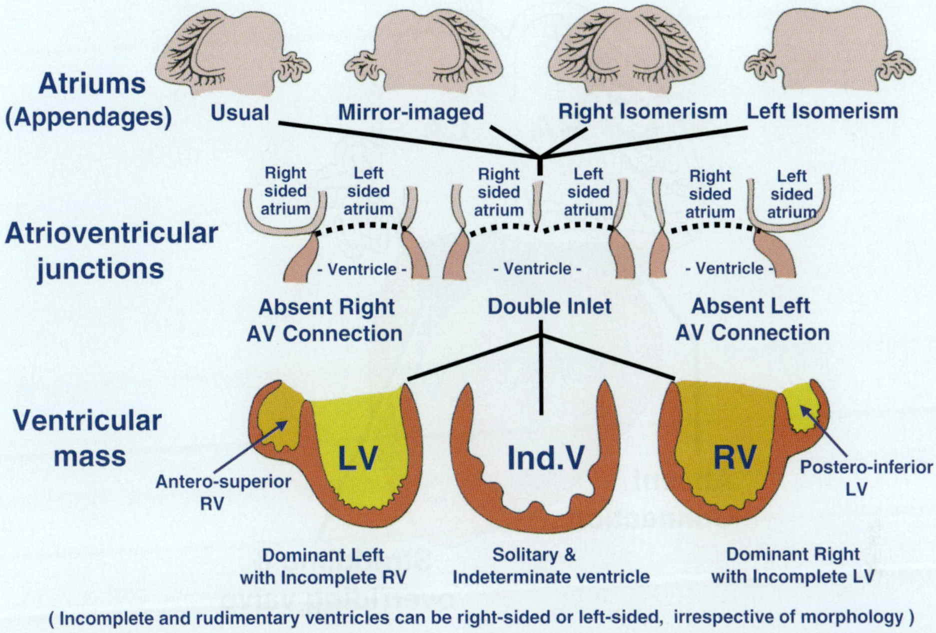

Figure 3.22 Diagram showing the three variants of univentricular connection across the atrioventricular junction, i.e. absent right, double inlet and absent left atrioventricular connections. These exist with any of the four types of atrial arrangements, and any of the three forms of ventricular morphology. The solitary and indeterminate ventricle is the rarest ventricular morphology. Most commonly, there are two ventricular chambers but one is larger and dominant. The smaller ventricle is also rudimentary since it lacks one or more of the three components of a normal ventricle.

The third group of connections is rare, but exists when one atrioventricular connection is absent and the solitary connection straddles and overrides the ventricular septum (Fig. 3.23). Such an arrangement, of necessity, is uniatrial but biventricular. It produces one variant of a double outlet atrium. Further variation depends on which connection is absent, and on the ventricular topology (Fig. 3.24). The morphology of the atrioventricular valves is independent of the junctional connections. There may be two atrioventricular valves, or a common valve. A common valve guards both atrioventricular junctions (Fig. 3.25). Where there are two valves, one may be stenotic, regurgitant, imperforate, straddling when its tension apparatus is attached on both sides of a septum, or overriding when the valvar orifice is positioned astride the septum (Fig. 3.25). When an atrioventricular valve is overriding, the heart is intermediate between having biventricular and univentricular connections (Fig. 3.26). Intermediate categories are not defined. If less than half the circumference of one valve overrides, then the connection is described as biventricular. The connection becomes univentricular when more than half of both atrioventricular connections are supported by the same ventricle. This is the so-called '50% rule'. Common valves

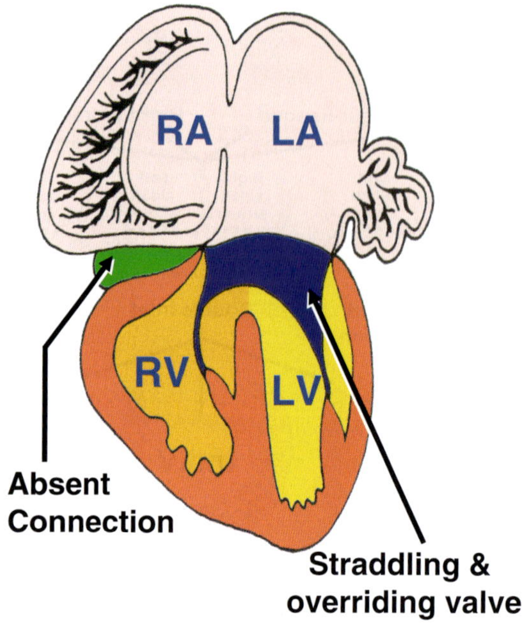

Figure 3.23 When there is straddling of an atrioventricular valve in the setting of absence of an atrioventricular connection, the arrangement can be described as uniatrial and biventricular.

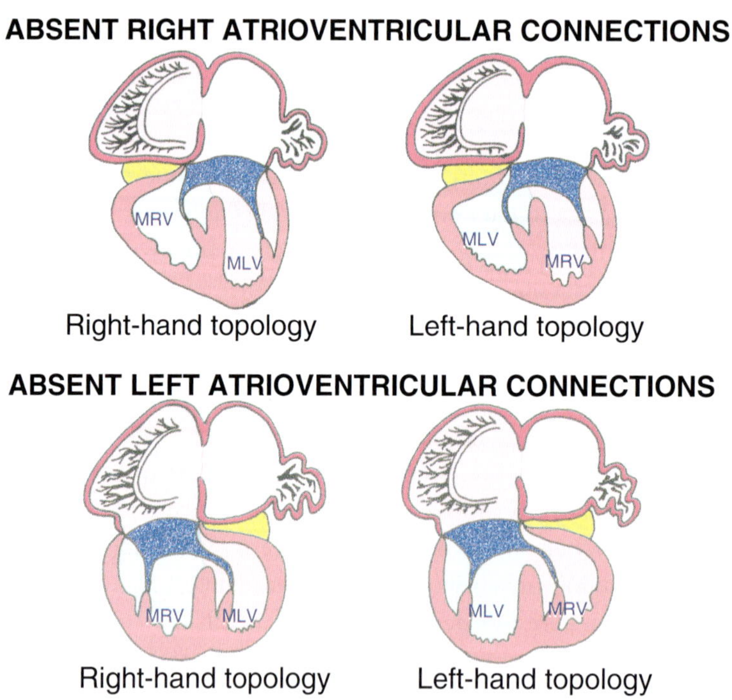

Figure 3.24 Double outlet atrium with variations in absent connections and ventricular topology.

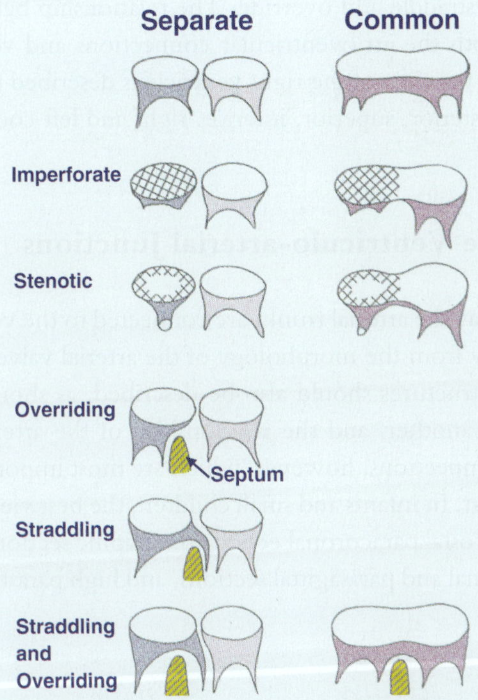

Figure 3.25 Schematic representation of the variations in morphology of the atrioventricular valves.

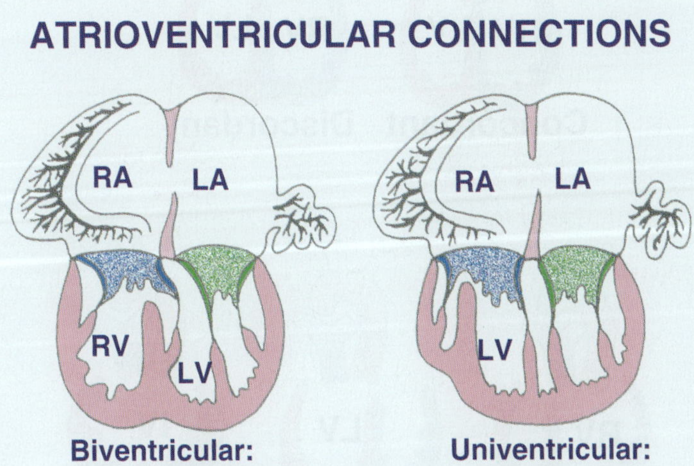

Figure 3.26 The type of atrioventricular connection is determined by the degree of override of the atrioventricular valve. The valve is assigned to the ventricle containing more than 50% of its circumference.

can also be stenotic or incompetent. They can be partially imperforate. Usually, but not always, they straddle and override. The relationship between the ventricles is independent of both the atrioventricular connections and ventricular topology. When necessary, the position of the right ventricle is described relative to the left in terms of anterior, posterior, superior, inferior, right and left coordinates.

Variations at the Ventriculo-arterial Junctions

Here, again, the way the arterial trunks are connected to the ventricular mass must be analysed separately from the morphology of the arterial valves. The morphology of the infundibular structures should also be described, as should the relationships of the valves to one another, and the relationships of the arterial trunks. It is the ventriculo-arterial connections, however, which are most important in determining flow through the heart. In infants and small children, the best views to establish these features are from subcostal paracoronal echocardiographic sections, supplemented by suprasternal paracoronal and parasagittal sections, and high parasternal short and long

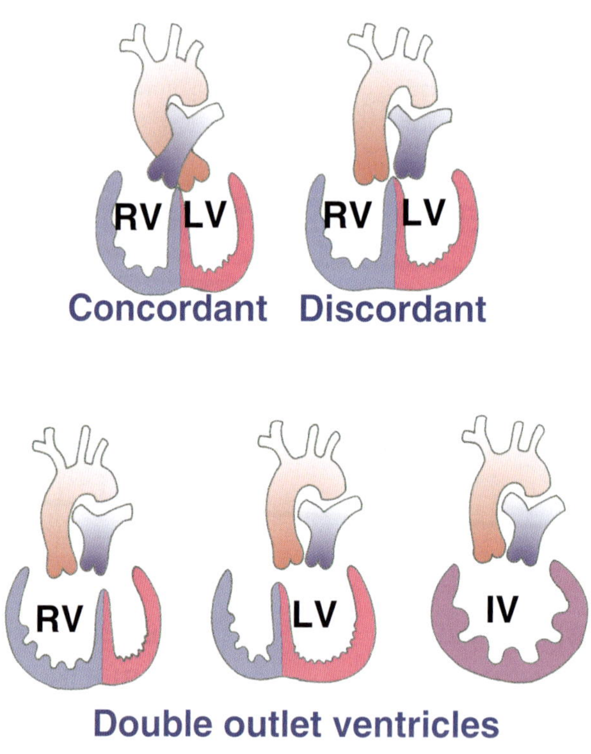

Figure 3.27 Diagram showing concordant and discordant ventriculo-arterial connections. Double outlet can be from the morphologically right (RV), left (LV) or indeterminate (IV) ventricle.

axis sections. When there are two arterial trunks, they can be connected to the ventricular mass in concordant or discordant fashion (Fig. 3.27). Alternatively, both trunks may arise from one ventricle, which may be of right, left or indeterminate morphology (Fig. 3.27). Overriding arterial valves are assigned to the ventricle supporting the greater part of their circumference using the 50% rule, again avoiding the need for intermediate categories. When only one arterial trunk is connected to the ventricular mass, then there is single outlet from the heart. This single outlet is usually via a common trunk, and is then guarded by a common arterial valve. It can be via a solitary trunk, or even via an aorta or a pulmonary trunk when it is not possible to locate the ventricular origin of the second, atretic, trunk.

Associated Malformations

The remainder of this book will be concerned with describing the morphological features, and their correlative clinical images, of the various lesions found within the heart. Such lesions can involve the great veins, the atriums, the ventricles and the great arteries. We will pay particular attention to septal defects, and to lesions which involve the atrioventricular and ventriculo-arterial junctions.

Position of the Heart

Thus far, we have not mentioned an abnormal position of the heart itself. This is because an unusual cardiac position is not an abnormality of cardiac morphology, although the two may coexist. A normal heart can itself be abnormally located. The cardiac position should be described separately from the cardiac morphology. The heart can, very rarely, occupy an extrathoracic position, so-called ectopia. More commonly, when abnormally positioned, it is located in the right chest rather than the left chest, or else is midline. Such a right-sided or left-sided position is independent of the location of the cardiac apex, which can also be to the right, to the left or directed to the middle. These combinations are best accounted for by using simple descriptive terms, rather than resorting to definitions which can vary markedly in their usage, such as 'dextrocardia'.

4

Isomeric Arrangement of the Atrial Appendages

It was Abernethy's description in 1793 of patients with multiple spleens, followed by Martin's observation early in the nineteenth century of congenital absence of the spleen and complex heart disease, which drew attention to the association of malformations of the spleen and the abdominal organs with congenital lesions within the heart. Since Ivemark's important contribution, it has become fashionable to describe patterns of cardiac malformations within the syndromes of asplenia and polysplenia. While the total absence of the spleen, or the presence of multiple spleens, is unlikely to be missed at autopsy, splenic status is much more difficult to establish in the clinical setting. It is now also recognised that the arrangement of the spleen does not correlate most constantly with atrial anatomy. In most instances, nonetheless, the 'asplenia syndrome' is associated with bilateral right sidedness of the bronchial tree, lungs and atrial appendages, an arrangement accurately called right isomerism. The 'polysplenia syndrome' is virtually always associated with bilateral left sidedness of the bronchi, lungs and the atrial appendages, thus giving left isomerism. It is the isomeric arrangement of the atrial appendages that is most important from the stance of the cardiologist since, in the sequential segmental approach for the diagnosis of congenital cardiac malformations, analysis starts with determining the morphological arrangement of the atriums. Within the atrium, it is the appendages that are the most constant components. Furthermore, their shape, and the particular morphology of their junction with the rest of the atrium, permit them always to be distinguished as morphologically right or left. As we have already described (see Chapter 3), this means that all hearts can be placed into one of four patterns of atrial arrangement. In this chapter, we are concerned with the cardiac manifestations of the two isomeric arrangements.

Recognition of Atrial Arrangement

In patients with isomeric atrial appendages, the arrangement of the rest of the heart is almost always abnormal. The venoatrial connections are particularly variable. The appendages, in contrast, retain their characteristic morphology, irrespective of their position. The morphologically right atrial appendage has a broad triangular shape and a wide junction with the rest of the atrial chamber. Significantly, in the presence of right isomerism, extensive pectinate muscles extend around both atrioventricular junctions to meet at the crux (Figs. 4.1 and 4.2). The morphologically left atrial appendage has a hooked and tube-like shape, with a narrow junction that is not marked by a terminal crest (Figs. 4.3 and 4.4). The pectinate muscles of the morphologically left appendage are much more limited in their extent. So, in the setting of left isomerism, they do not reach to the crux on either side, leaving smooth posterior vestibules bilaterally. It is easy in the autopsied heart, therefore, to recognise the presence of bilateral morphologically right appendages, and to distinguish them from either bilateral morphologically left appendages, or from the usual (solitus) and mirror-imaged (inversus) arrangements.

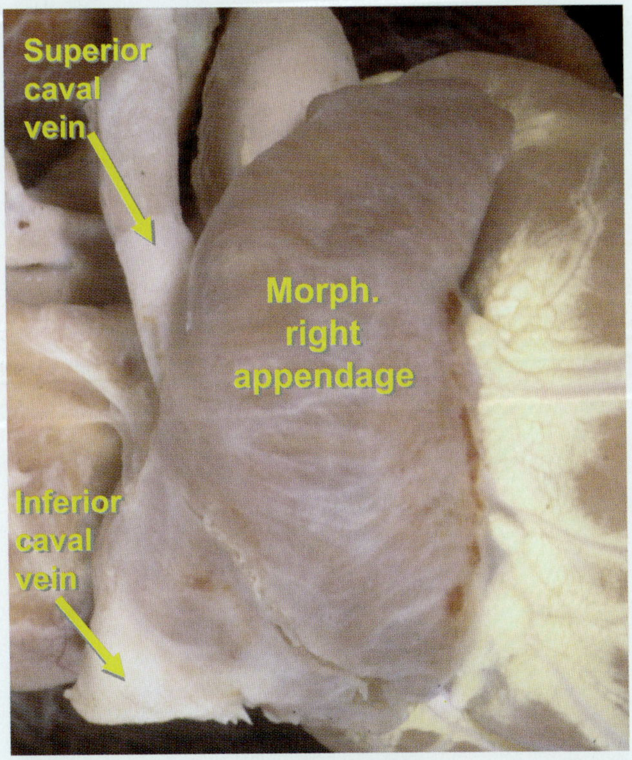

Figure 4.1 The external aspect of the morphologically right atrial appendage shows the pectinate muscles visible through its thin wall.

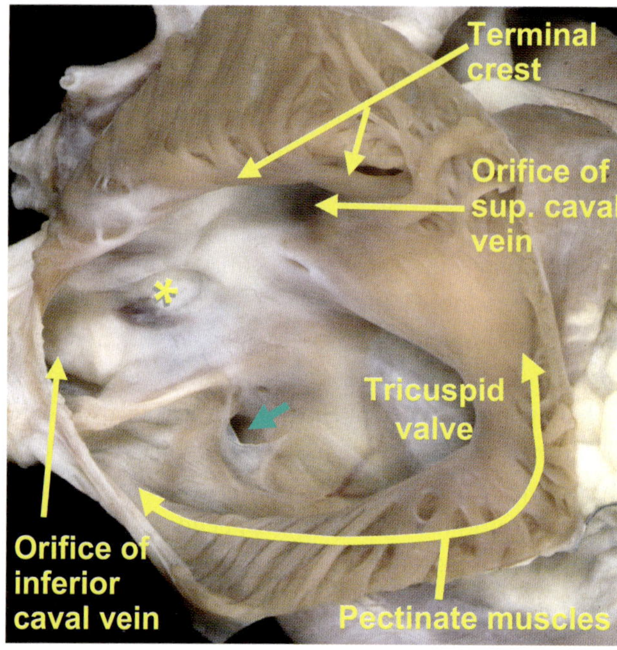

Figure 4.2 The morphologically right atrial appendage opened to display the array of pectinate muscles arising from the terminal crest. * = oval fossa; green arrow = coronary sinus.

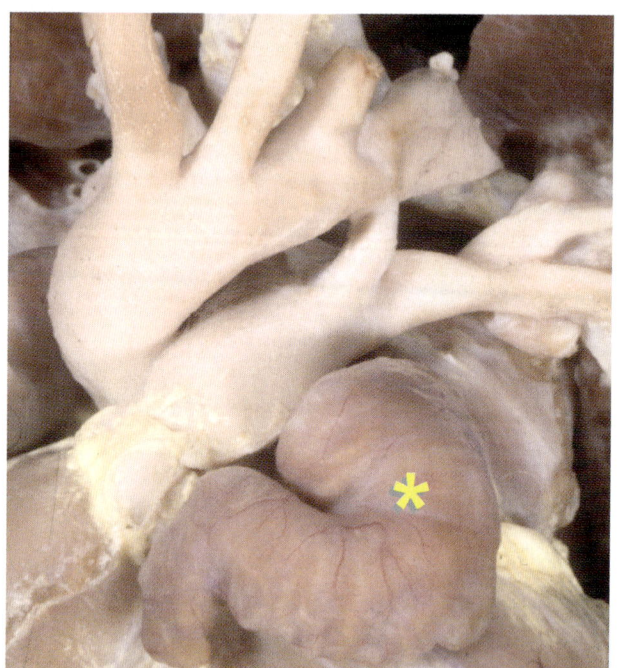

Figure 4.3 The morphologically left atrial appendage (*) is finger-like.

Atrial Anatomy

There are bilateral terminal crests in the presence of right isomerism. As may be expected, a groove marks the epicardial aspect of each terminal crest and, within the terminal grooves, there are bilateral sinus nodes. In the majority of patients both superior caval veins connect bilaterally to the atrial roof (Fig. 4.5). The venous return

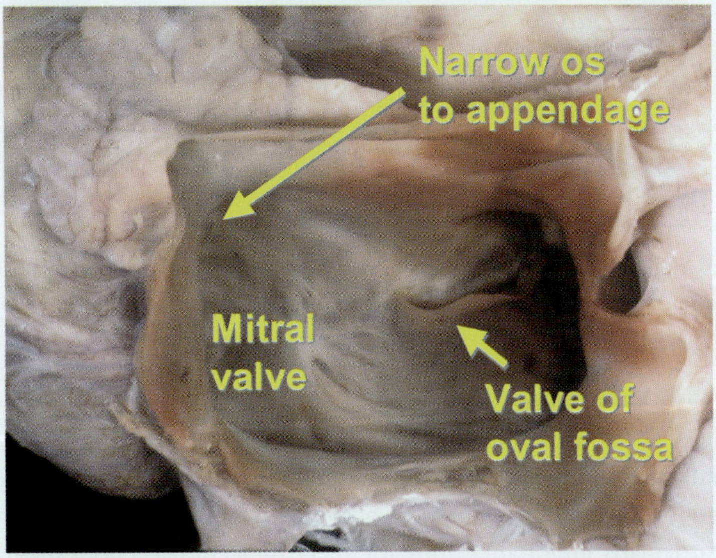

Figure 4.4 The internal aspect of the left atrium shows a smooth wall.

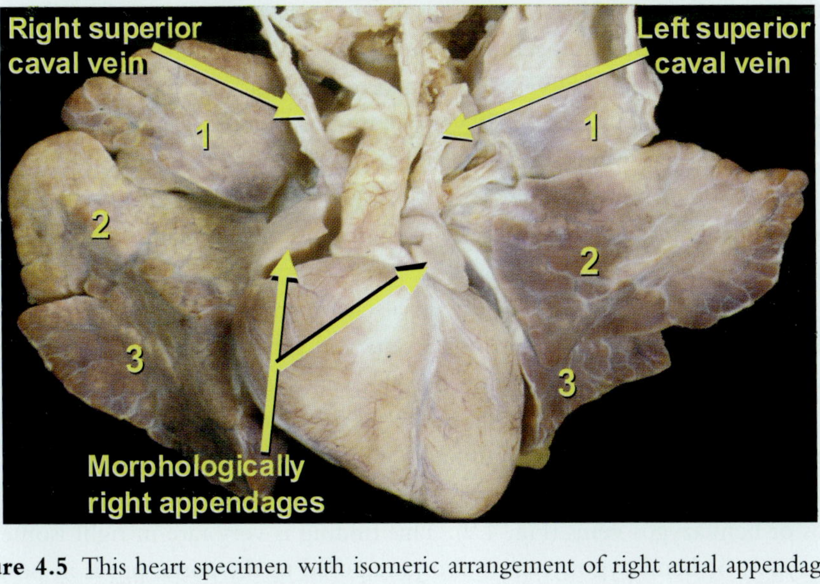

Figure 4.5 This heart specimen with isomeric arrangement of right atrial appendages has corresponding trilobed lungs bilaterally.

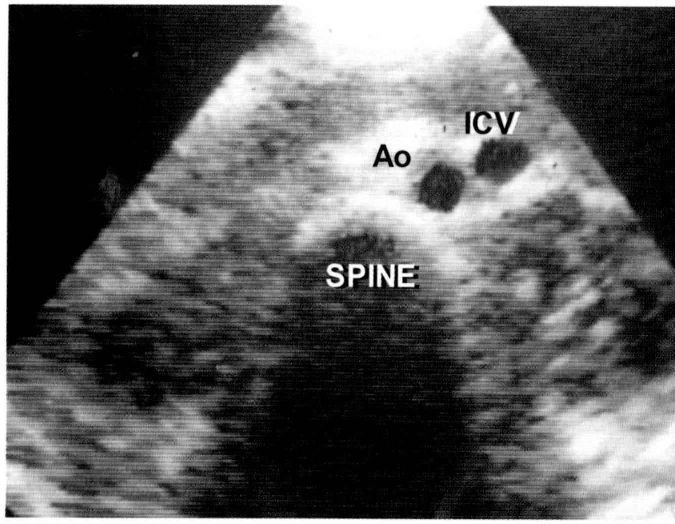

Figure 4.6 Subcostal horizontal section at the level of T12 showing juxtaposition of the aorta and inferior caval vein in the abdomen of a patient with isomeric arrangement of right atrial appendages. The inferior caval vein is anterior to the aorta.

from the heart itself is direct, with no formation of a coronary sinus in the atrioventricular grooves. Connection of the inferior caval vein to the atriums, whether right- or left sided, is almost always present. Another important marker of right isomerism is the juxtaposition, within the abdomen, of the aorta and inferior caval vein (Fig. 4.6). This is a particularly important feature for the cross-sectional echocardiographer, and is almost constantly present. Typically, at least some of the hepatic veins join the intrahepatic caval vein, although there may be partially anomalous hepatic drainage to either of the atriums. Also significant is the necessary occurrence of totally anomalous pulmonary venous connections. These connections are anatomically abnormal even should the pulmonary veins be joined to the heart. In the majority of cases, however, the anomalous pulmonary veins drain to a supracardiac or infracardiac site. When the pulmonary veins are connected to the heart, the connection is usually via a midline confluence situated in the roof of a common atrium (Fig. 4.7). The atrial septum is usually just a cord-like strand in right isomerism (Fig. 4.8). An intact atrial septum is very rare.

In contrast to right isomerism, the atrial chambers in hearts with isomerism of the left atrial appendages lack terminal crests and grooves. Bilateral superior caval veins are often still present, but then one frequently drains via the coronary sinus, although the sinus can also be absent in hearts with isomeric left appendages. The most characteristic feature of patients having left isomerism is interruption of the suprarenal course of the inferior caval vein, with the venous return passing via the azygos or hemiazygos veins (Fig. 4.9). This finding is very rare in right isomerism. The azygos, or hemiazygos, vein is also juxtaposed to the aorta, but is in posterior position (Fig. 4.10). When there is azygos continuation, the hepatic veins are often

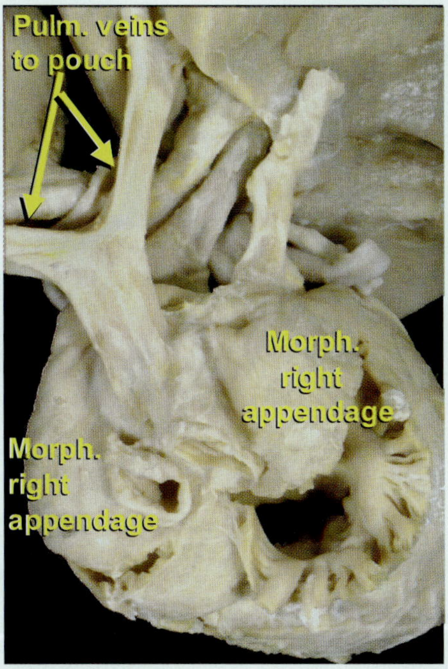

Figure 4.7 This heart specimen with isomeric arrangement of right atrial appendages is viewed from the back. It shows the pulmonary veins from both lungs entering a pouch that opens to the left-sided atrium.

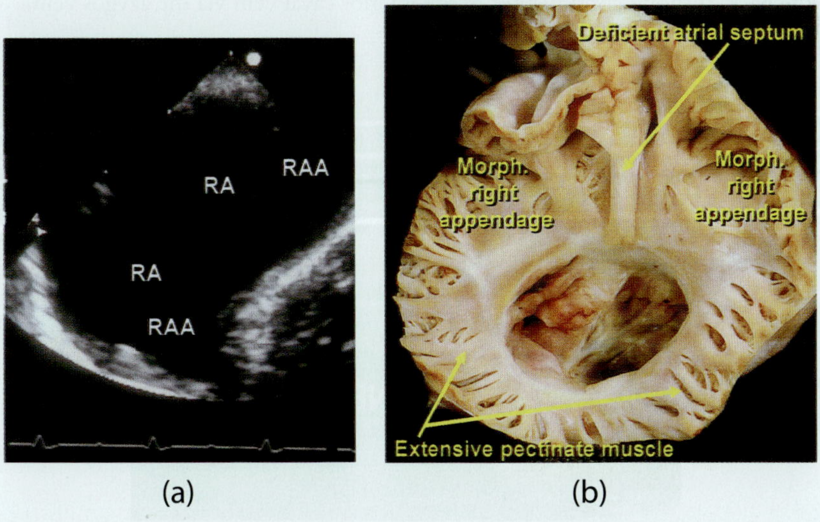

Figure 4.8 (a) Transoesphageal echocardiogram in right isomerism showing deficient atrial septum in a patient with isomeric arrangement of right atrial appendages. (b) Heart specimen with isomeric arrangement of right atrial appendages is displayed to show bilaterally extensive pectinate muscles and deficiency of the atrial septum.

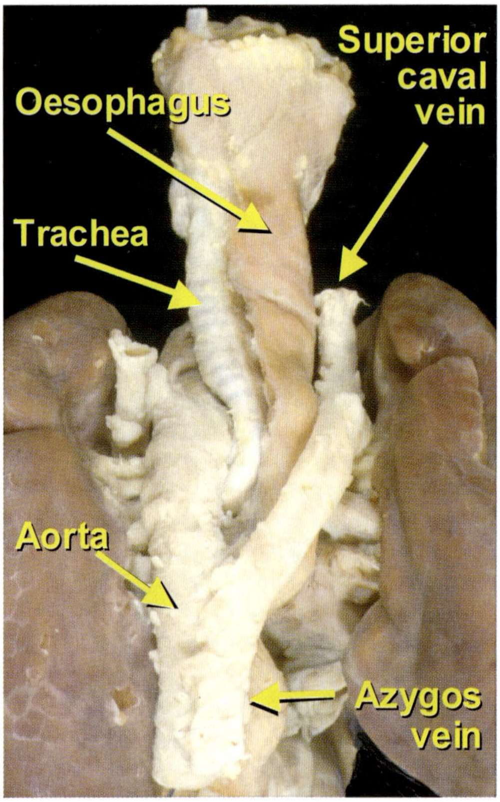

Figure 4.9 This specimen with isomeric arrangement of left atrial appendages is viewed from the back. It shows continuation of the inferior caval vein via the azygos vein.

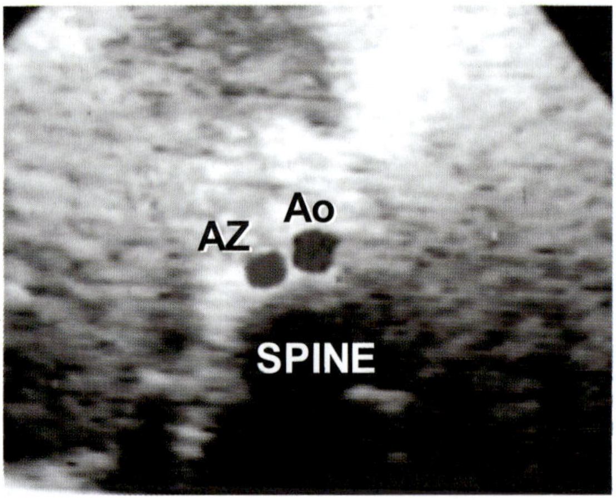

Figure 4.10 Subcostal horizontal section at level of T12 showing juxtaposition between abdominal aorta and azygos (AZ) vein. Note the posterior location of the azygos vein relative to the aorta in this case of isomeric arrangement of the left atrial appendages.

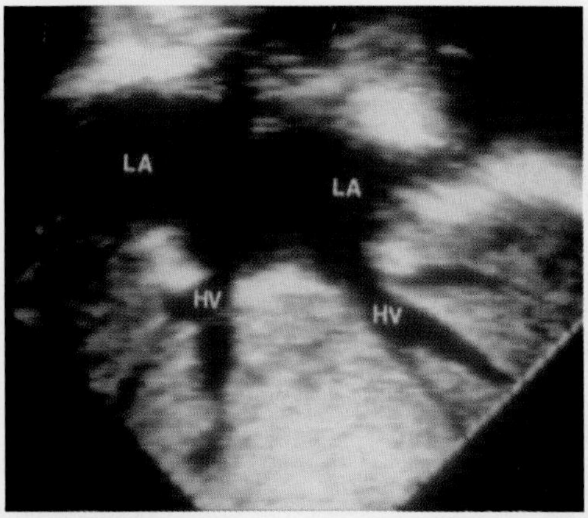

Figure 4.11 Subcostal paracoronal echocardiographic section of a patient with isomeric arrangement of left atrial appendages. The hepatic veins drain into a suprahepatic confluence.

connected bilaterally to the atriums. A suprahepatic confluence of the hepatic veins can be identified in a good number of cases, nonetheless, and, on occasion, this can drain the inferior caval vein also (Fig. 4.11). The conjunction of aorta and azygos vein, therefore, is less valuable as a clinical marker for left isomerism than is the aorto-caval juxtaposition for right isomerism. The atrial septum tends to be better formed in left than in right isomerism. The septal surface, nonetheless, lacks the typical rim of the oval foramen. The pulmonary veins are connected to the atriums in anatomically normal fashion even when two veins each join to right-sided and left-sided atriums, respectively. All four veins draining to one or the other atrium, however, is by no means uncommon.

The Atrioventricular Junctions

In hearts with isomeric atrial appendages, the atriums can connect to the ventricular mass in either biventricular or univentricular fashion. In those with biventricular connections, it is necessary to specify both the type of isomerism present, and the topological pattern of the ventricular mass. Only in this way is it possible to provide a full description (see Chapter 3, Figs. 3.19 and 3.20). Ventricular topology is important since it determines the distribution of the atrioventricular conduction tissues. A normally positioned atrioventricular node is the rule with right hand topology, while an anterior node, or dual nodes, are found with left hand topology. Such biventricular connections are, of necessity, also ambiguous (Fig. 4.12). They are more commonly seen in hearts with left than with right isomerism. Univentricular atrioventricular connections, particularly double inlet, occur with some frequency in

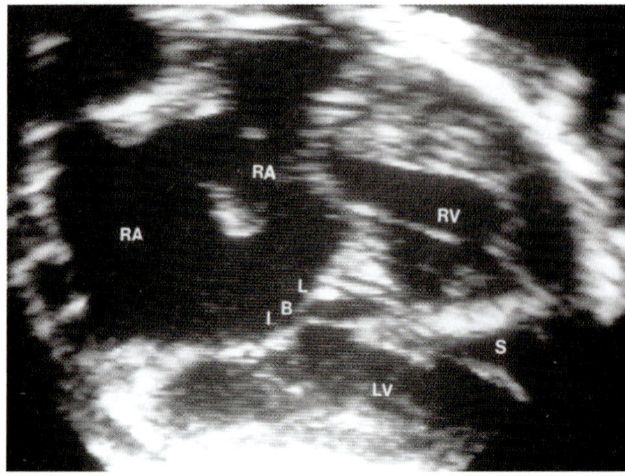

Figure 4.12 Subcostal four-chamber section in isomeric arrangement of the right atrial appendages and biventricular atrioventricular connections with left hand pattern ventricular topology. The left-sided right ventricle is characterised by multiple cordal insertions to the septum.

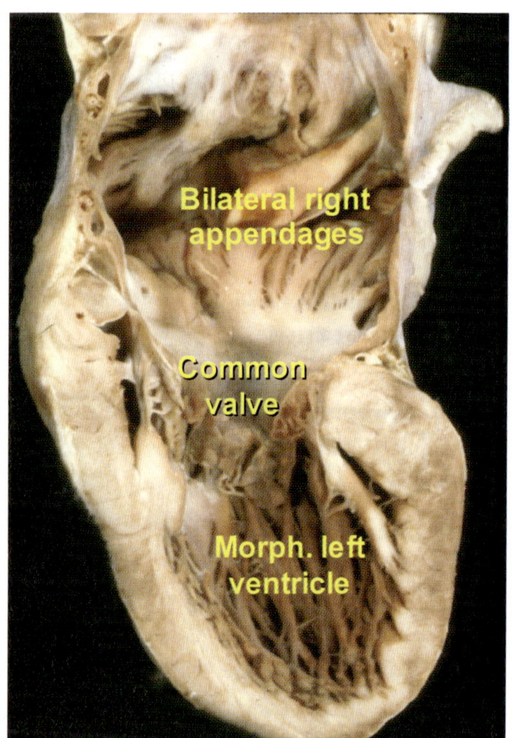

Figure 4.13 This heart sectioned longitudinally shows isomeric arrangement of the right atrial appendages with double inlet atrioventricular connections to a morphologically left ventricle. A common valve guards the atrioventricular junction.

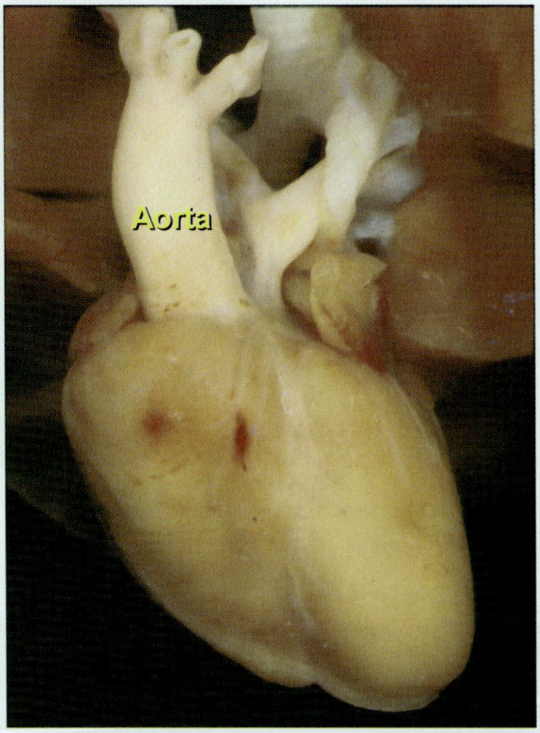

Figure 4.14 This heart with isomeric arrangement of the right atrial appendages is associated with pulmonary atresia.

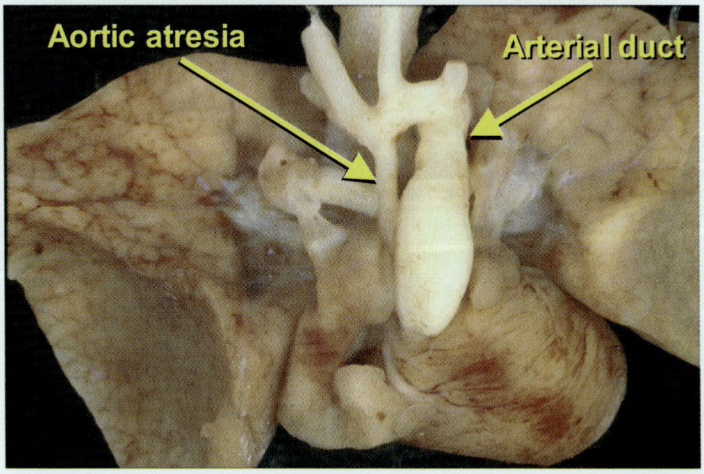

Figure 4.15 A specimen of isomeric arrangement of the left atrial appendages associated with aortic atresia.

right isomerism. The ventricular mass can then take any possible form (Fig. 3.22). A common valve guarding the atrioventricular junctions, with either an atrioventricular

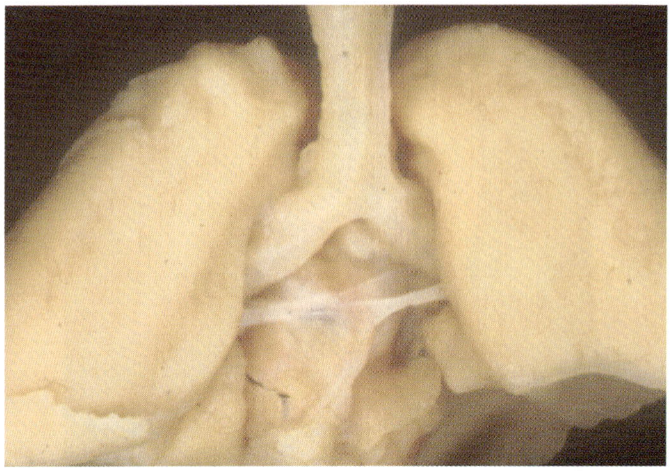

Figure 4.16 A specimen with isomeric arrangement of the right atrial appendages viewed from behind shows bilaterally short main bronchi.

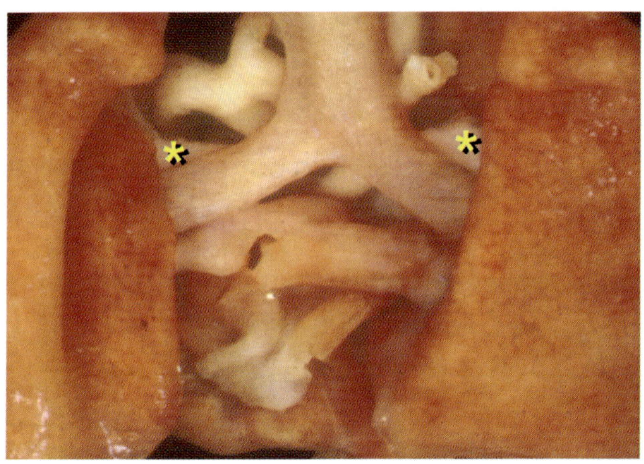

Figure 4.17 This specimen with isomeric arrangement of the left atrial appendages seen from behind shows bilaterally long main bronchi. The pulmonary arteries (*) supplying the lower lobes pass above the bronchi.

septal defect or double inlet connection, is found in between two-thirds and three-quarters of hearts with left or right isomerism (Fig. 4.13).

Ventriculo-arterial Junctions

Any combination of ventriculo-arterial connections can be anticipated. Few patients with right isomerism, however, have concordant ventriculo-arterial connections, whereas concordant connections are found in about two-thirds of those with left isomerism. Discordant connections, and double outlet from the right ventricle, are much more common in right isomerism. Significantly, pulmonary obstruction, stenosis or atresia, is present in the majority of cases with right isomerism, but is seldom seen in left isomerism (Fig. 4.14). On the other hand, obstruction to aortic flow, produced by lesions such as coarctation or tubular hypoplasia, is more common in left isomerism (Fig. 4.15).

Summary

Although the combination of lesions found in patients with isomeric atrial appendages can be daunting, there is nothing complex about understanding them if the cardiac structure is analysed in sequential manner. The cardiac defects are characteristic, and can be anticipated from the nature of the isomerism. Thus, the presence of totally anomalous pulmonary venous connection is to be expected when the heart lacks any morphologically left atrial structures. It is absence of the inferior caval vein, with azygos continuation, that is characteristic of the majority of, but not all, the hearts lacking morphologically right atrial structures. In this context, although the morphology of the spleen is of only limited value as an indication of cardiac morphology, it is always important to recognise its absence, since this increases the susceptibility to clinical infection. The best inferential guide to the presence of isomerism of the atrial appendages, nonetheless, is the discovery of an isomeric arrangement of the bronchial tree (Figs. 4.16 and 4.17).

5

Normal Septal Structures

To appreciate the arrangement of the septums within the heart, we must first provide a clear distinction between septal and parietal structures. A septum separates the cavities of adjacent chambers, and can be removed without disturbing the walls of the heart itself. A parietal structure, in contrast, separates the inside from the outside of the heart. Removal of a parietal wall, therefore, creates a hole in the margins of the heart (Fig. 5.1). When defined in this fashion, three major cardiac septums can be distinguished — the atrial septum separating the cavity of the right from that of the left atrium, the atrioventricular septum located between the right atrium and the left ventricle, and the ventricular septum interposed between the cavities of the ventricles.

The Atrial Septum

The atrial septum is made up largely of the flap valve of the oval fossa, together with the thickened anterior rim of the fossa which abuts on the muscular atrioventricular sandwich (Fig. 5.2). The so-called 'septum secundum' is formed almost exclusively by the infolded atrial walls between the connections of the superior caval vein to the right atrium and the right pulmonary veins to the left atrium. Such infoldings (Fig. 5.3) are not septal structures within the definitions given above. Similarly, the so-called sinus septum, found postero-inferiorly, is no more than the fold separating the openings of the inferior caval vein and the coronary sinus (Fig. 5.2). Antero-superiorly, this fold and the inferior rim of the oval fossa are directly continuous with the muscular atrioventricular sandwich, which we previously described incorrectly as a septal component (see below).

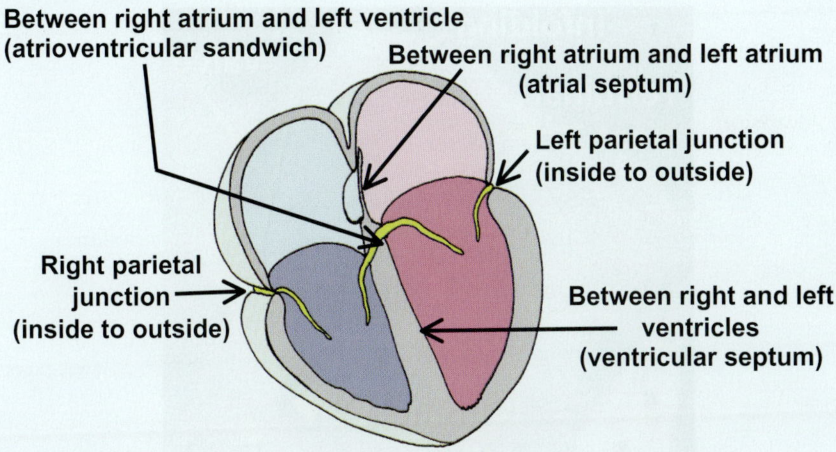

Figure 5.1 Schematic representation of a four-chamber section to show parietal versus septal structures.

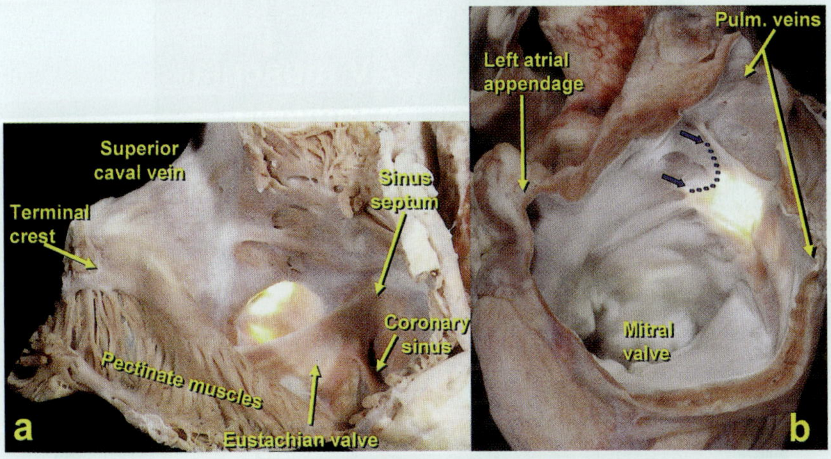

Figure 5.2 (a) This view of the right atrium shows the atrial septum 'enface' with the valve of the oval fossa transilluminated. The Eustachian valve guarding the orifice of the inferior caval vein is particulary extensive in this heart. (b) This view of the left atrium shows the valve transilluminated marking the extent of the oval fossa. The small arrows indicate the edge of the valve (dotted line), which can be probed from the right atrium in cases with probe patency of the oval fossa.

The Atrioventricular Sandwich

Appreciation of the location of the atrial and ventricular septal structures is essential for the understanding of septal defects. In the normal heart, with separate right and left atrioventricular junctions, the outflow tract of the aorta interposes between the larger part of the orifice of the mitral valve and the ventricular septum (Fig. 5.4).

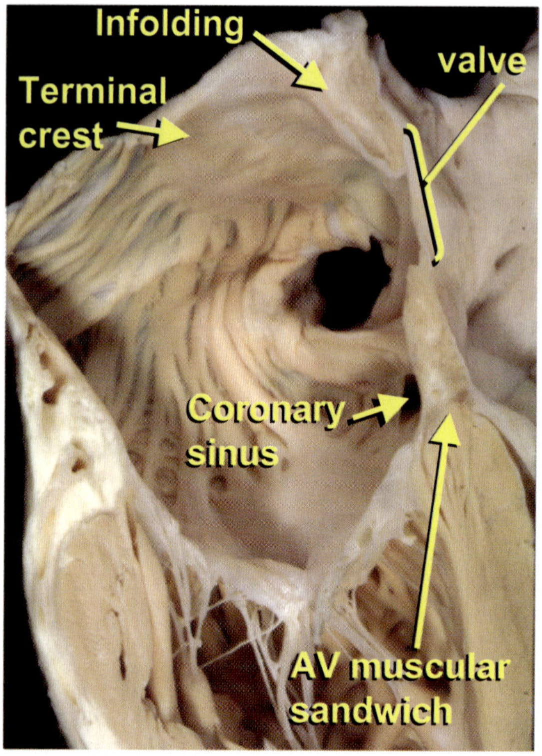

Figure 5.3 This section shows the infolding of the right atrial wall that forms the rim of the oval fossa.

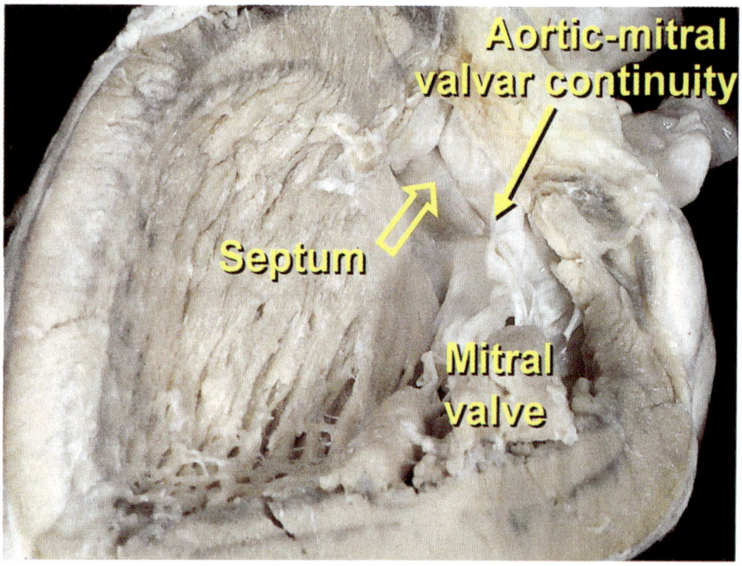

Figure 5.4 This window dissection of the left ventricle shows the aortic outflow tract (open arrows) passing between the septal surface and the mitral valve.

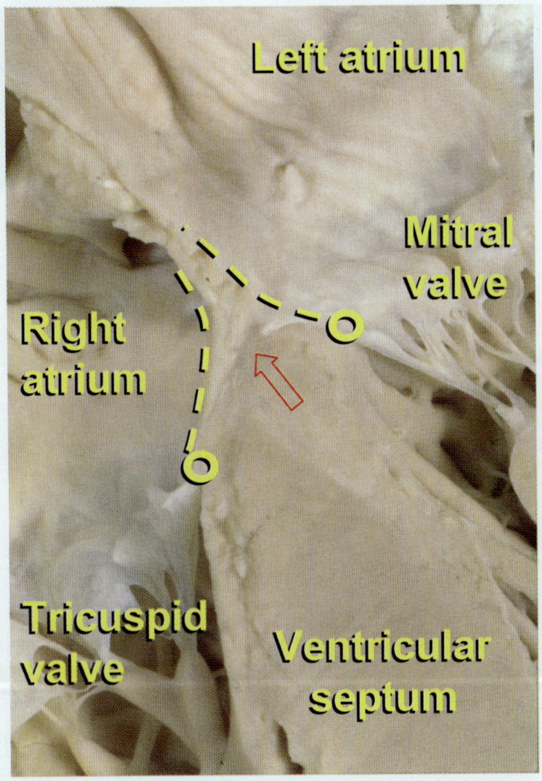

Figure 5.5 This four-chamber cut displays the higher attachment of the mitral valve relative to the tricuspid valve (o-o). The crest of the muscular ventricular septum (arrow) is in atrioventricular location, between right atrium and left ventricle. Structurally, however, it is capped by overlying atrial musculature (broken lines) and epicardial fibro-fatty tissues.

In the posterior aspect of the diverticulum thus formed, the hingepoint of the mitral valve is offset relative to that of the tricuspid valve. In this area, therefore, there is overlapping of the right atrial vestibule and the crest of the ventricular septum. The arrangement produces an area that is atrioventricular in location, being positioned between the right atrium and the left ventricle, but is a composite of atrial musculature, epicardial fat and ventricular musculature. Antero-superiorly, the open sandwich is closed by the central fibrous body (Fig. 5.5). This fibrous area forms the medial wall of the subaortic outflow tract, being the confluence of the rightward margin of the area of fibrous continuity between the leaflets of the aortic and mitral valves and another a plate of fibrous tissue that separates the right and left sides of the heart. The plate-like component, therefore, is a true septal structure, specifically the membranous septum (Fig. 5.6). The tendon of Todaro, the fibrous structure formed by the junction of the Eustachian and Thebesian valves, extends through the inferior rim of the oval fossa and inserts into the atrial aspect of this central fibrous body. The membranous septum itself is crossed on its right-sided aspect by the hingepoint of the septal leaflet of the tricuspid valve (Fig. 5.7). This divides the

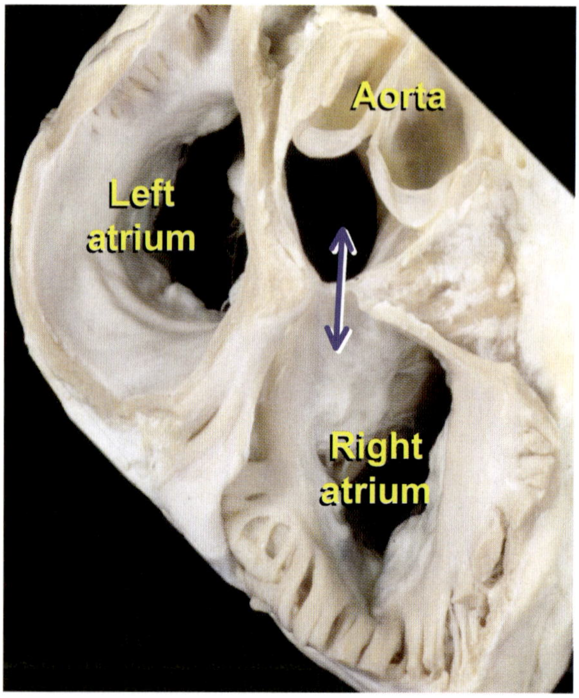

Figure 5.6 Removal of the non-coronary aortic leaflet and sinus in this specimen shows the location of the membranous septum (↔) between the aortic root and the right atrium.

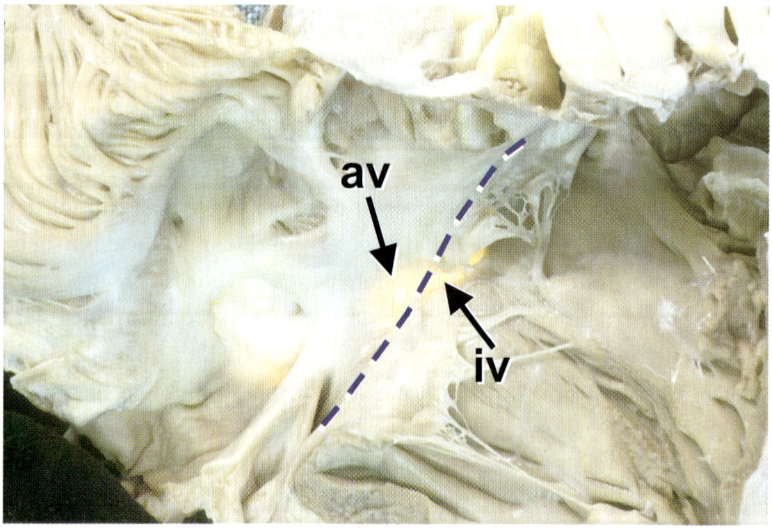

Figure 5.7 The right atrium and ventricle displayed with transillumination of the membranous septum. The hingeline (- - -) of the tricuspid valve divides the membranous septum into atrioventricular (av) and interventricular (iv) components.

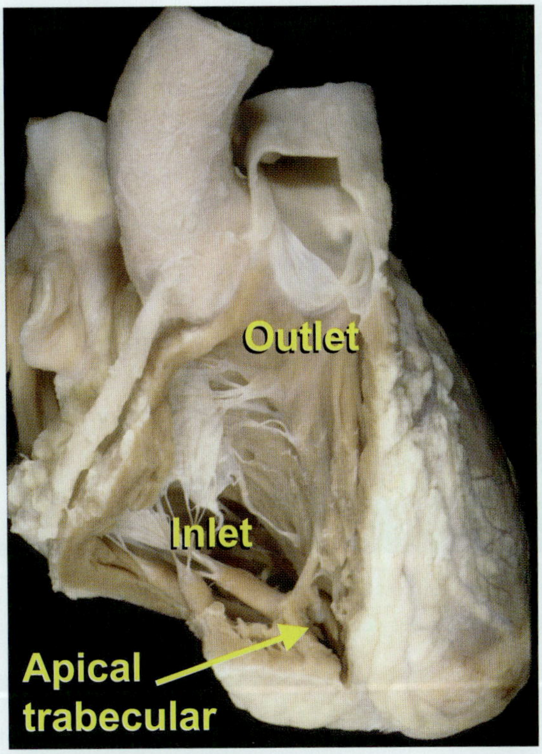

Figure 5.8 The three components of the right ventricle are shown in this dissection.

membranous septum into atrioventricular and interventricular components. Thus, whilst the membranous septum is exclusively fibrous, the atrioventricular sandwich is made up of layers of muscle enclosing epicardial fat and fibrous tissue (Figs. 5.5 and 5.6).

The Ventricular Septum

The septal structures separating the ventricular cavities are made up almost exclusively of muscle, albeit that the small interventricular component of the membranous septum is also, self-evidently, a ventricular septal component (Fig. 5.7). This fibrous component, in fact, can be considered as the central part of the septum, with the muscular septum radiating out from this point to separate the ventricular cavities. In the past, we tended to draw arbitrary lines on the right ventricular surface of the septum, arguing that it could be divided into inlet, apical trabecular and outlet components (Fig. 5.8). We now know that this approach was simplistic. In reality, such lines divide the right ventricle itself into its component parts. But, because of the deeply wedged origin of the subaortic outflow from the left ventricle, the muscular septum separates the inlet of the right ventricle mostly from the outlet of the left

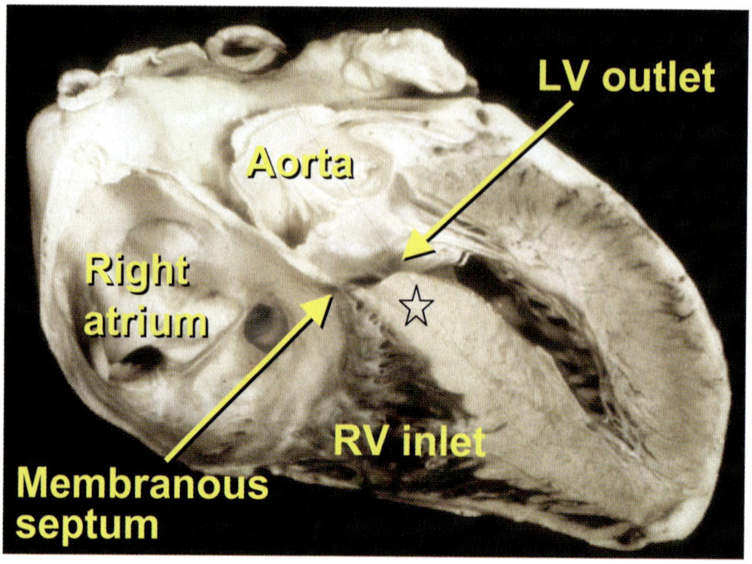

Figure 5.9 This simulated subcostal long axis section demonstrates the part of the ventricular septum (☆) that is situated between the right ventricular (RV) inlet and left ventricular (LV) outlet.

ventricle (Fig. 5.9). And, because of the free-standing subpulmonary infundibulum, only a very small part of the right ventricular outlet is a true muscular outlet septum (Fig. 5.8). In the normal heart, this outlet part of the septum cannot be distinguished from the rest of the muscular septum. For all these reasons, therefore, it is best to analyse the normal ventricular septum simply in terms of its muscular and membranous components (Fig. 5.7). As discussed, nonetheless, it is entirely appropriate to analyse the ventricles themselves in terms of inlet, apical trabecular and outlet components (Fig. 5.8).

6

Interatrial Communications

Deficiencies in the atrial septum permitting an interatrial shunt are, at first sight, amongst the simplest of congenital cardiac malformations. A hole within the atrial septum is an integral part of the foetal circulation, being necessary to permit the richly oxygenated inferior caval venous blood to reach the left side of the heart, and thence the developing brain. Most interatrial communications represent persistence of this arrangement. They are real defects in the atrial septum (Fig. 6.1). This is not true of the less common morphological defects, which permit shunting of blood between the atriums. The phenotypic feature of these less common variants is that they are outside the confines of the true atrial septum. They are appropriately described as interatrial communications but they are not true atrial septal defects.

The Normal Interatrial Septum

As we have just discussed, the atrial septum is made up of the tissues that separate the cavity of the right atrium from that of the left. In the normal heart, a surprisingly small area of the atrial walls qualifies for this description. In essence, the tissue separating the atriums is solely within and inferior to the rims of the oval fossa. As long as the floor of the fossa, the so-called flap valve, overlaps its rim, and left atrial pressure is higher than the right, there will be no interatrial shunting (Fig. 6.2). This is true regardless of whether the flap valve is fused to the rims of the fossa. In a significant proportion of the normal population, even up to the ninth decade, the flap valve and rim of the fossa remain unfused, producing a probe-patent oval foramen. This arrangement is of haemodynamic significance only in the unusual situation in which right atrial pressure exceeds left. This sometimes occurs with pulmonary vascular

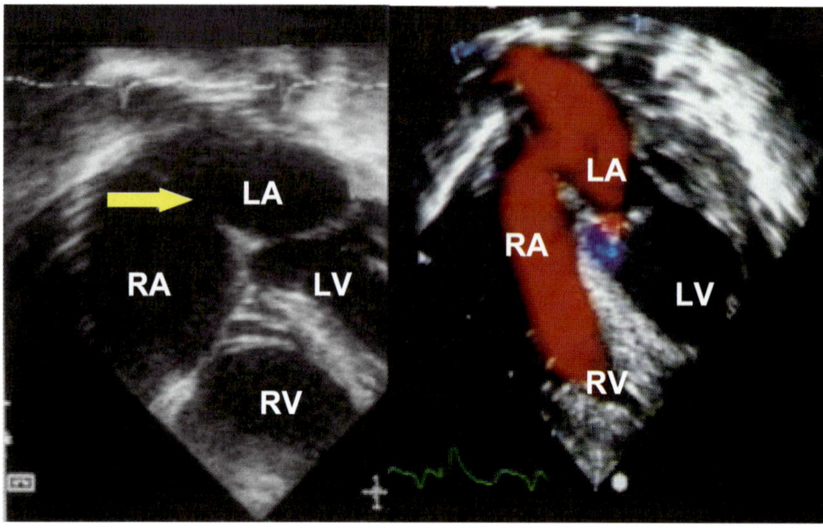

Figure 6.1 Echocardiogram demonstrating an oval fossa defect in subcostal view.

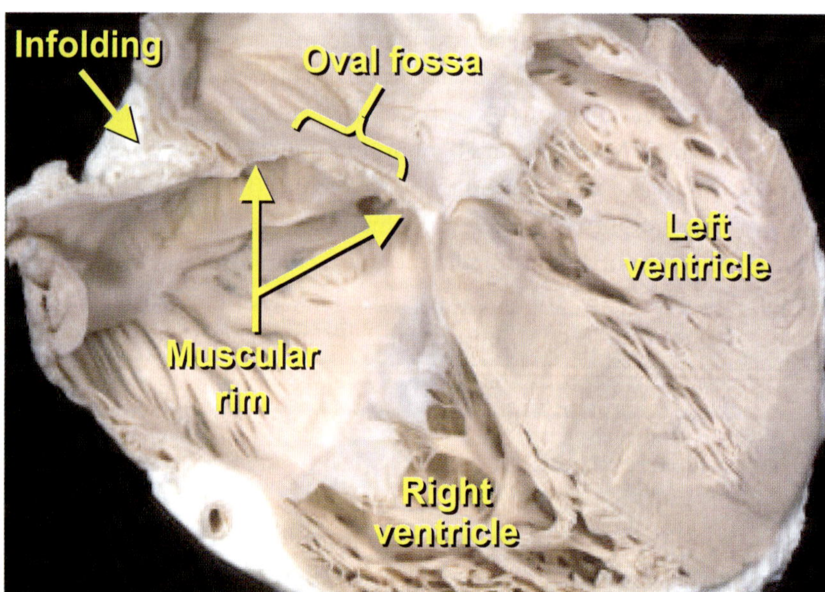

Figure 6.2 This four-chamber section shows the valve of the oval fossa adherent to the left side of its muscular rim. The pale areas are the ingress of epicardial fat within the rim.

disease. The significance of such a probe-patent oval foramen in the aetiology of some forms of cerebral embolisation is as yet unclear. At first sight, it might also be thought that the rims of the oval fossa are also part of the atrial septum. Indeed, the superior rim is often called the 'septum secundum'. Sectioning the heart shows that, in reality, the superior rim is simply the infolded atrial walls. It is possible to

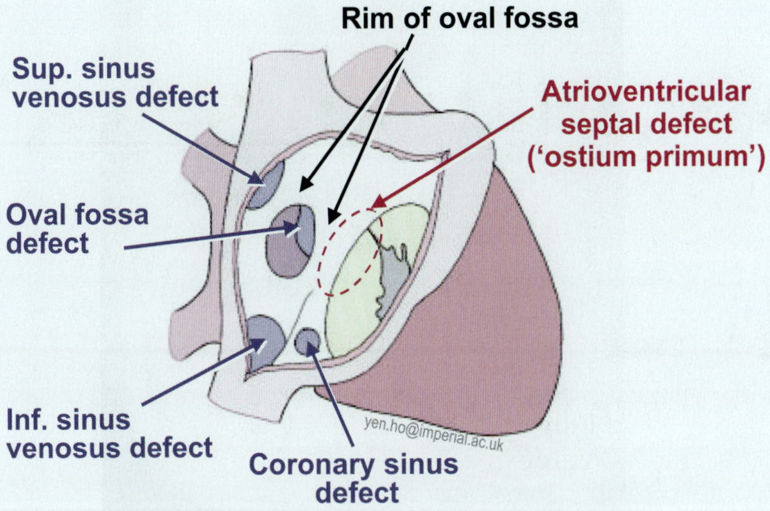

Figure 6.3 Only deficiencies within the oval fossa are true defects of the atrial septum. The locations of other interatrial communications are shown in this diagram.

pass a needle from the right to left atrium through this rim, but only by traversing the fat-filled extracardiac space (Fig. 6.2). The inferior rim of the oval fossa, in contrast, is an extensive muscular buttress supporting the base of the flap valve. This is a true septum. It is then continuous with the area where the cavity of the right atrium is separated from that of the left ventricle because the mitral valve is attached more proximally than the tricuspid valve. As explained in the previous chapter, this arrangement produces an atrioventricular sandwich (Chapter 5, Fig. 5.5). The so-called 'ostium primum' defects occupy this area of the septum (Fig. 6.3). They permit interatrial communications, but are atrioventricular rather than atrial septal defects. The anterior wall of the coronary sinus is also continuous with the inferior margin of the oval fossa. As the sinus extends into the left atrioventricular junction, nonetheless, it becomes a free-standing structure within the left atrioventricular groove, having its own muscular walls discrete from those of the left atrium (Fig. 6.4).

Echocardiographic display of the atrial septum is best made using the subcostal four chamber section. Short axis sections of the aortic root obtained either from the subcostal right oblique or parasternal short axis views can also be used.

Defects within the Oval Fossa

In the neonatal period, anything which produces congestive cardiac failure can result in dilation of the right atrium. This, in turn, can stretch the rims of the oval fossa. The stretched fossa may not then be overlapped by the flap valve, producing

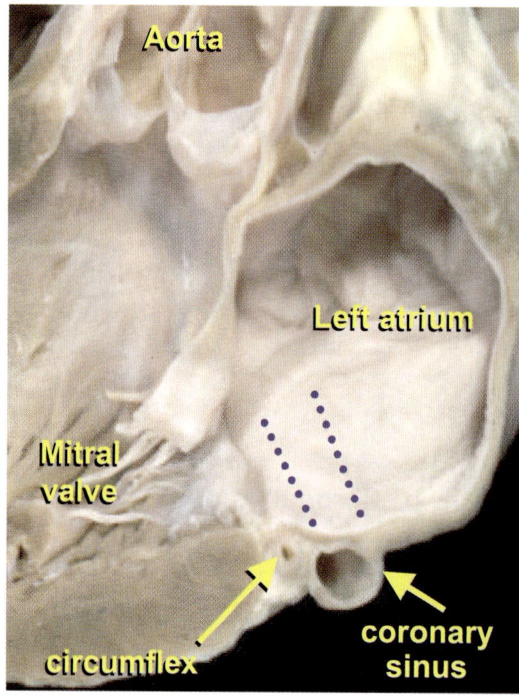

Figure 6.4 This longitudinal section through the left ventricular outflow tract and the left atrium shows the location of the coronary sinus in the left atrioventricular groove and its rightward course (between dotted lines) along the epicardial aspect of the left atrium.

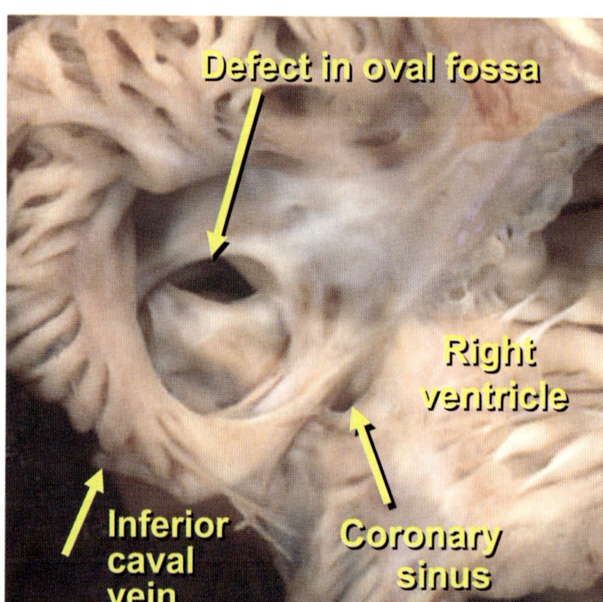

Figure 6.5 This heart shows a defect in the oval fossa.

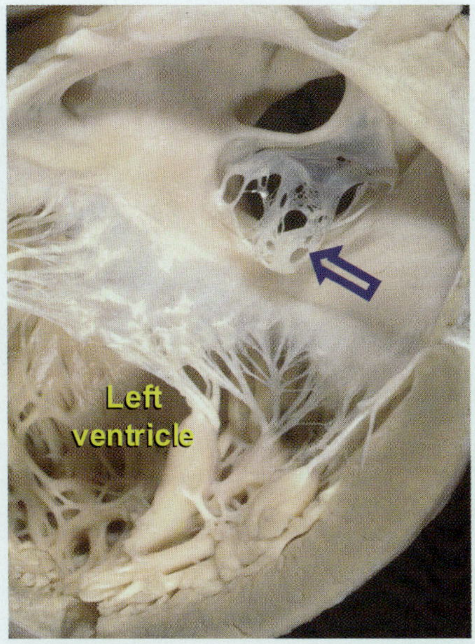

Figure 6.6 This flap valve of the oval fossa is aneurysmal and filigreed (arrow).

the potential for an interatrial shunt. This type of lesion will correct itself when the dilation itself is corrected. It should not, therefore, be considered as an atrial septal defect. This mechanism is the cause of some of the so-called spontaneous closures of atrial septal defects reported with some frequency over the neonatal period. True septal defects within the oval fossa are found when the flap valve does not overlap the rim even when there is no atrial dilation. This can be because the flap valve is too small, or because it has a hole in it (Fig. 6.5). The flap valve can sometimes be completely absent. When the valve is perforate, the holes can be so numerous that there is a filigreed network across the area of the fossa (Figs. 6.6 and 6.7). When the flap valve is deficient postero-inferiorly, the defect can extend into the mouth of the inferior caval vein. The caval vein can then drain predominantly into the left atrium. When the flap valve is perforate or deficient, it is unlikely that a defect will close spontaneously, although some cases are documented when aneurysmal expansion of the floor of the fossa has closed a pre-existing atrial septal defect.

The Sinus Venosus Defect

This much less common congenital lesion, making up perhaps one-eighth of interatrial communications excluding 'primum' defects, can only be understood properly when it is realised that it is not a defect of the atrial septum (Fig. 6.8). Found almost always within the mouth of the superior caval vein, but rarely in the mouth of the inferior caval vein, the defect usually exists because the caval vein has biatrial connections, overriding the rim of the oval fossa so as to produce an extraseptal interatrial

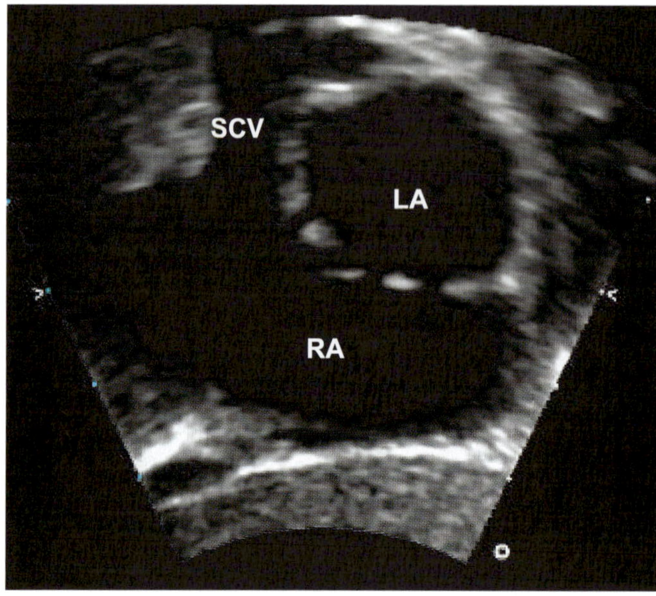

Figure 6.7 Subcostal section showing multiple defects in the oval fossa.

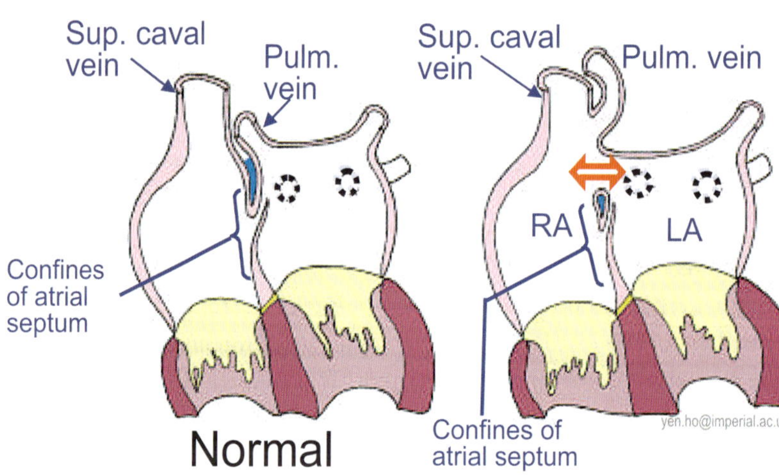

Figure 6.8 The superior sinus venosus defect (double headed arrow) is located outside the confines of the true atrial septum.

communication (Fig. 6.9). Most frequently, the pulmonary veins from part of the right lung are also involved, being anomalously connected to the superior caval vein. This defect should not be diagnosed echocardiographically unless it can be positively shown that the interatrial communication is outside the confines of the oval fossa (Fig. 6.10).

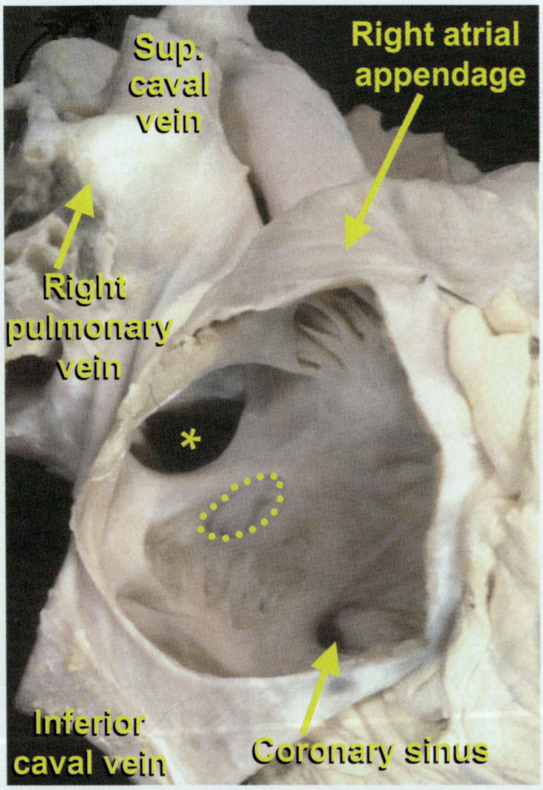

Figure 6.9 This view into the right atrium shows the orifice of the superior caval vein in the roof of the superior sinus venosus defect (*) while the superior rim of the oval fossa (dotted oval) forms its inferior border.

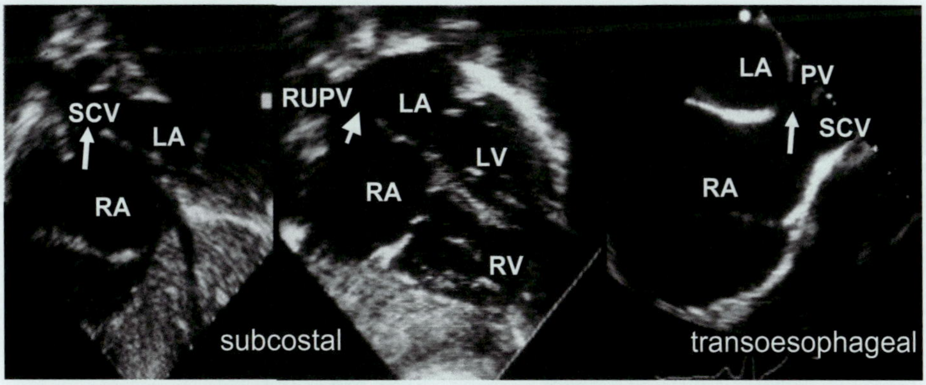

Figure 6.10 Subcostal paracoronal sections showing a superior sinus venosus defect (arrows) with overriding of the superior caval vein and right upper pulmonary vein. The oval fossa is intact. The transoesophageal echocardiogram is a vertical (parasagittal) section which again shows overriding of the superior caval and right upper pulmonary veins.

The Coronary Sinus Defect

This is the rarest type of interatrial communication, although the rarity may, in part, reflect an unawareness of its precise morphology. In essence, any communication between the cavities of the coronary sinus and left atrium will produce an interatrial communication through the mouth of the coronary sinus. In the mildest form, this exists as a simple fenestration or multiple fenestrations (Fig. 6.11). In

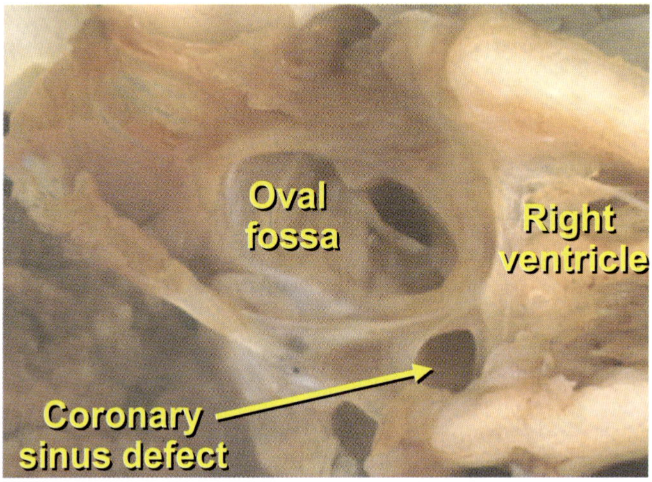

Figure 6.11 A hole at the anticipated location of the orifice of the coronary sinus leads directly to the left atrium.

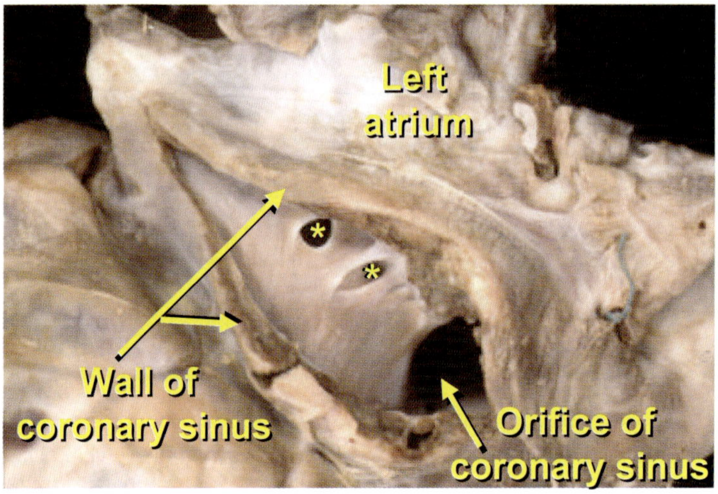

Figure 6.12 The coronary sinus has been opened along its inferior wall to show a large orifice that leads to the right atrium. Two small fenestrations (*) in its superior wall communicate with the left atrium.

the most extreme form, the entirety of the walls normally separating the cavities is lacking, and the mouth of the coronary sinus forms a large defect (Fig. 6.12). This extreme form is usually found when a left superior caval vein connects to the roof of the left atrium between the opening of the appendage and the orifices of the left pulmonary veins. In this situation, there are often filigreed remnants of the wall of the sinus running across the postero-inferior wall of the left atrium. Such an arrangement is termed unroofing of the coronary sinus. In this setting, it is important to establish whether there is a communicating vein superiorly between the right and left caval venous systems. When such a communication is present, the defect can be repaired by tying the left superior caval vein and patching the mouth of the sinus. When it is not, the surgeon must reconstruct the left atrium to connect the left caval vein with the mouth of the coronary sinus. When the coronary sinus defect exists without a left sided superior caval vein, then the mouth of the sinus can be closed.

7

Atrioventricular Septal Defects

These hearts have as their phenotypic feature total absence of the normal arrangement of the atrioventricular sandwich, and are unified in having a common atrioventricular junction.

What Is the Normal Atrioventricular Septum?

The atrioventricular sandwich of the normal heart separates the right atrium from the left ventricle. As explained in Chapter 5, this is not a true septum. It exists because the attachment of the septal leaflet of the tricuspid valve is more towards the ventricular apex than is the corresponding attachment of the mitral valve (Fig. 7.1). This is the feature that the echocardiographer describes as off-setting of the valvar leaflets evident on subcostal and parasternal four-chamber sections (Fig. 7.2). Postero-inferiorly, invagination of the fibro-fatty tissues from the epicardium separates the atrial from the ventricular myocardium at the area described as the cardiac crux. Anterosuperiorly, fibro-fatty tissues give way to atrial musculature directly overlying the central fibrous body. The true atrioventricular septum is fibrous, and is an integral part of the central fibrous body (Fig. 7.3). It is the part of the membranous septum that is superior to the attachment of the septal leaflet of the tricuspid valve, and thus separates the right atrium from the subaortic outflow tract. In the normal heart, because the aortic root is wedged between it and the septum, the mitral valve has a very limited septal attachment. Furthermore, the mural leaflet of the normal mitral valve guards two-thirds of the circumference of the left atrioventricular orifice.

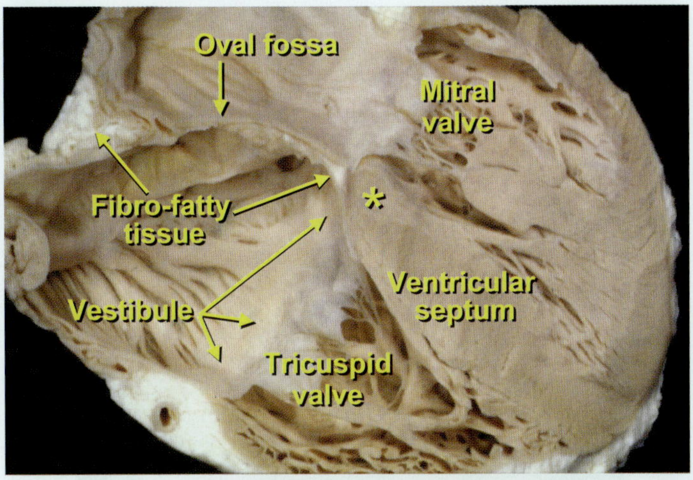

Figure 7.1 This four-chamber cut through a normal heart shows the offset arrangement between tricuspid and mitral valves, which produces the atrioventricular 'sandwich' of vestibular wall, fibro-fatty tissue and crest of the muscular ventricular septum (*).

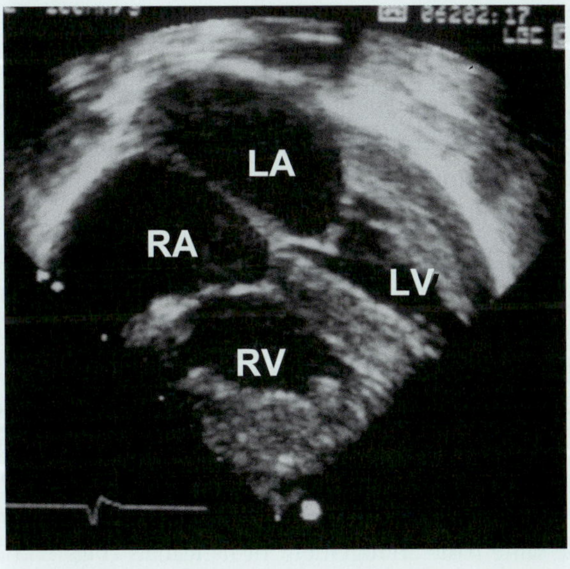

Figure 7.2 Subcostal parasternal echocardiogram showing normal valvar offset in the four-chamber plane.

The Consequences of Defective Atrioventricular Septation

Exceedingly rarely, hearts exist with the absence only of the atrioventricular component of the membranous septum. Such lesions, therefore, are better described as atrioventricular membranous septal defects with separate right and left

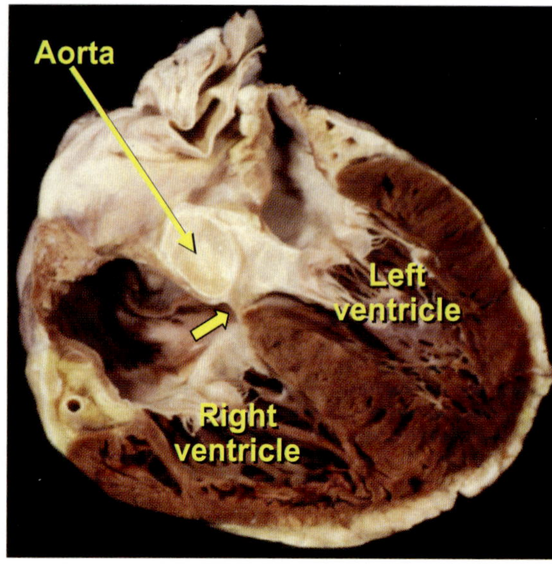

Figure 7.3 This five-chamber cut includes the aortic root and the atrioventricular component of the membranous septum (arrow).

atrioventricular junctions. Apart from the hole at the anticipated site of the membranous septum, the structure of these hearts is normal. They do not have a 'common atrioventricular canal'. The hearts we group together as atrioventricular septal defects have absence of both the membranous septum and muscular atrioventricular sandwich. The absence of these septal parts then markedly changes the configuration of the atrioventricular junctions and the ventricular mass. In such hearts, the aorta is no longer wedged between the mitral and tricuspid valves. Instead, the aortic valve is positioned anteriorly to a common atrioventricular junction (Fig. 7.4 — upper). This common junction is guarded by a characteristic atrioventricular valve. In the majority of hearts, the valve has a common atrioventricular orifice, and is made up of five leaflets. In a minority, the so-called 'ostium primum' defects, the common valve is divided into separate orifices for the right and left ventricles (Fig. 7.4 — lower). Whether the valve has one orifice, or separate right and left orifices, it has the same basic arrangement of its leaflets (Figs .7.5 and 7.6). There are two leaflets attached exclusively within the right ventricle. These are broadly comparable with leaflets of the normal tricuspid valve. They are found anterosuperiorly and inferiorly (or murally). The other leaflets of the common valve have no counterpart in the normal heart. One leaflet is solely within the left ventricle, being located along the lateral aspect of the left atrioventricular junction. It is the mural leaflet. It is different from the mural leaflet of the normal mitral valve because it guards less than one-third of the overall circumference of the left junction (Fig. 7.7). The other two leaflets are attached by a tension apparatus in both ventricles. They are the superior and inferior bridging leaflets. It is the presence

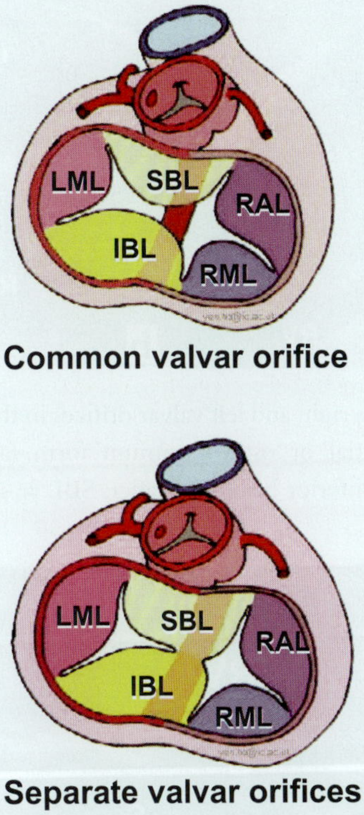

Figure 7.4 Diagram showing the common atrioventricular junction in hearts with atrioventricular septal defect. The junction is guarded by a valve with common orifice (upper panel) or separate right and left valvar orifices (lower panel). The common valve has five leaflets. Two of them, the superior and inferior bridging leaflets, are shared by both ventricles. Fusion between the bridging leaflets divides the common valvar orifice into two discrete orifices. IBL = inferior bridging leaflet, LML = left mural leaflet, RAL = right antero-superior leaflet, RML = right mural leaflet, SBL = superior bridging leaflet.

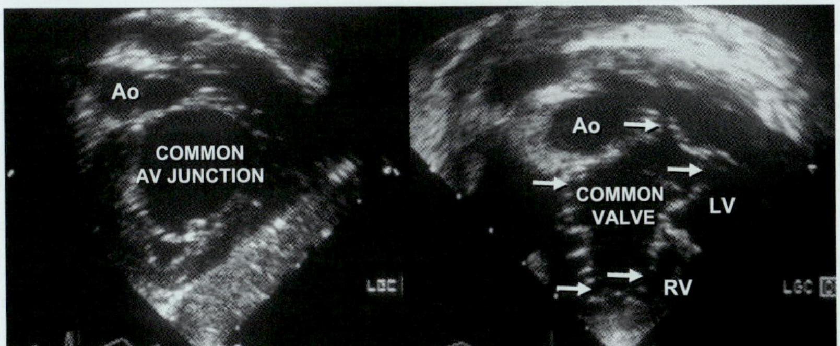

Figure 7.5 Subcostal left oblique short axis echocardiogram demonstrating the common atrioventricular junction in a case of atrioventricular septal defect with common valvar orifice. Note that there are five leaflets. The arrows indicate the 'commissures'.

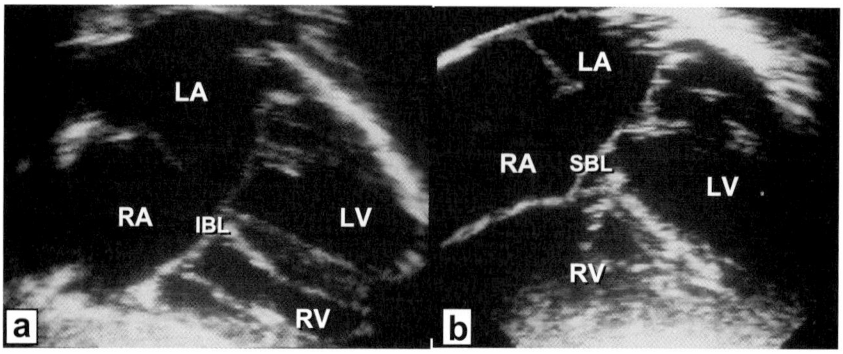

Figure 7.6 There are separate right and left valvar orifices in this case of atrioventricular septal defect — the so-called 'partial' or 'ostium primum' form. (a) subcostal and (b) parasternal four-chamber planes. IBL = inferior bridging leaflet; SBL = superior bridging leaflet.

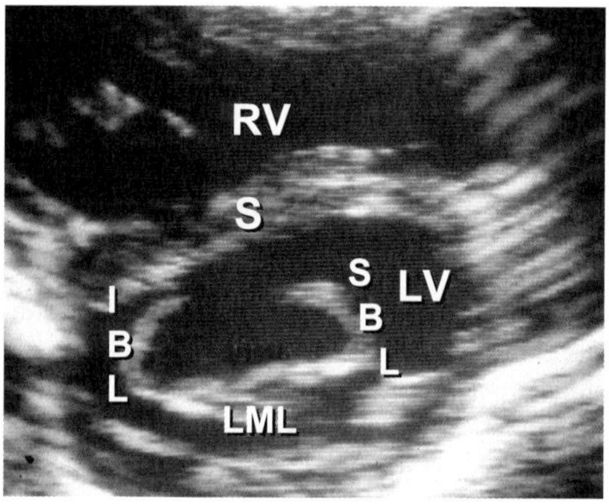

Figure 7.7 Echocardiogram showing the left ventricular valve with the characteristic configuration of three leaflets in parasternal short axis section. IBL = inferior bridging leaflet, LML = left mural leaflet, S = septum, SBL = superior bridging leaflet.

of a tongue of leaflet tissue between the two bridging leaflets that may separate the valve into separate right and left orifices (Figs. 7.8 and 7.9). Echocardiographically, it is the subcostal four-chamber view that demonstrates the inferior bridging leaflet, while the parasternal and apical four-chamber sections permit visualisation of the superior bridging leaflet. Irrespective of the presence of separate orifices, or a common orifice, the left component of the valve guarding the common atrioventricular junction has three leaflets (Fig. 7.7), while the right component has four leaflets. The zone of apposition between the left ventricular components of the bridging leaflets is part of the valvar orifice although it is often described erroneously as a 'cleft' in the aortic (or anterior) leaflet of a normal mitral valve. The papillary muscles supporting the leaflets of the left valve, furthermore, are markedly

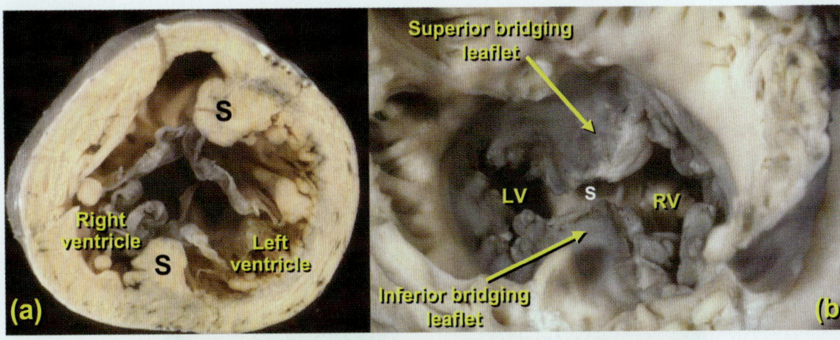

Figure 7.8 (a) This section viewed from the cardiac apex shows the common atrioventricular junction. S = septum. (b) This specimen viewed from the atrial aspect shows the five leaflets of the atrioventricular valve. The superior and inferior bridging leaflets have not fused and the crest of the ventricular septum is visible through the gap.

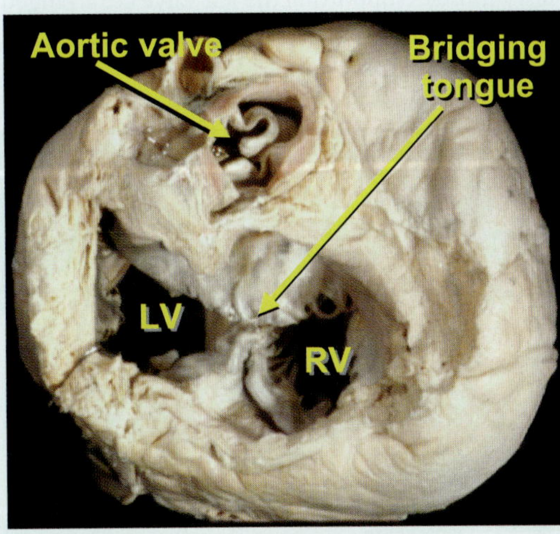

Figure 7.9 A tongue of leaflet tissue connects the bridging leaflets to form separate right and left valvar orifices.

different in orientation from those supporting the normal mitral valve, as is the arrangement of the leaflets themselves (Figs. 7.10 and 7.11). In addition to the abnormalities of the atrioventricular junction, the ventricular mass in patients with atrioventricular septal defects shows marked disproportion between its inlet and outlet dimensions. In the normal heart, these dimensions are more-or-less the same. In atrioventricular septal defects, the outlet dimension is much longer than the inlet (Fig. 7.12). This disproportion, and the unwedged position of the subaortic outflow tract (Figs. 7.13 and 7.14), result in the left ventricular outlet being much narrower in atrioventricular septal defects than in normal hearts. All atrioventricular septal defects have these anatomical features in common, namely a common

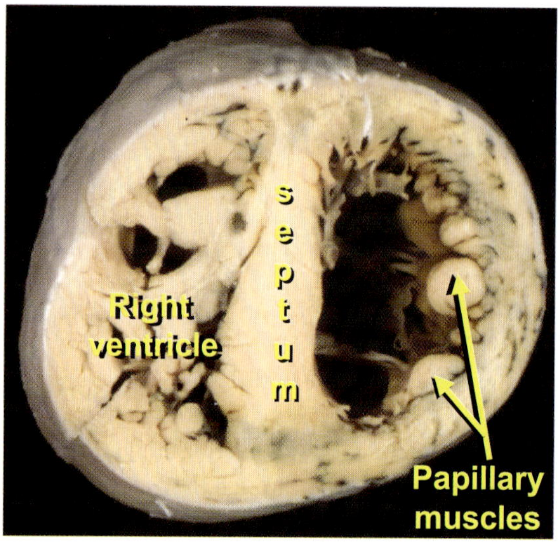

Figure 7.10 The papillary muscles supporting the left valve are arranged in superior–inferior locations in this heart with atrioventricular septal defect.

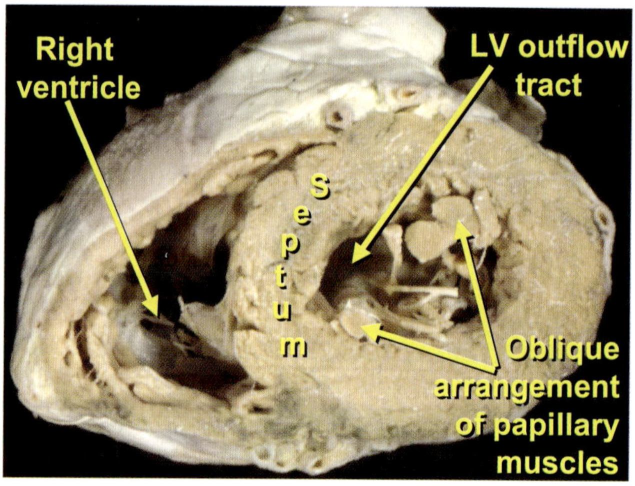

Figure 7.11 This cut through a normal heart in attitudinal orientation shows the oblique arrangement of the papillary muscles supporting the mitral valve.

atrioventricular junction, unwedging of the aorta, a left atrioventricular valve with three leaflets, a narrowed subaortic outflow tract, and disproportion between the inlet and outlet dimensions of the ventricular septum. Not all defects, however, are alike in their other anatomical features. The significant variability concerns, first, the arrangement of the leaflets of the effectively common atrioventricular valve and, second, the anatomical potential for shunting through the atrioventricular septal defect.

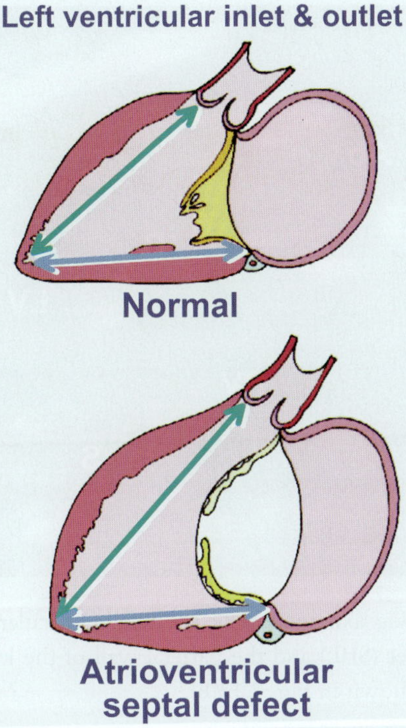

Figure 7.12 The outlet dimension is much longer than the inlet dimension in hearts with atrioventricular septal defect.

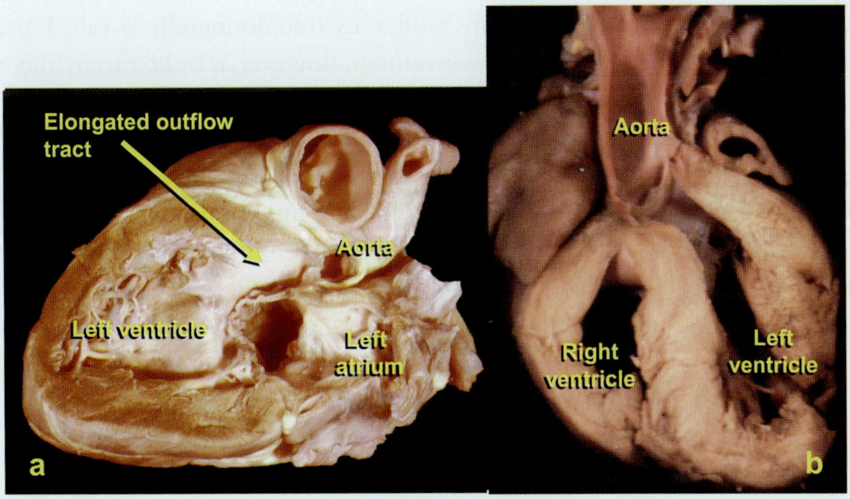

Figure 7.13 (a) This longitudinal section approximating to the parasternal long axis view shows the curved and elongated left ventricular outlet. (b) This longitudinal cut made antero-superior to the four-chamber plane shows the passage from the left ventricle to the aorta resembling a dog's leg.

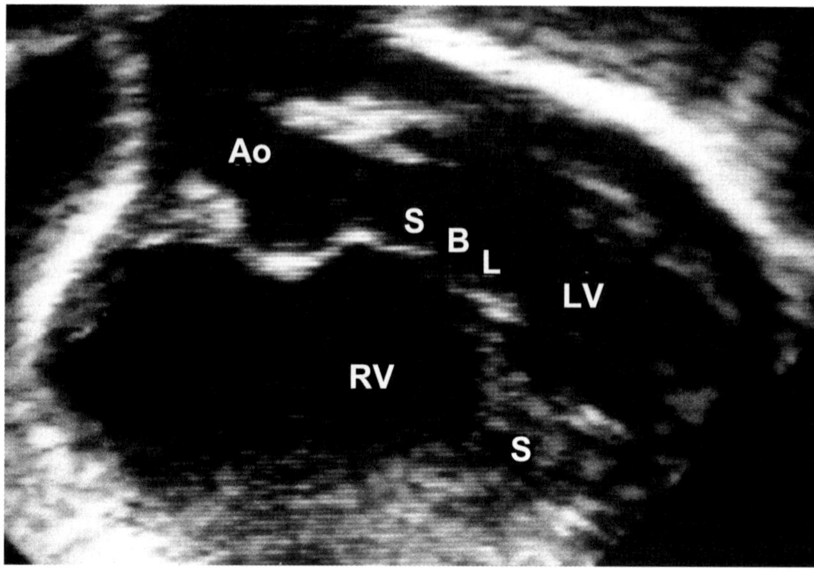

Figure 7.14 Subcostal long axis section of the left ventricular outflow tract formed by the superior bridging leaflet (SBL) and the parietal wall of the left ventricle cut in a plane resembling the specimen shown in Fig. 7.13(b).

Variability of the Atrioventricular Valve

The common atrioventricular valve may have a single orifice or separate right and left orifices (Fig. 7.4). This feature is often used to distinguish so-called 'partial' defects from 'complete' defects. This convention, however, is by no means universal, since some prefer to distinguish these variants on the basis of the level of shunting (see below). This, inevitably, results in the description of 'intermediate' categories, which can, in turn, lead to the creation of truly formidable alpha-numeric classifications. We prefer to avoid attempts at 'pigeon holing', and simply describe the arrangement of the atrioventricular valves and the potential for shunting as separate features of each heart.

Variability of Shunting through the Defect

This depends upon the relationship between the bridging leaflets of the common valve, and the connecting tongue if present, and the atrial and ventricular septal structures (Fig. 7.15). If the bridging leaflets and tongue are firmly attached to the crest of the ventricular septum, then all shunting through the defect will be at atrial level (Fig. 7.16). If, in contrast, the leaflets are attached to the underside of the atrial septum, then shunting will occur only at the ventricular level. If the leaflets

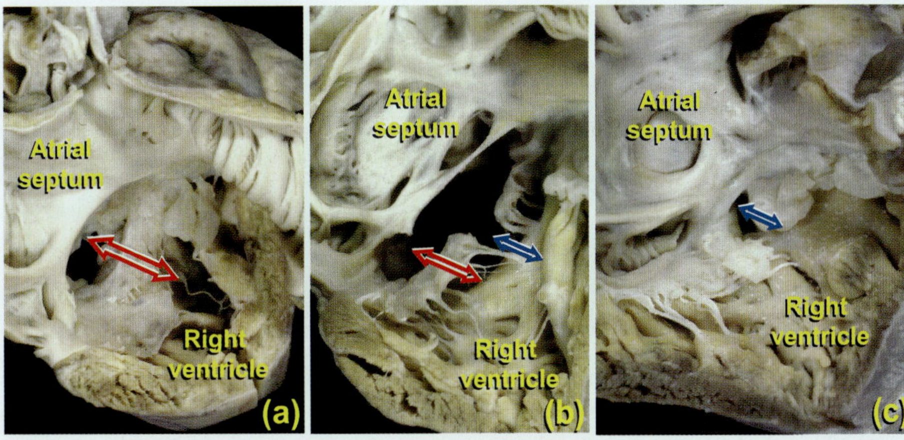

Figure 7.15 The arrangements of the valvar leaflets relative to the septum results in variations in levels of shunting. These three hearts show the atrioventricular septal defect from the right side. (a) The bridging leaflets have fused together. Adherence of the leaflets to the crest of the ventricular septum leaves shunting at the atrial level. This example is the so-called 'ostium primum defect'. Note that the atrial septum at the oval fossa is intact. (b) The superior and inferior bridging leaflets are not fused together nor are they adherent to the septal crest. This arrangement leaves shunting at atrial and at ventricular levels (arrows). (c) The bridging leaflets are adherent to the free margin of the atrial septum, leaving the level of shunting at the ventricular level.

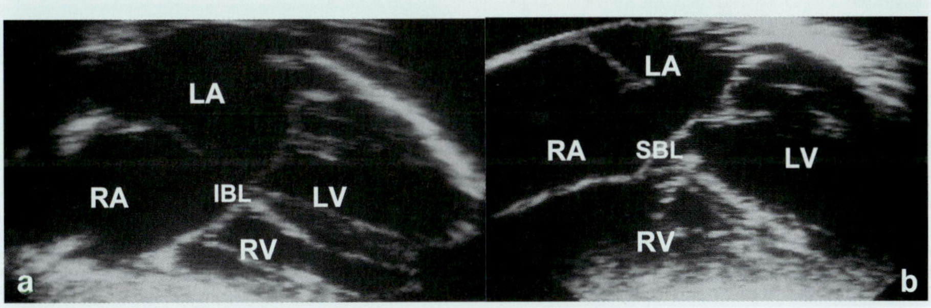

Figure 7.16 Echocardiograms showing interatrial shunting in a case with separate right and left valvar orifices. (a) Subcostal four-chamber view displays the inferior bridging leaflet (IBL) and (b) parasternal four-chamber view shows the superior bridging leaflet (SBL).

are attached to neither the atrial nor ventricular septal structures, i.e. the so-called floating leaflets, shunting will occur at both atrial and ventricular levels (Fig. 7.17). The amount of shunting at the ventricular level will depend in part on the haemodynamic conditions, but also on the extent of tethering of the bridging leaflets to the ventricular septum by tendinous cords.

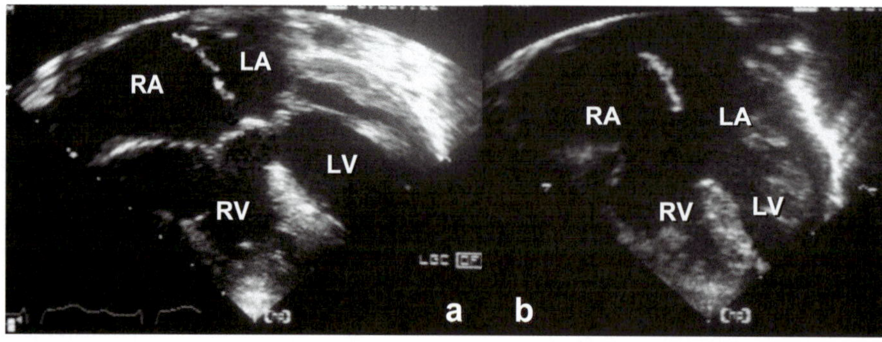

Figure 7.17 Parasternal four-chamber section of a case with common valvar orifice showing the 'primum' defect and interventricular component. During ventricular systole (a) and diastole (b) with shunting at atrial and ventricular levels.

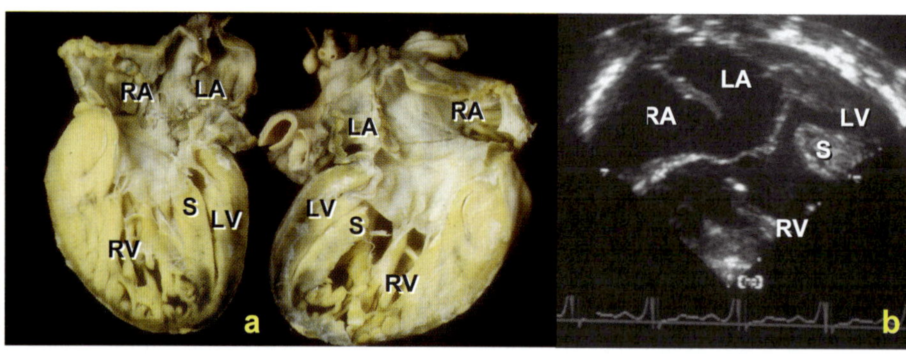

Figure 7.18 (a) A heart specimen with atrioventricular septal defect sectioned in the four-chamber plane to show dominance of the right chambers. (b) Parasternal four-chamber section of an atrioventricular septal defect with common valve orifice and dominance of the right ventricle. The overriding of the atrioventricular valve is more than 75% into the right ventricle. This may also be described as double inlet right ventricle in terms of atrioventricular connections.

The Structure of the Ventricular Wall

Another crucial clinical feature reflects the way in which the common atrioventricular junction is shared between the ventricles. Usually there is a balanced arrangement. Problems can arise, however, if the junction is committed predominantly to one or the other ventricle, giving the so-called right or left ventricular dominant patterns. Those are readily diagnosed by the echocardiographer (Fig. 7.18).

8

Ventricular Septal Defects

Ventricular septal defects are by far the commonest congenital cardiac malformation. Despite this, there is no consensus about the best way to describe their morphological features. Conflict between the various classifications that have been proposed has led to much confusion. A simple and easily understandable way of describing ventricular septal defects is essential, since they frequently occur with other defects, such as complete or congenitally corrected transposition. They are an integral part of tetralogy of Fallot, double outlet ventricles and common arterial trunk. Ventricular septal defects also occur in 'isolation', nonetheless, and the descriptions of the morphology of such 'isolated' defects must be equally applicable to those which occur in the more complex settings.

Terminology

The size of the defect is important, since this determines the haemodynamic consequences. The location of the defect within the ventricular septum is equally important, particularly to the surgeon, since this indicates its proximity to the atrioventricular conduction tissues. The relationship of the defect to valvar structures will provide an indication of its likelihood of spontaneous closure. The classification we use takes note of all these features, and is particularly useful to echocardiographers.

What are the margins of a ventricular septal defect? The answer to this question is not as obvious as it may seem. It is not a problem when there is a simple hole in the muscular ventricular septum (Figs. 8.1 and 8.2). All the margins of such a hole are, more-or-less, in the same plane, and are readily identified from either the right or left ventricular aspects. Problems arise when the defect is at the edge of the muscular

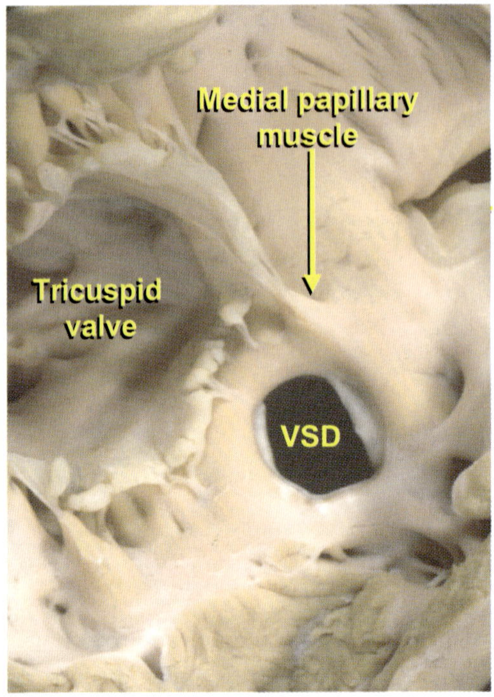

Figure 8.1 This muscular ventricular septal defect is located in the trabecular portion of the right ventricle.

ventricular septum, particularly when the ventricular septum is then overridden by the orifices of either an atrioventricular or arterial valve. The margins of the defect can then be different when viewed from the right or left ventricular side (Fig. 8.3). Some echocardiographers may choose to describe the leaflets of the overriding valve as the roof of the defect. The surgeon, however, closes the defect by placing a patch on its right ventricular margins. For this reason, it is the right ventricular margin on which we concentrate when describing these defects.

When describing the location of a defect, we first consider its margins and, then, the way it opens into the right ventricle. The normal ventricular septum is mostly composed of muscle, but has a small fibrous portion, the membranous septum (Fig. 5.7). There are no clear demarcations within the muscular septum but, from the right ventricular side, it can be divided into an inlet part close to the tricuspid valve, an apical trabecular component and an outlet part adjoining the subpulmonary infundibulum (Fig. 8.4). In the normal heart, the left ventricular outlet is the centrepiece of the heart. Because of this, the so-called 'inlet' septum in reality separates the inlet of the right ventricle from the outlet of the left ventricle. Furthermore, the outlet septum, that part of the septum separating the subarterial outlets, is miniscule in the normal heart (Figs. 8.5 and 8.6). For these reasons, it is best to describe defects as opening to the inlet, apical trabecular or outlet components of the right ventricle

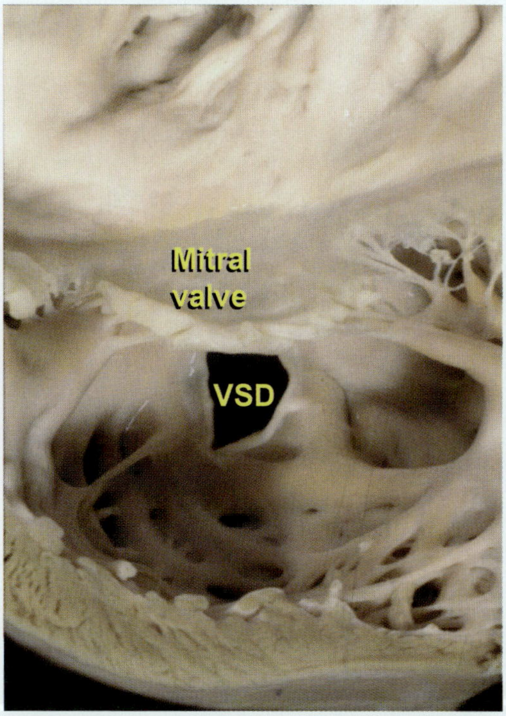

Figure 8.2 The left ventricular view of the defect shown in Fig. 8.1 demonstrates the margins in one plane.

(Fig. 8.4), or as being confluent when they are large and open to more than one component.

All ventricular septal defects can be placed into one of three groups according to their borders (Fig. 8.7). They are, first, those that have a completely muscular border, and hence muscular defects. Second, those that have, as part of their border, fibrous tissue comprising the junction between valvar leaflets and the central fibrous body or membranous septum. We call these perimembranous defects. Third, those that have as part of their border fibrous continuity between the leaflets of the arterial valves, or else are overridden by a common arterial valve. These defects are doubly committed and juxta-arterial.

Muscular Defects

Ventricular septal defects that have completely muscular borders can be situated anywhere within the septum. They can still be subdivided into those opening to the inlet, the trabecular or the outlet components of the right ventricle. Muscular defects can be multiple or may coexist with perimembranous or juxta-arterial defects. Muscular defects opening to the inlet of the right ventricle are, to a large extent,

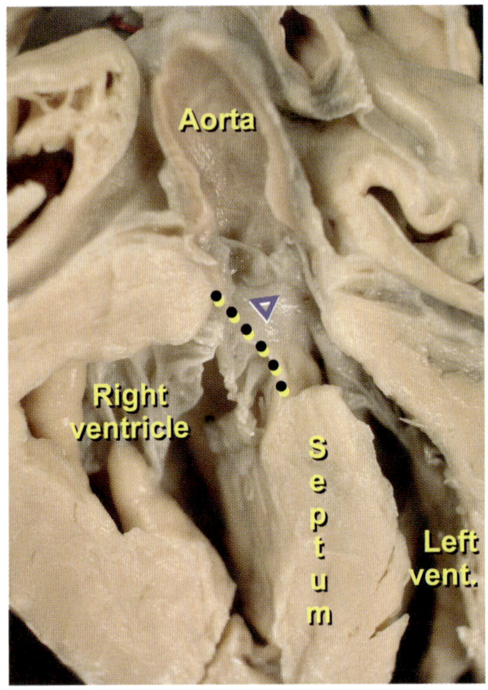

Figure 8.3 This section through the long axis of a heart with a perimembranous ventricular septal defect shows the aortic valve in the 'roof' of the defect. The right ventricular margin (dotted line) is the border of the defect that the surgeon patches. The triangle indicates the area of fibrous continuity between tricuspid, aortic and mitral valves.

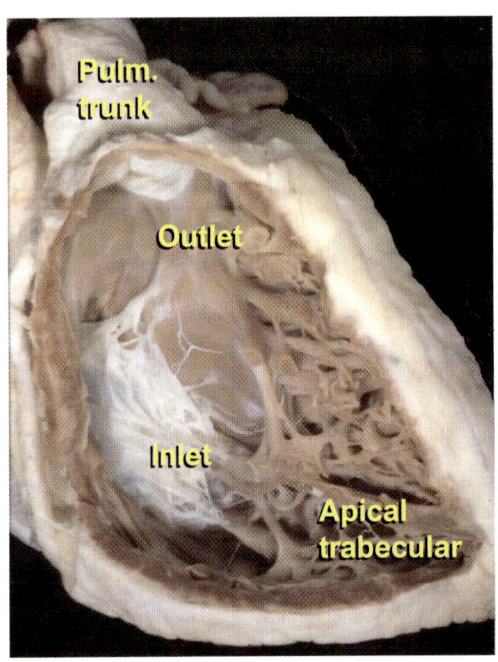

Figure 8.4 The inlet, outlet and trabecular components of the right ventricle.

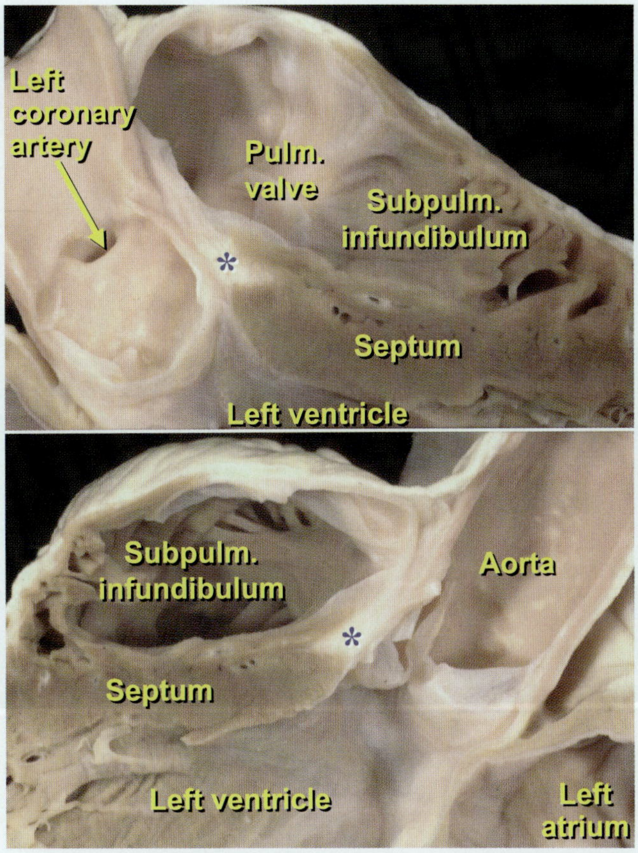

Figure 8.5 Two halves of a specimen sectioned in the simulated parasternal long axis plane to show the pulmonary valve elevated by a muscular infundibulum and the lack of a discrete outlet septum in the normal heart. Epicardial fat (*) fills the space between the subpulmonary infundibulum and the aortic valve.

covered by the septal leaflet of the tricuspid valve (Figs. 8.8 and 8.9). Differentiation between these defects and perimembranous defects opening into the right ventricular inlet is crucial to the surgeon. The ventricular conduction tissue passes anterosuperior to the muscular defect, whereas it is always postero-inferior to perimembranous defects (Fig. 8.10). In hearts where an inlet muscular defect coexists with a perimembranous defect, the conduction tissue passes in the muscle bar between the two (Fig. 8.11).

Multiple small defects may exist between the trabeculations of the apical septum, giving a 'Swiss-cheese' appearance. These may close by growth or hypertrophy of the trabeculations. When found to either side of the septomarginal trabeculation, muscular defects tend to be larger (Fig. 8.12). Their borders are unrelated to the conduction tissue, but the distal bundle branches may be difficult to avoid. Muscular defects opening to the right ventricular outlet are usually small, and tend to close spontaneously. The mechanism involved may be growth of the surrounding muscle, prolapse of the aortic valve leaflet or, possibly, deposition of fibrous tissue

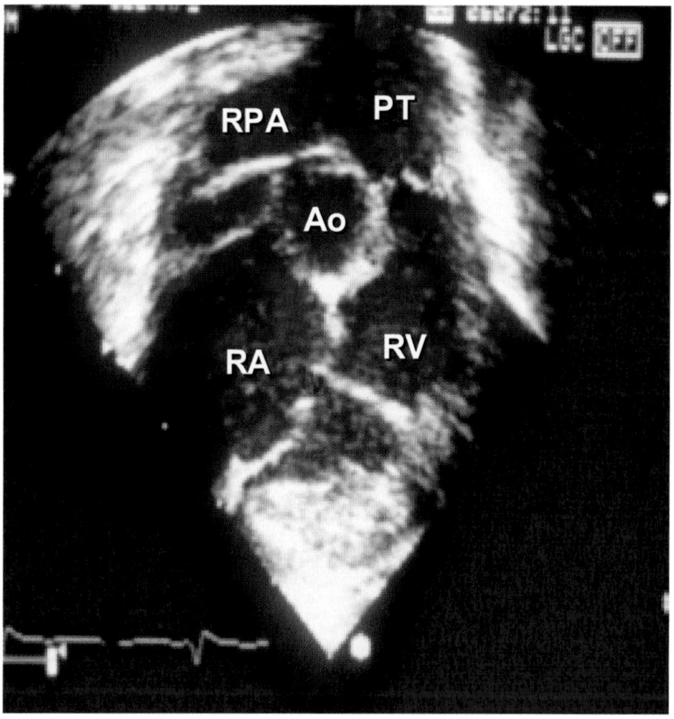

Figure 8.6 Echocardiogram of a normal heart in subcostal right oblique section shows the lack of an outlet septum.

around their margins. The conduction tissue is usually remote from the defect, being protected by the muscle at the postero-inferior border.

Perimembranous Defects

These defects are not simply holes in the membranous septum. Such a hole would be small indeed. The membranous septum is the meeting point of the three parts of the right ventricular aspect of the septum. Defects found here can extend to open into any or all parts of the right ventricle. They can, therefore, be classified as opening to the ventricular inlet, trabecular or outlet parts (Fig. 8.13), depending on which part of the muscular septum is most involved. Confluent defects are those in which the defect opens into more than one part of the right ventricle, for instance a defect large enough to open into both the inlet and outlet components (Fig. 8.14). A perimembranous defect that opens into the inlet component beneath the tricuspid valve has, in its postero-inferior margin, an area of fibrous continuity between the mitral and tricuspid valves (Figs. 8.15 and 8.16). The aortic valve

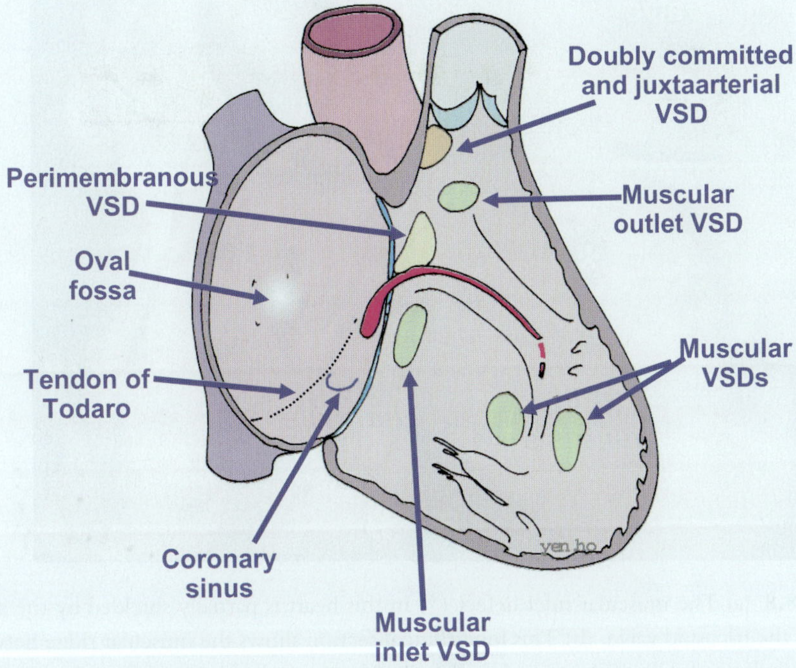

Figure 8.7 Morphologically, ventricular septal defects (VSD) are categorised into muscular defects and perimembranous defects. The doubly committed and juxta-arterial defects are bordered by the adjoining leaflets of the aortic and pulmonary valves. The nature of their postero-inferior borders allows further categorisation into muscular and perimembranous types.

and the central fibrous body make up the superior border. The medial papillary muscle is anterior and cephalad to these defects. They can have a large postero-inferior extension. These defects have been described as 'isolated atrioventricular canal' type defects. This is misleading, since the hearts have none of the features of deficiency of the atrioventricular muscular sandwich, and do not have a common atrioventricular junction. Perimembranous defects that extend towards the cardiac apex are described as trabecular perimembranous defects. The medial papillary muscle is located at the apex of the defect. The septal leaflet of the tricuspid valve is often cleft. If the cleft is adherent to the margins of the defect then these holes can permit shunting between the left ventricle and the right atrium, giving an impression of absence of the atrioventricular membranous septum (Fig. 8.17). True deficiency of the atrioventricular membranous septum is very rare. It can be identified from conventional four-chamber sections.

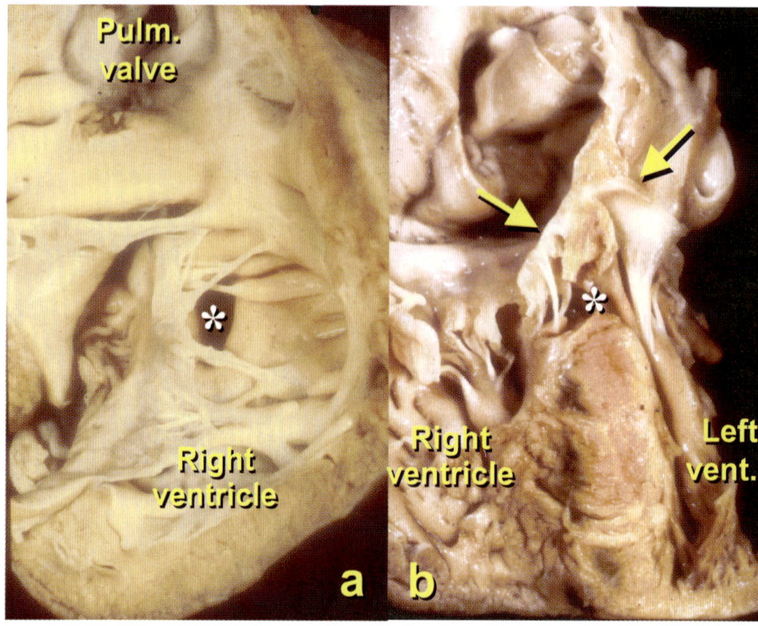

Figure 8.8 (a) The muscular inlet defect (*) in this heart is partially shielded by the septal leaflet of the tricuspid valve. (b) This longitudinal section shows the muscular ridge between tricuspid and mitral valves. The offset (small arrows) between the hinges of the atrioventricular valves is preserved.

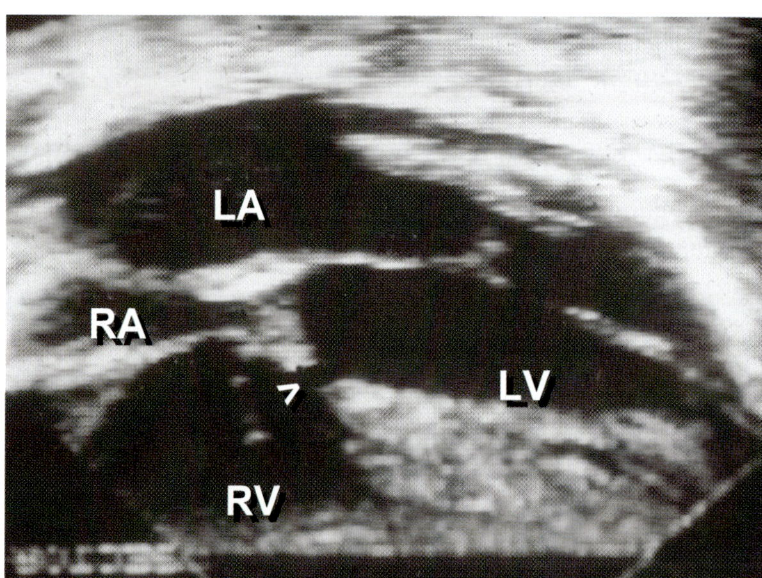

Figure 8.9 Subcostal four-chamber section showing a muscular inlet ventricular septal defect (>) and normal offsetting of the atrioventricular valves.

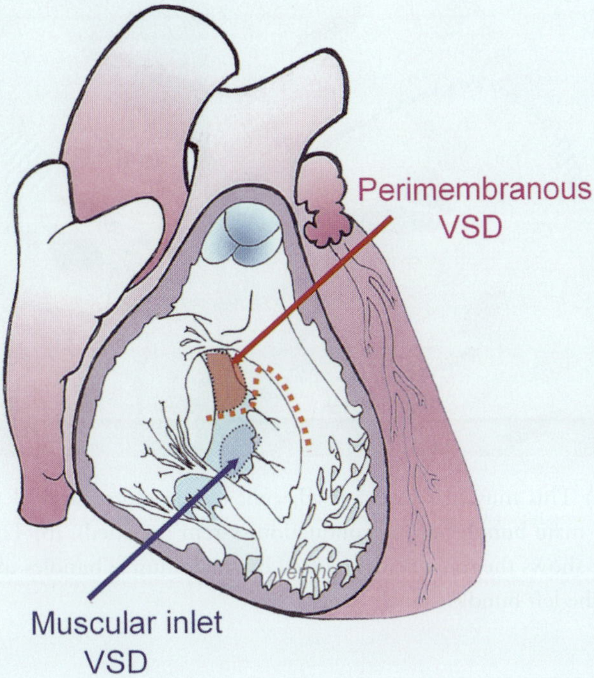

Figure 8.10 Diagram comparing the location of the atrioventricular conduction bundle (dotted line) in hearts with perimembranous and muscular defects in the inlet portion of the right ventricle.

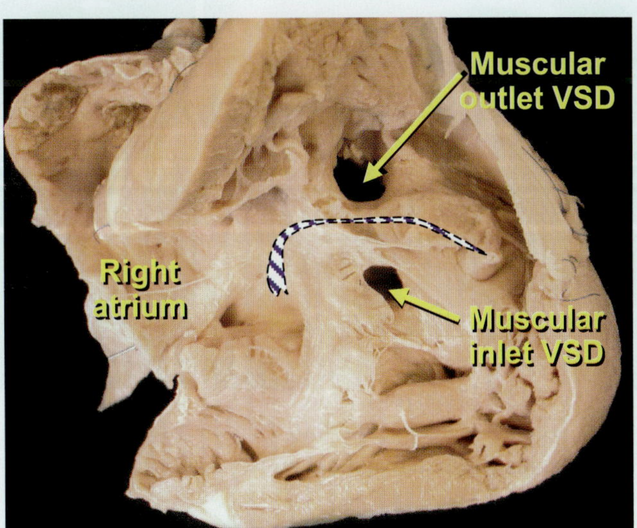

Figure 8.11 When a muscular inlet defect coexists with an outlet, the conduction bundle (hatched) is within the muscle bar between the two defects.

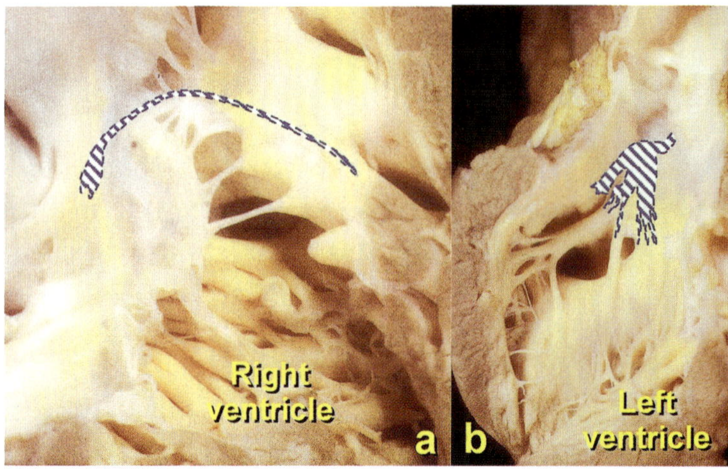

Figure 8.12 (a) This muscular defect is adjacent to the septomarginal trabeculation and distant from the main bundles of the conduction system (hatched). (b) The septal aspect of the left ventricle shows the same defect crossed by small muscle bundles that carry the distal ramification of the left bundle branch (hatched).

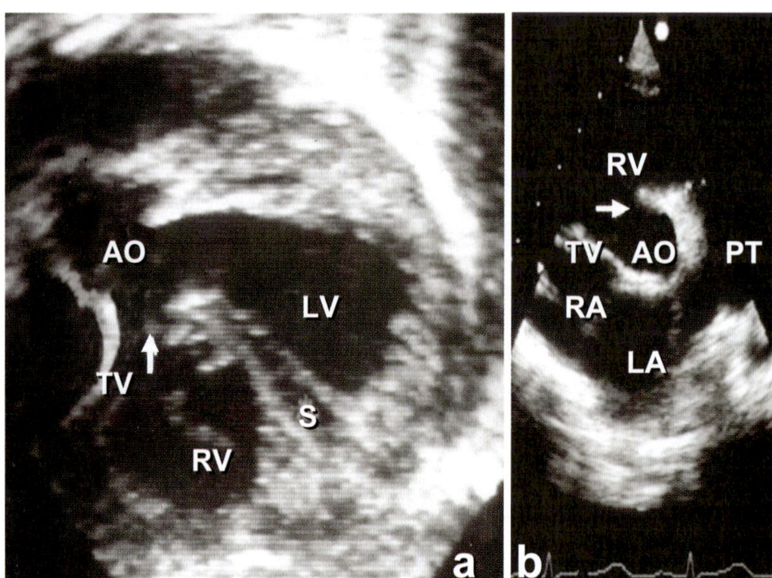

Figure 8.13 Echocardiograms showing perimembranous outlet ventricular septal defect in (a) subcostal long axis and (b) parasternal short axis sections.

Defects that open into the right ventricular outlet are rarely due to a deficiency of the true outlet septum, which, as we have said, is exceedingly small in the normal heart. More usually there is malalignment between the outlet septum and the muscular ventricular septum, associated with overriding of an arterial valve. When

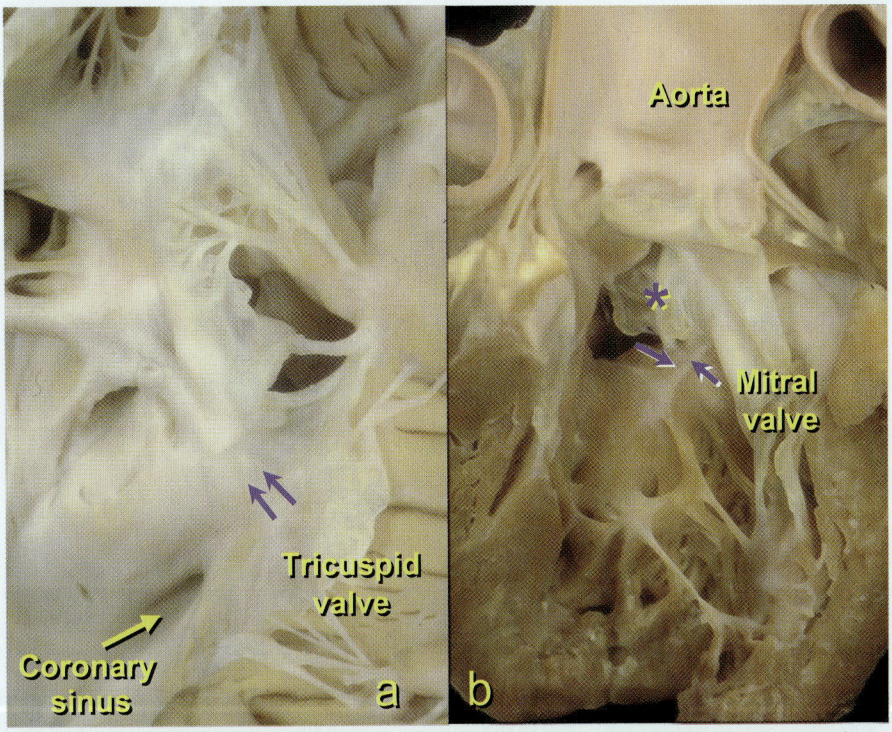

Figure 8.14 (a) This perimembranous defect excavates into the outlet and inlet portions of the right ventricle. The septal leaflet of the tricuspid valve partially covers the defect. The postero-inferior margin (blue arrows) carries the atrioventricular conduction system. (b) The left ventricular view shows its fibrous border with the tricuspid valve (*) visible through the hole. The grey streak (between blue arrows) is the fibrous sheath containing the atrioventicular bundle.

such malalignment is present, the outlet septum is a clearly defined structure that is easily seen (Fig. 8.18). Defects with malalignment of the outlet septum into the left ventricular outflow tract tend to be associated with obstructive lesions, such as tubular hypoplasia in the aortic arch. Those with malalignment to the right ventricle tend to produce subpulmonary obstruction, as in tetralogy of Fallot. The basic distribution of the atrioventricular conduction tissue is the same for all 'isolated' perimembranous defects. As it passes through the central fibrous body, the conduction axis is related to the postero-inferior rim of the defect (Fig. 8.10). The atrioventricular node is situated in its normal position at the apex of the triangle of Koch (Fig. 8.19). The nodal triangle may be displaced posteriorly when there is an extensive inlet defect. The only exception to this rule in hearts with concordant atrioventricular connections is when there is overriding and straddling of the leaflets of the tricuspid valve (Figs. 8.20 and 8.21). Different rules apply, however, when there are abnormal atrioventricular connections.

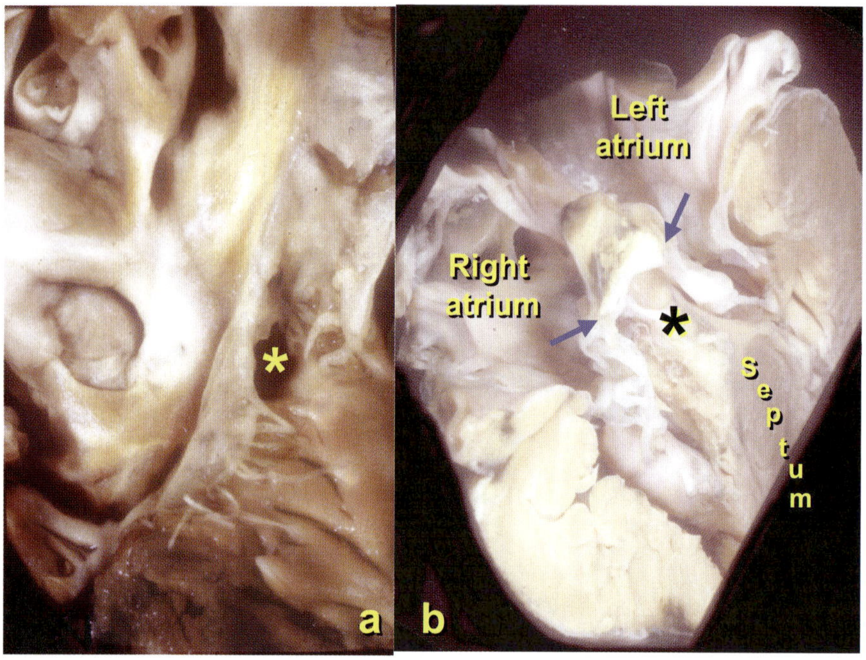

Figure 8.15 (a) This right ventricular view shows the defect (*) excavating into the inlet portion. Its postero-inferior border is the fibrous continuity between tricuspid and mitral valves. (b) This long axis section shows the hinges (blue arrows) of the tricuspid and mitral valves in the 'roof' of the defect.

Since they are close to the septal leaflet of the tricuspid valve, small inlet or trabecular perimembranous defects may be closed by adhesion of the leaflet to the defect or be plugged by aneurysmal tags of fibrous tissue, usually derived from the leaflet of the tricuspid valve (Fig. 8.22). These are often described as 'aneurysms of the membranous septum', but it is rare for any remnant of the membranous septum to be involved in the aneurysmal process. Defects involving malalignment of the outlet septum are unlikely to close, as are extensive inlet defects, particularly when there is overriding of the tricuspid valve.

Doubly Committed and Juxta-arterial Defects

The essential feature of these defects is fibrous continuity between the leaflets of the pulmonary and aortic valves, or presence of a common arterial valve. This is because the outlet septum and the 'septal' component of the subpulmonary infundibulum are both absent. Frequently one, and often both, arterial valves override the trabecular septum (Fig. 8.23). Prolapse of the aortic valve is commonly seen, and can contribute to closure of the defect, but may also cause aortic regurgitation (Fig. 8.24). The

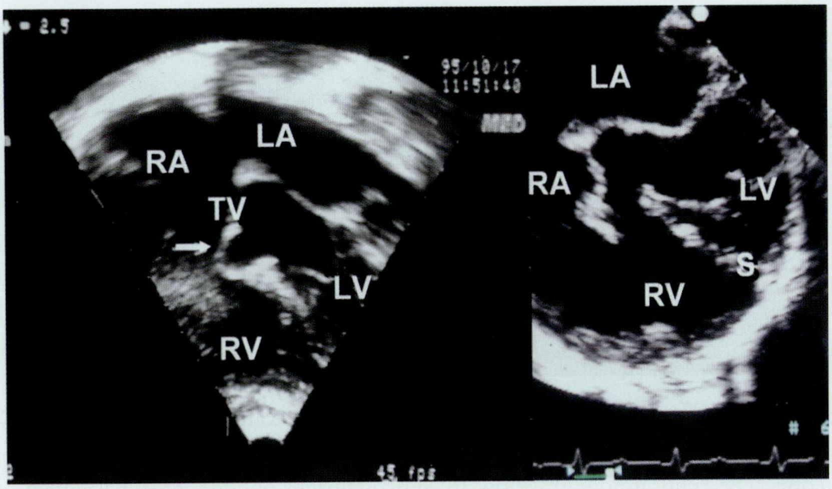

Figure 8.16 Parasternal four-chamber sections from perimembranous ventricular septal defects with (a) aneurysm derived from tricuspid valve and (b) without significant tricuspid valve tissue tags. The mitral and tricuspid valves are in fibrous continuity and have lost their usual offset relationships in each case.

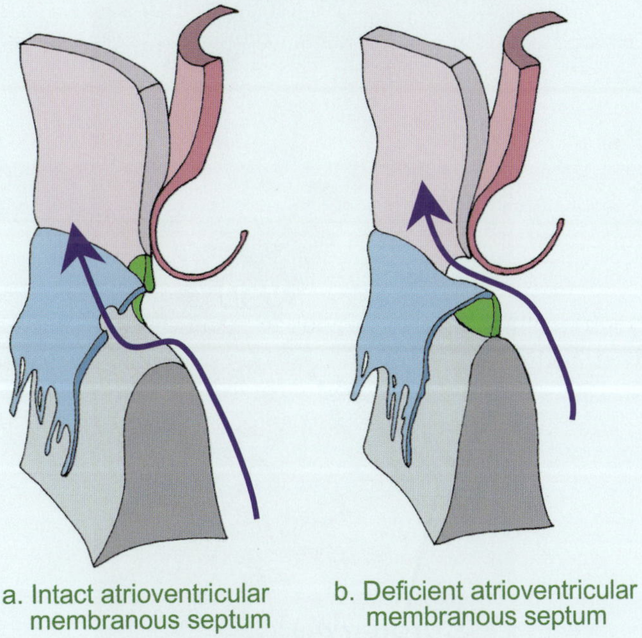

Figure 8.17 Deficiency in the septal leaflet of the tricuspid valve in the region of a ventricular septal defect can give the impression of absence of the atrioventricular component of the ventricular septal defect. (a) A defect in the septal leaflet existing with a ventricular septal defect and intact atrioventricular membranous septum. (b) True left-ventricular–right-atrial communication due to deficiency of the atrioventricular membranous septum is very rare.

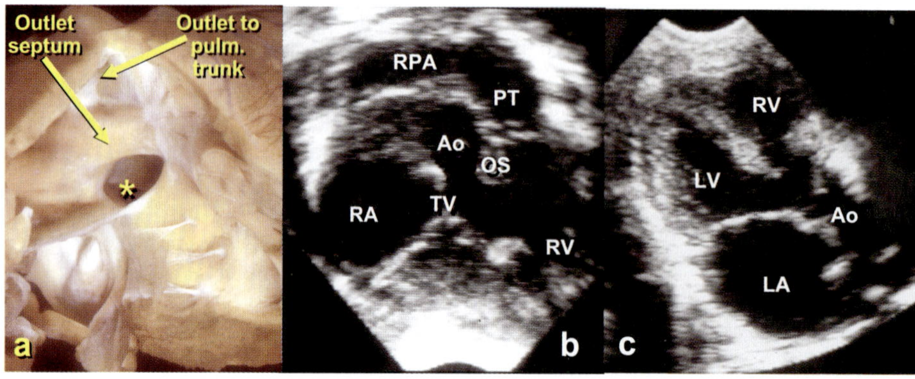

Figure 8.18 This perimembranous defect excavates (*) towards the outlet portion. There is a distinct outlet septum in the right ventricle but it has not produced subpulmonary obstruction. The echocardiograms show (b) subcostal right oblique with malaligned outlet septum and (c) parasternal long axis view showing overriding of the aorta, which may or may not be present in every case.

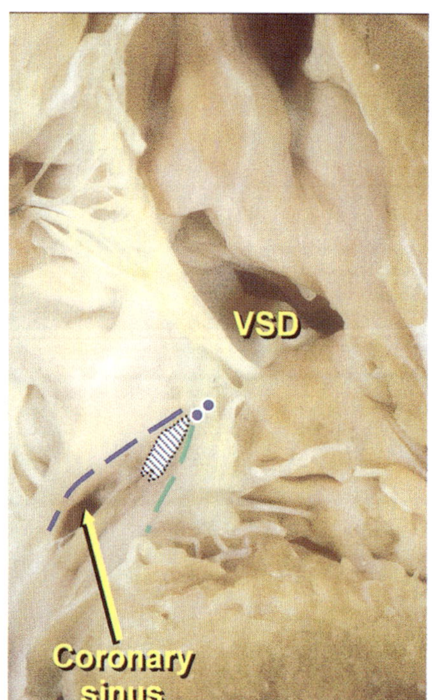

Figure 8.19 The atrioventricular node (hatched area) is located in the triangle of Koch which is demarcated by the attachment of the tricuspid valve (green line) anteriorly and the sinus septum containing the tendon of Todaro (blue line) posteriorly. The penetrating atrioventricular bundle of His (dots) passes through the fibrous body at the postero-inferior margin of the perimembranous septal defect (VSD).

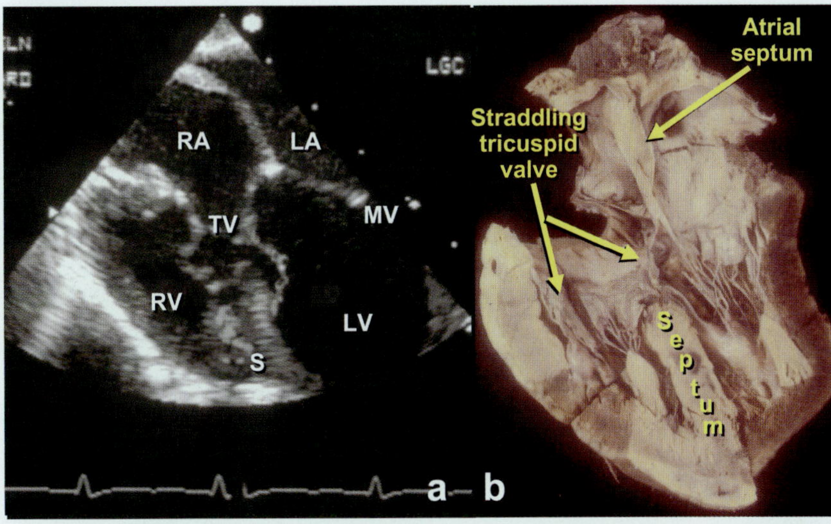

Figure 8.20 (a) Parasternal four-chamber view with a large perimembranous ventricular septal defect with overriding and straddling of the tricuspid valve and a small right ventricle. S = septum. (b) This heart specimen sectioned in the corresponding plane shows insertions of the tricuspid valve into both ventricles. The ventricular septum is malaligned.

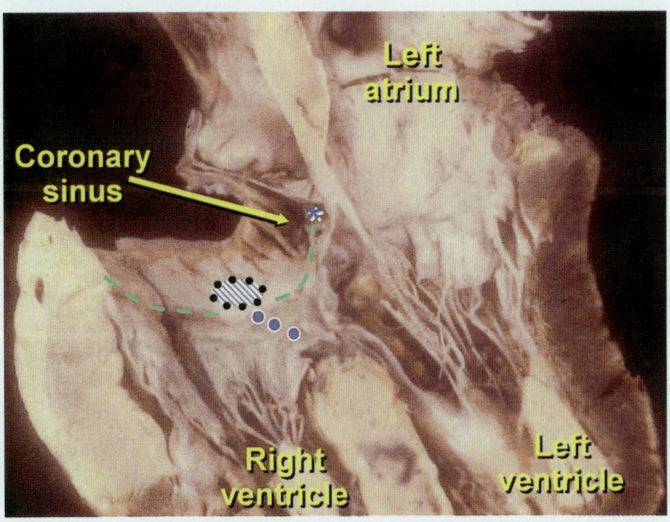

Figure 8.21 The atrioventricular conduction system is displaced to the right when there is rightwards deviation of the ventricular septum away from the cardiac crux. The node at the apex of Koch's triangle (*) is unable to connect with the ventricular conduction tissues (dotted line). Instead, the connecting node (hatched area) is located at the atrioventricular junction (broken line) where the ventricular septum meets the hinge line of the tricuspid valve.

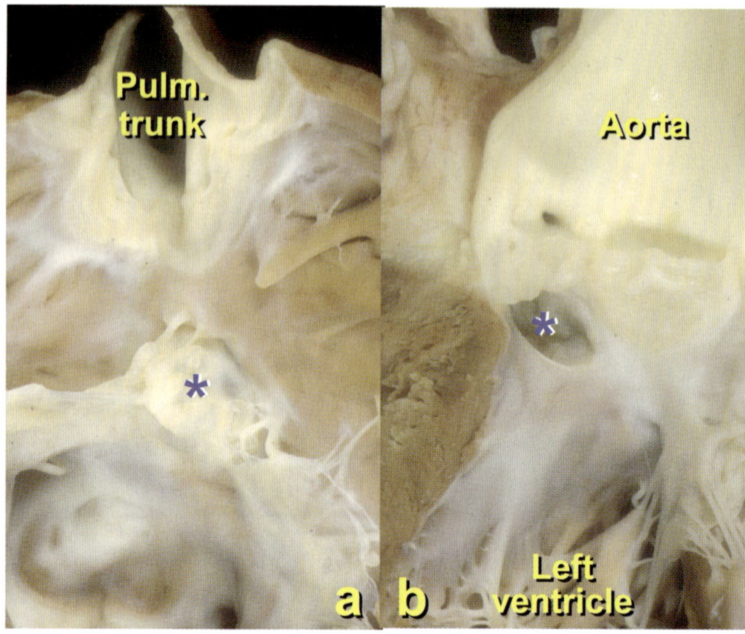

Figure 8.22 (a) The leaflet of the tricuspid valve has closed the septal defect (*). (b) A depression in the left ventricle marks the site of a previous defect.

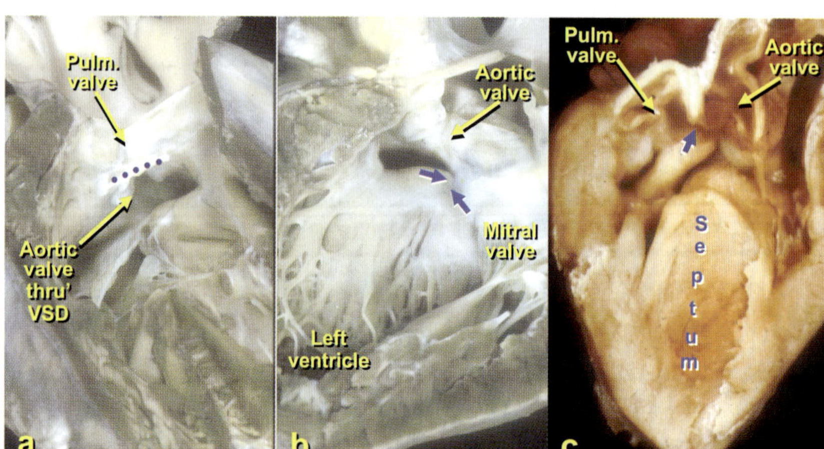

Figure 8.23 (a) The doubly committed and juxta-arterial defect is bordered by the aortic and pulmonary valves. The valvar leaflets are in fibrous continuity through a raphe (dots). There is no muscular outlet septum. (b) The left ventricular view shows its postero-inferior margin and relationship to the atrioventricular conduction bundle (between blue arrows). (c) This long axis section shows fibrous continuity (blue arrow) between aortic and pulmonary valves.

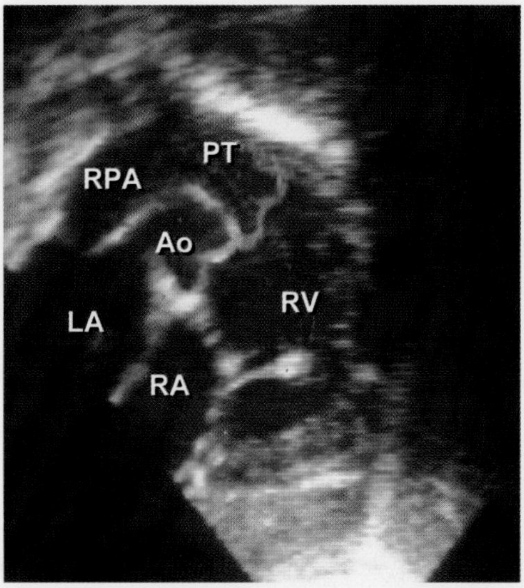

Figure 8.24 Subcostal right oblique view of a doubly committed and juxta-arterial ventricular septal defect.

postero-inferior margin of the defect may be muscular, in which case it does not contain the conduction tissue (Fig. 8.23). If the defect extends far enough postero-inferiorly, so that there is fibrous continuity with the central fibrous body, it becomes perimembranous. The conduction tissue is then closely related to the margin at this point.

9

The Ventricular Outflow Tracts

Obstructions within the outflow tracts of the ventricles are generally considered at three levels: subvalvar, valvar and supravalvar. The nature of subvalvar obstruction reflects the morphology of the outflow tract of the specific ventricle, so that patterns vary markedly in the right and left ventricles. The morphological nature of the obstruction, nonetheless, shows the same pattern in each ventricle irrespective of whether the ventriculo-arterial connections are concordant or discordant. The variants producing subvalvar obstruction can then be distinguished as discrete anatomical entities. In contrast, the valvar and supravalvar forms have similar patterns in both right and left ventricles. Furthermore, when approached anatomically, the valvar and supravalvar variants merge into a continuum. The understanding of these variants of stenosis lies in a precise appreciation of the nature of formation and structure of normal arterial valves, a topic which, perhaps surprisingly, remains poorly understood. For this reason, we will review the anatomy of the normal aortic and pulmonary valves, together with their supporting structures in the normal heart, before considering mechanisms of obstruction of the ventricular outlets.

Normal Valvar Anatomy

When most clinicians consider arterial valves, be they surgeons, physicians, radiologists or pathologists, they almost always refer to a 'valvar ring'. This term, to us, conjures the picture of a complete collagenous ring encircling the ventricular outflow tract, and supporting the valvar leaflets. Close examination of the structure of the arterial valves, however, reveals that there is no structure fulfilling such a concept of a 'valvar ring'. Even histological sections fail to reveal a fibrous structure which is both annular and supports the hinges of the leaflets of the arterial valves. Instead, if an arterial valve is dissected to show its component parts (Fig. 9.1), removal of the leaflets reveals a crown-shaped arrangement with three points. The valvar leaflets are attached to the arterial wall along the arcs between the points, and to the supporting ventricular structures at the base of each scoop. Thus, each leaflet has a low point and two high points of attachment (Fig. 9.2). These lines of attachment to the ventricular and arterial walls constitute the haemodynamic ventriculo-arterial junction. When the valve is closed, they mark the extent of the ventricular cavity. The high points of adjacent leaflets meet to form the peripheral extent of the valvar commissures. Commissures are, literally, the zones of apposition of adjacent leaflets. In reality, therefore, each commissure extends from the arterial wall to the centre of the valve

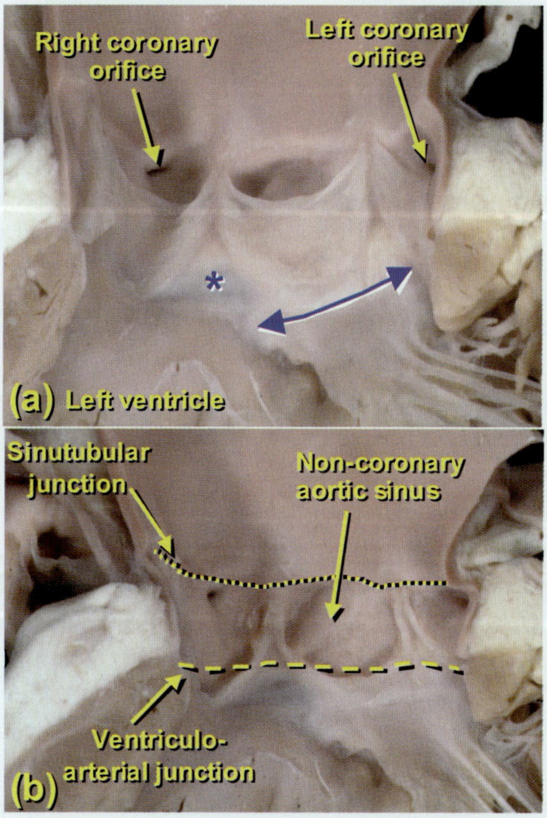

Figure 9.1 (a) The aortic valve is displayed by opening it through an incision made in the left coronary aortic sinus. The leaflets are hinged in semilunar fashion. The aortic outflow tract in the normal heart is muscular on one side, being the ventricular septum and the left ventricular wall, and fibrous on the other side where the aortic and mitral valves are in continuity (double headed arrow). Note the site of the membranous septum (*). (b) Removal of the aortic leaflets shows the semilunar hingelines crossing the ventriculo-arterial junction. The hingelines peak at the level of the sinutubular junction.

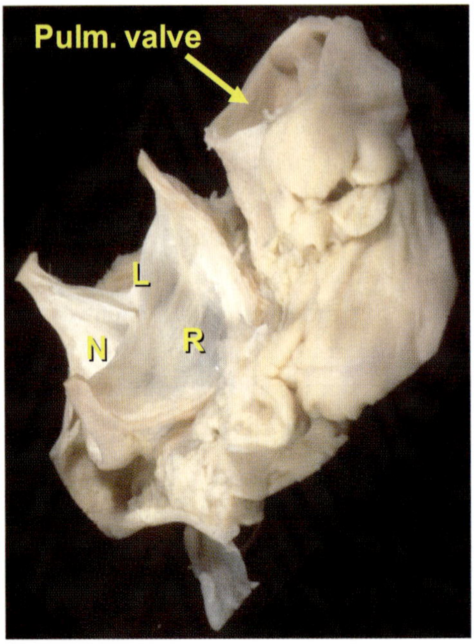

Figure 9.2 The three-pronged coronet arrangement of the aortic valve is evident when the sinuses are removed. The right (R), left (L) and non-coronary (N) leaflets are shown.

(Fig. 9.3). It is a gross oversimplification of valvar function to define the commissure as only the peripheral end of this zone of coaptation.

When examining an arterial valve from above, in other words from its arterial aspect, a true ring can be constructed by joining together the three peripheral extents of the commissures. This ring has an anatomical foundation when seen in longitudinal section, being the commissural ridge, or arterial bar, which is the distinct waist between the sinusal and tubular parts of the arterial trunk (Fig. 9.4). Another 'ring' can then be constructed by joining the nadirs of attachment of the leaflets within the ventricular outflow tracts. This circle is probably the most frequent point of reference used by cardiac surgeons when describing the 'annulus'. Anatomically, it is the least sound in terms of representing a collagenous circle. It is an exclusively muscular ring within the right ventricle (Figs. 9.5 and 9.6), and is partly muscular and partly fibrous in the left ventricle (Fig. 9.7). Importantly, there is then a further ring within the outflow tracts of both ventricles. It is not obvious, but is most marked anatomically when revealed by dissection. This is the region over which the wall of the arterial trunk is attached to the supporting structures of the ventricles and is the true anatomic ventriculo-arterial junction (Figs. 9.1 and 9.6). There is marked discrepancy between this anatomical junction and the locus forming the haemodynamic junction between the ventricle and arterial trunk. The discrepancy between the two junctions means that part of the wall of the arterial trunk is, in haemodynamic terms, ventricular, while parts of the ventricle are subjected to arterial pressures. There are three areas

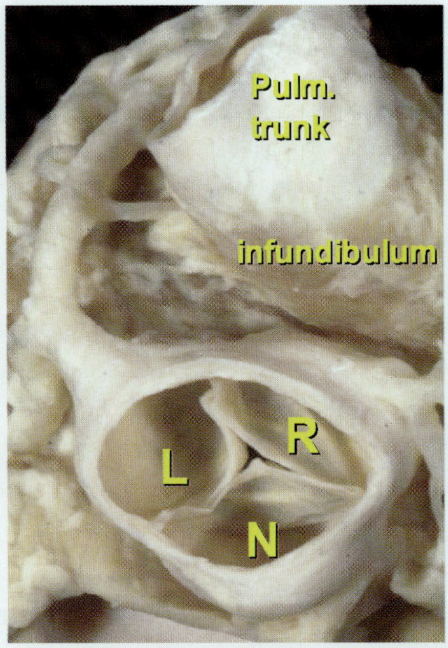

Figure 9.3 This view of the aortic valve shows the leaflets apposing from the periphery towards the centre of the valvar orifice. The two sinuses nearest to the pulmonary trunk are the left (L) and right (R) coronary sinuses. The third sinus (N) is non-adjacent and non-coronary.

of arterial wall incorporated within the ventricle. These are the apical parts of the arcs described above as forming the crown-like arrangement of the valvar supporting mechanisms (Fig. 9.2). As can be seen in Fig. 9.1, these fibrous triangles protrude from, and are supported by, the ventricular musculature, or else, in the left ventricle, the fibrous skeleton. Being in communication with extracardiac space, these areas, which are thin-walled in comparison to the rest of the arterial wall, are potential sites for the formation of aneurysms. The parts of the ventricle that become arterial are found at the troughs of each valvar leaflet, where the line of attachment dips below the anatomical ventriculo-arterial junction (Figs. 9.6 and 9.8).

Valvar Stenosis

It follows from the descriptions of the normal valve that, for a valve to open appropriately, the three leaflets must be free along the entire edges of their zones of apposition, that is the areas where they abut the adjoining leaflets. They must also be sufficiently mobile to fall back into the sinuses of Valsalva during ventricular systole. The pathological mechanisms that disturb this sequence, producing valvar stenosis, involve, first, fusion of the leaflets along the zones of opposition. Such fusion starts from the peripheral attachment at the sinutubular junction, and extends towards the

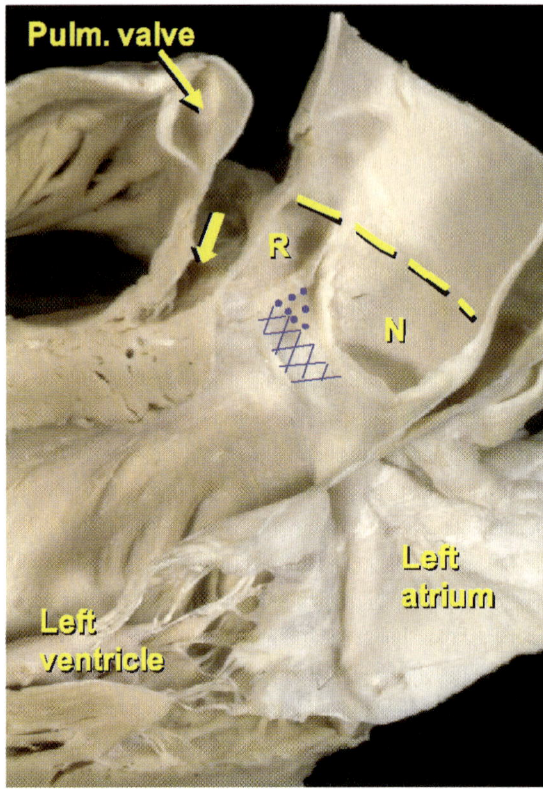

Figure 9.4 This section simulating the parasternal long axis plane shows the sinutubular junction (broken line) marking the border between the tubular and sinusal portions of the aortic wall. The interleaflet triangle (dotted area) between the right (R) and non-coronary (N) sinuses adjoins the membranous septum (hatched area). Note that there is no discrete outlet septum in the normal heart. Epicardial tissues (arrow) interpose between the subpulmonary infundibulum and the aortic root.

centre of the valvar orifice (Fig. 9.9). Second, the free edges of the leaflets become adherent to the arterial wall at the level of the sinutubular junction, a process termed tethering (Fig. 9.10). This process also 'pinches' in the arterial trunk at the level of the sinutubular junction. This appearance is often catalogued as representing supravalvar stenosis — in reality, it is the narrowing of the outflow tract at the level of the distal attachments of the valvar leaflets. The third process is one of thickening of the leaflets, thus reducing their mobility (Fig. 9.11). Even in those valves said to have two leaflets, or even a solitary leaflet, examination of the subvalvar arrangement of the sinuses reveals that, initially, most were developed on the basis of a three-leaflet template, but that fusion of the zones of opposition occurred during foetal life.

Stenosis of the aortic valve accounts for about one-twentieth of congenital malformations of the heart. The intrinsically stenotic aortic valve is one often considered to have a single leaflet, with a single commissure and an eccentric orifice like a keyhole,

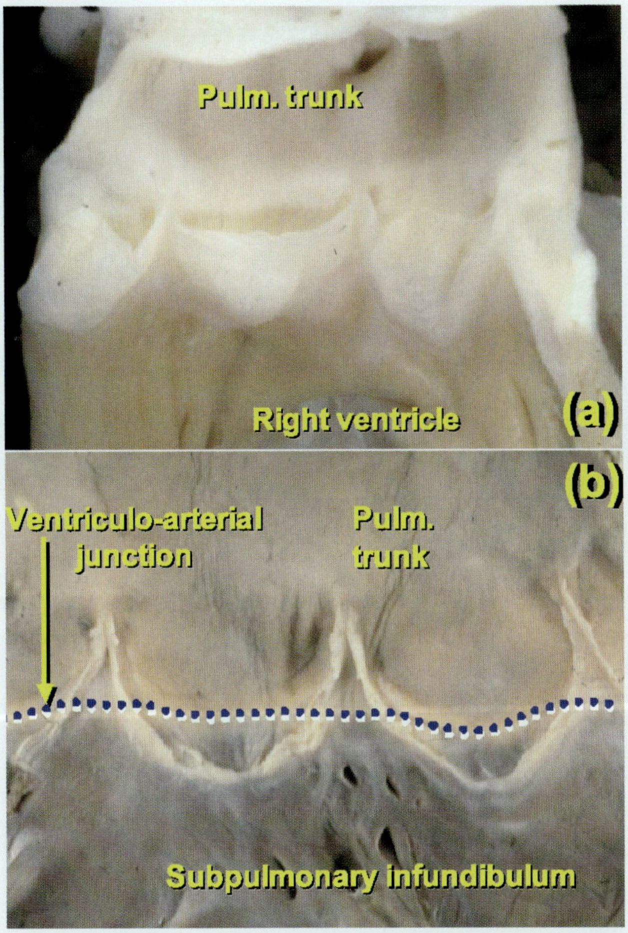

Figure 9.5 (a) The pulmonary valve is supported by a complete cone of muscle, the infundibulum. (b) Removal of the valvar leaflets show the semilunar hingelines enclosing segments of infundibular wall within the sinuses. The dotted line indicates the junction between ventricular structures and the wall of the pulmonary trunk.

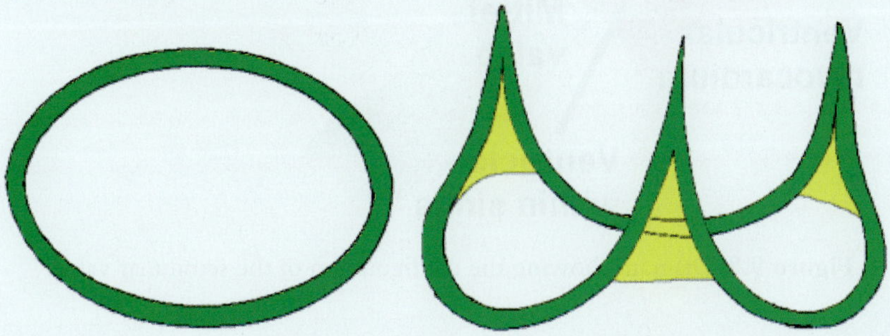

Figure 9.6 The leaflets of semilunar valves are hinged along arcs not to a circular ring.

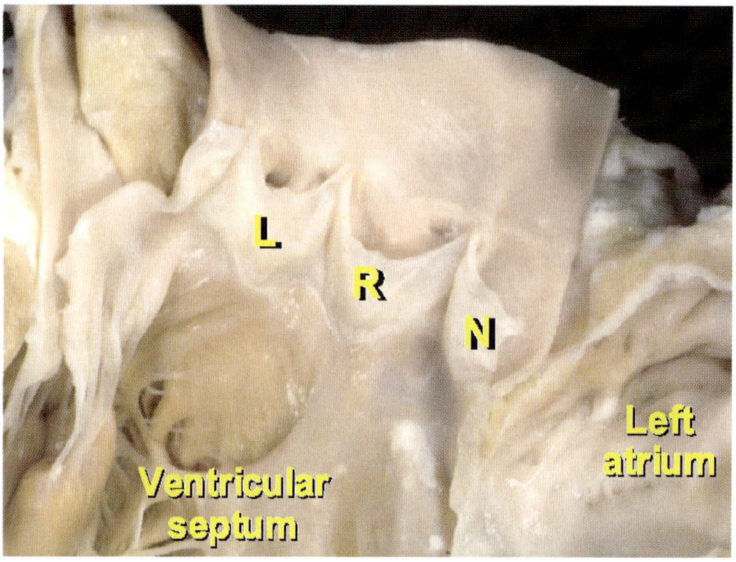

Figure 9.7 This aortic valve is displayed by cutting through the aortic ('anterior') leaflet of the mitral valve to show the part fibrous and part muscular nature of the aortic outflow tract. L, N, R are left, non-, and right aortic sinuses, respectively.

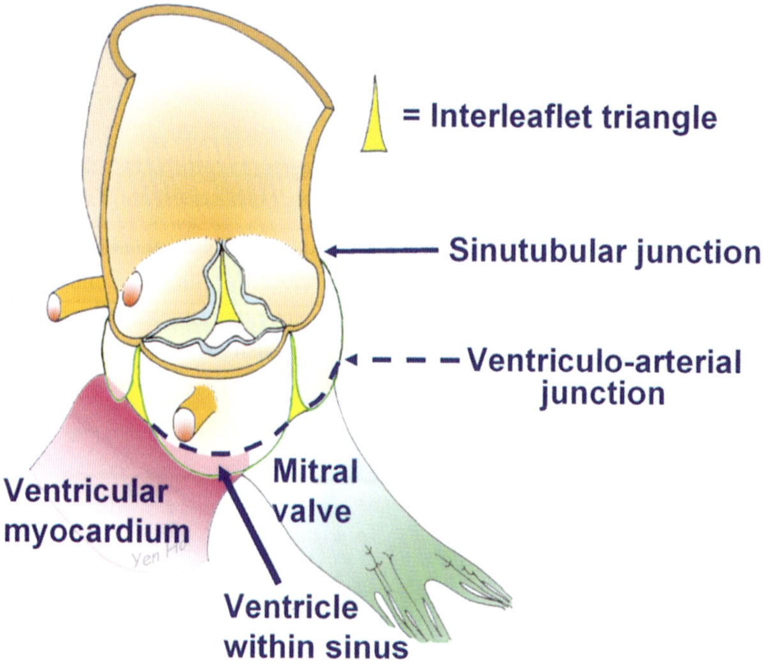

Figure 9.8 Diagram showing the configuration of the semilunar valve.

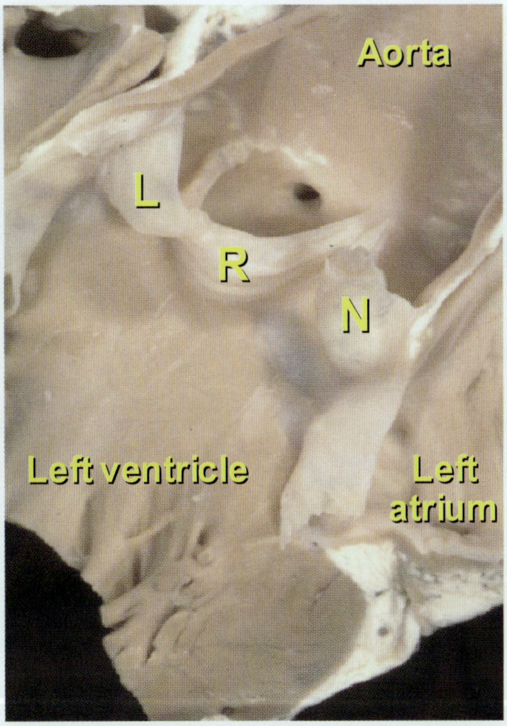

Figure 9.9 Fusion between left (L) and right (R) coronary leaflets produces aortic stenosis in this heart.

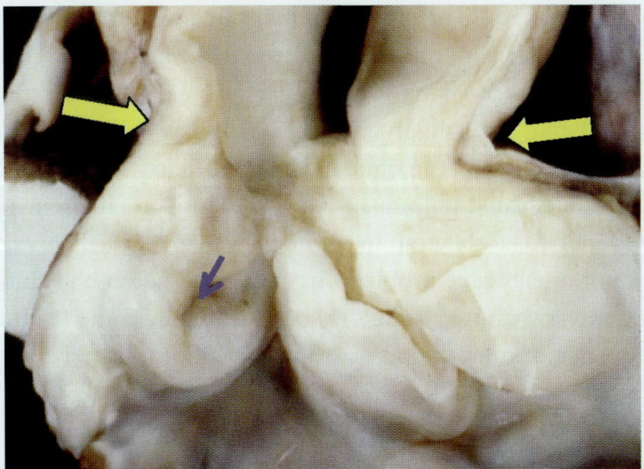

Figure 9.10 This is a case of so-called supravalvar aortic stenosis showing narrowing at the sinutubular junction (large arrows) with pocket-shaped leaflets that are thickened. The free-edges of the leaflets are limited. The margin of the left coronary leaflet is adherent to the sinutubular junction. A tiny hole (small arrow) allows communication with the left coronary artery, which has been 'isolated' from the circulation.

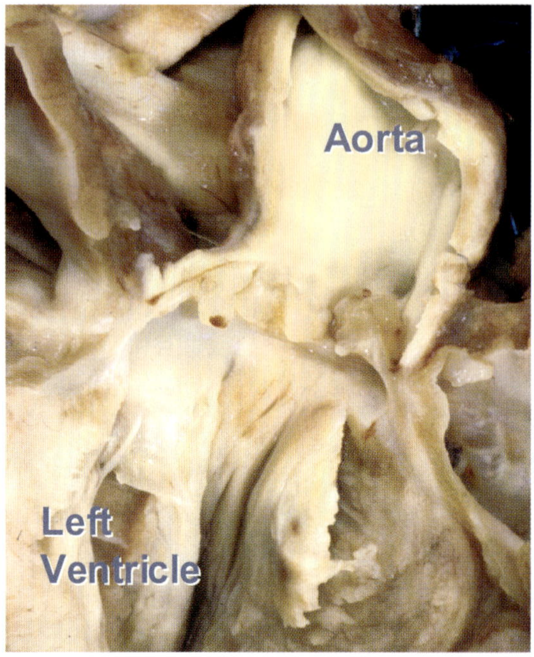

Figure 9.11 Valvar stenosis in this heart is due to thickening of the leaflets.

or one that is dome-shaped and lacks commissures. The so-called unicuspid, unicommissural variant is seen most frequently in critical stenosis of infancy, but is formed on the basis of fusion of zones of apposition in a valve with three leaflets (Fig. 9.12). Interestingly, the persisting commissure points to the mitral valve. This feature of an eccentric orifice is not observed in the pulmonary valve (Fig. 9.13), 'unicommissural' pulmonary valves being exceedingly rare. This fact may well reflect the differences in infundibular morphology of the right and left ventricles. The domed variant is the commonest cause of isolated pulmonary valvar stenosis in children. In others, two leaflets can be identified, as they can in the aortic valve. The valve with two leaflets, however, does not usually give problems in childhood because it is not intrinsically stenotic. Aortic valves with two leaflets (Fig. 9.14) usually come to attention in later life as a consequence of calcification, prolapse or endocarditis. The leaflets in such valves can be arranged in either left–right positions, or antero-posterior orientations. In the left–right variant, a coronary artery arises from each sinus, and a raphe is usually present in the right leaflet. Both coronary arteries arise from the anterior sinus in the antero-posterior variant. In this type, the raphe is usually in the anterior leaflet. The raphe represents fusion of a putative zone of apposition during foetal development. Although stenosis of the valve with two leaflets usually occurs in later life, mucoid dysplastic changes can occur in the leaflets. The swollen leaflets can then cause valvar stenosis earlier in life. Valves with three leaflets are seldom stenotic during childhood unless affected by mucoid dysplasia. They typically become stenotic much later in

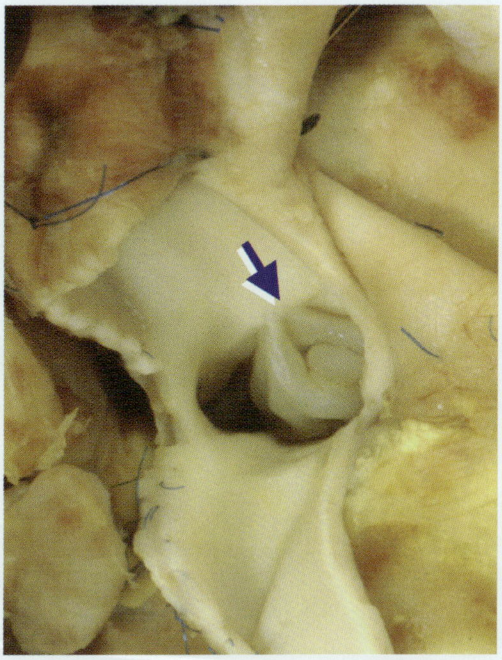

Figure 9.12 This unicuspid and unicommissural aortic valve has an eccentric keyhole orifice.

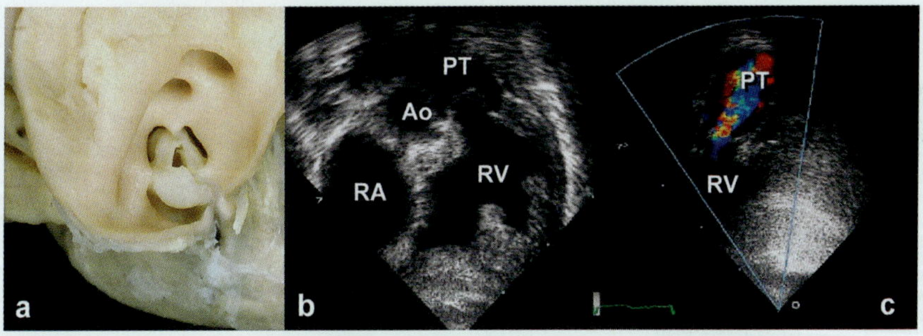

Figure 9.13 (a) This dome-shaped pulmonary valve has a central orifice. The three commissures are at the periphery. (b) Subcostal right oblique section in critical pulmonary valve stenosis shows a dome-shaped and dysplastic valve. (c) Parasternal anterior section with a narrow colour flow jet passing through the pulmonary valve. There is severe right ventricular hypertrophy.

life as a consequence of fusion and calcification of the zones of apposition of the leaflets, producing the entity known as senile isolated calcific stenosis (Fig. 9.15).

Pulmonary stenosis constitutes up to one-twelfth of congenital cardiac malformations. Its most common substrate is found at the level of the valvar leaflets. Isolated stenosis of the valve in pulmonary position is most frequently seen with a trifoliate arrangement. These valves are usually dome shaped. In most, evidence

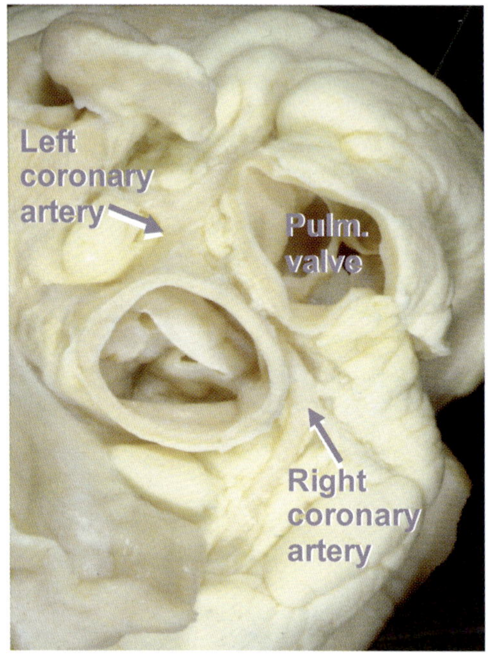

Figure 9.14 The aortic valve has two leaflets. Both leaflets are thick and stiff.

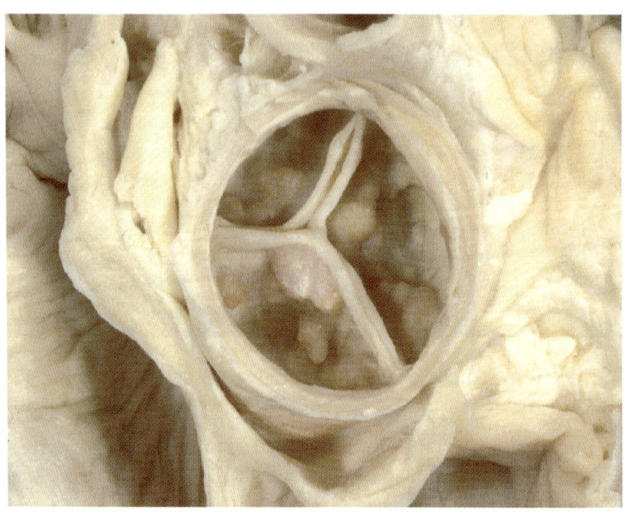

Figure 9.15 The leaflets of this aortic valve are rigid with large nodules of calcification.

of fusion of the leaflets can be seen from the periphery of the dome towards the centre. The fused margins are amenable to surgical division or balloon dilation. In others, especially in neonates presenting with a pin-hole orifice, the dome is smooth, with evidence of the initial zone of apposition only at the periphery (Fig. 9.13). As in the aortic valve, dysplasia causing cauliflower-like excrescences can also cause

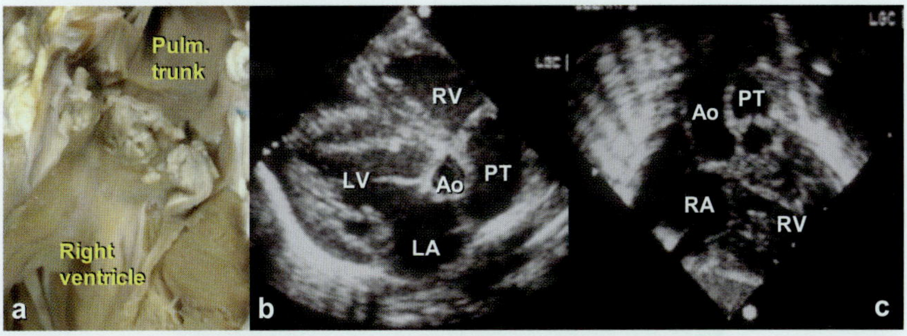

Figure 9.16 (a) All three leaflets of this pulmonary valve are irregular and thick. (b) Echocardiogram in parasternal long axis view of the right ventricles showing extensive hypertrophy of the septomarginal trabeculation and dysplastic and stenotic pulmonary valve. (c) This is the corresponding right oblique section showing extensive right ventricular hypertrophy.

obstructions in a pulmonary valve with three leaflets (Fig. 9.16). This is commonly observed in patients with Noonan's syndrome. Dysplastic valves are less amenable to either balloon dilation or surgical repair than those with simple fusion along the zones of opposition. Another variant of valvar stenosis, albeit usually categorised as supravalvar, is the so-called hourglass pattern. This is the result of tethering of the peripheral ends of the zones of apposition to the arterial wall, with corresponding reduction in the orificial diameter at the level of the sinutubular junction. The openings between the edges of the leaflets and the sinuses of Valsalva are narrowed, while the sinuses themselves become dilated and bottle-shaped. Post-stenotic dilation of the arterial wall above the ridge enhances the hourglass appearance. Attempts at dilating these valves by balloon angioplasty will probably result in rupture of the arterial wall. Surgical division of the free edges of the leaflets, with liberation of the tethering to the arterial wall, which enables the circumference of the sinutubular junction to widen, may be a better option. This pathological mechanism has its counterpart in the aortic valve, with this variant again usually being considered to represent supravalvar aortic stenosis (Fig. 9.17). As emphasised above, from the anatomical point of view, stenosis at the sinutubular junction is, effectively, valvar stenosis. The other recognised variants of supravalvar stenosis, the membranous and the tubular types, are much rarer (Figs. 9.18 and 9.19). They do involve the arterial trunk rather than the sinutubular junction, and are appropriately described as being supravalvar.

Subvalvar Pulmonary Stenosis

Most frequently, the substrate of obstruction is in the immediately subvalvar area of the right ventricular outflow tract. In congenitally malformed hearts, this is usually seen in association with a ventricular septal defect. The outlet septum as, for

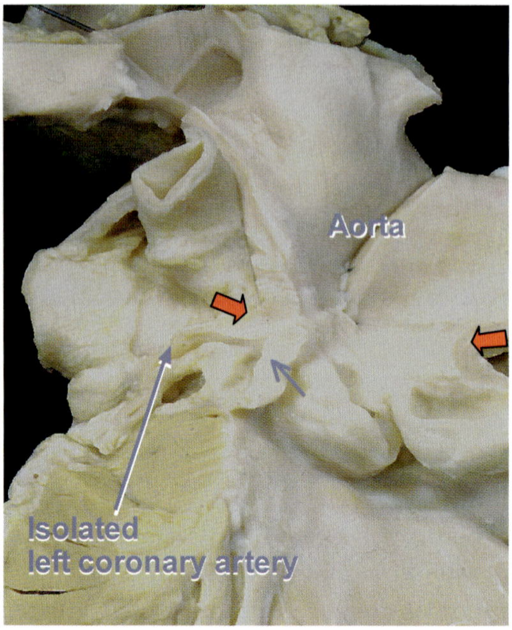

Figure 9.17 This heart also shown in Fig. 9.10 has an hourglass appearance of the aorta with the 'waist' at the sinutubular junction (block arrows). A small aperture in the left coronary leaflet (small arrow) is the only entrance to the aortic sinus.

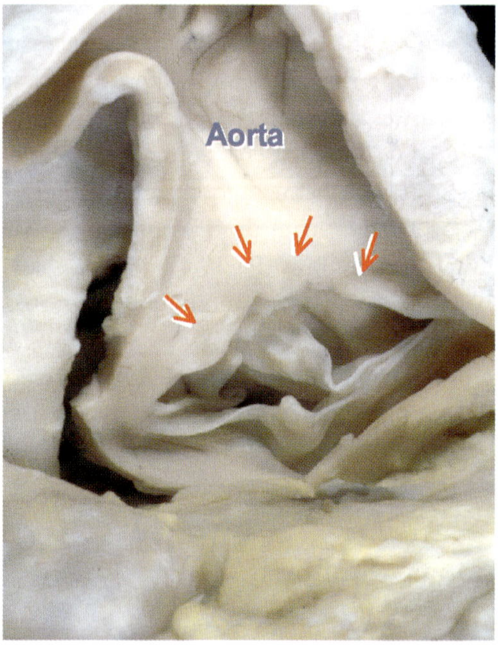

Figure 9.18 A fibrous membrane (small arrows) just above the sinutubular junction protrudes into the aortic lumen.

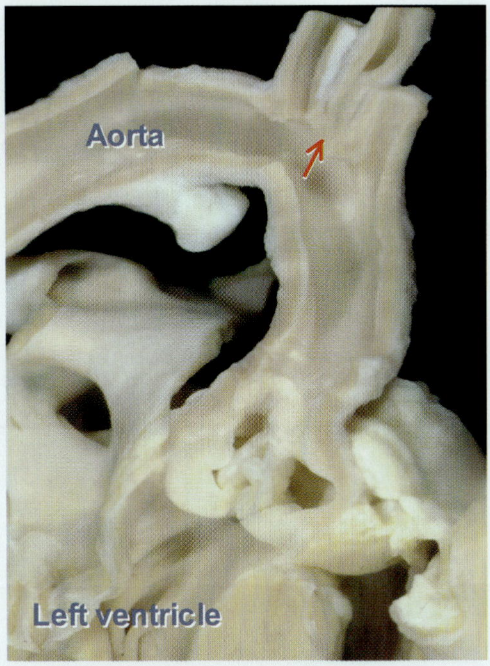

Figure 9.19 The aortic wall is thick uniformly. The arteries arising from the aortic arch are also affected. The origin of the left common carotid artery is occluded (arrow).

instance, in hearts with tetralogy of Fallot, is well defined and is likely to become hypertrophied, thus contributing to the infundibular narrowing. Tubular muscular obstruction of the subpulmonary outflow tract is unusual except when there is an associated septal defect. Isolated obstruction of the outflow tract can also be produced by an anomalous muscle bundle, usually a hypertrophied septoparietal trabeculation. This pattern is often called 'two chambered right ventricle'. Even rarer as a cause of subpulmonary obstruction is the finding of pouches of accessory tricuspid valvar tissue that prolapse into the outflow tract during systole, or accessory valvar leaflets derived from the tricuspid valve that have attachments directly in the outflow tract. Such fibrous windsocks can also be derived from the valvar tissues guarding the openings of the inferior caval vein or coronary sinus within the right atrium (Fig. 9.20), or from an aneurysmal membranous septum.

Subvalvar Aortic Stenosis

Several morphological types of subvalvar stenosis exist in the left ventricular outflow tract. The so-called shelf lesion is commonest. It is usually a crescentic shelf of fibrous tissue on the ventricular septum, just below the aortic valve, often extending on to the aortic leaflet of the mitral valve (Fig. 9.21). Although often described as

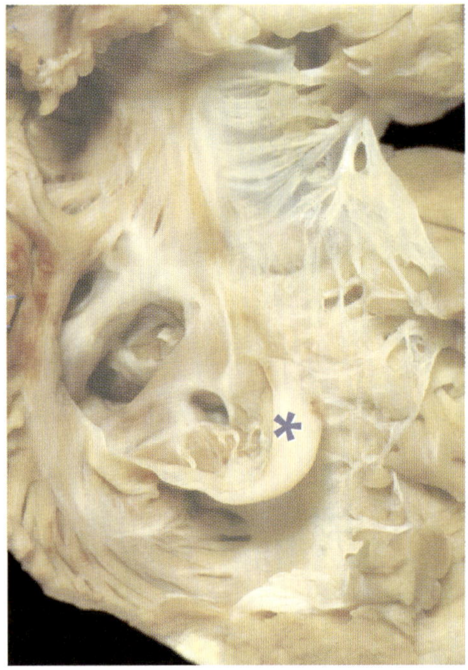

Figure 9.20 This view of the right atrium and right ventricle shows a pouch (*) extending between the Eustachian and tricuspid valves.

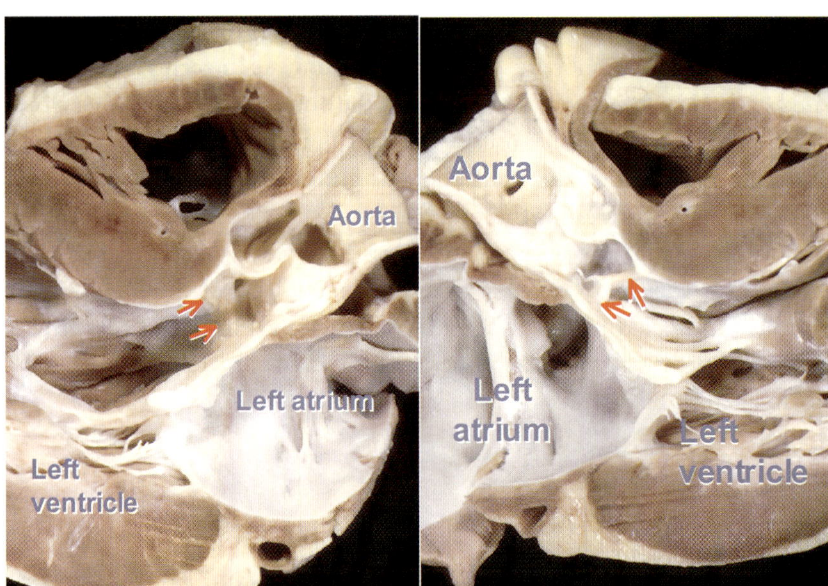

Figure 9.21 This heart sectioned in simulated parasternal long axis plane shows a fibrous shelf (small arrows) beneath the aortic valve.

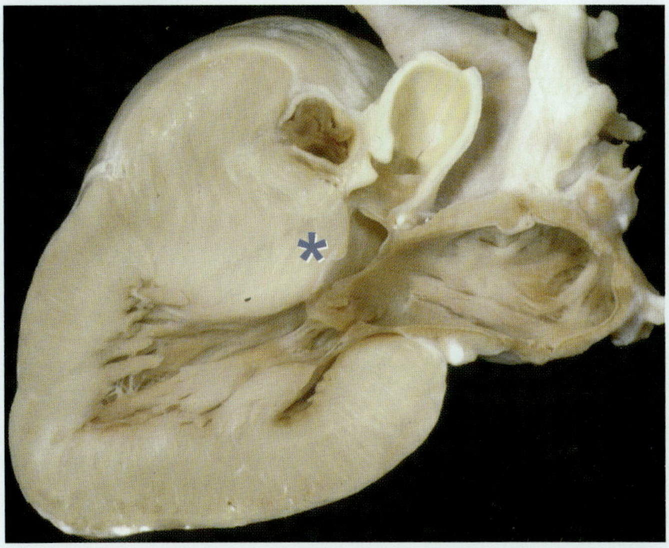

Figure 9.22 This case with glycogen storage disease shows septal hypertrophy (*) compromising the left ventricular outlet.

'membranous', this lesion is hardly ever found in the form of a membrane. The tunnel lesion involves a length of the outflow tract. It is usually due to hypertrophy of the septal myocardium causing a bulge to protrude into the outflow tract (Fig. 9.22). A thick layer of fibrous tissue may be superimposed upon the bulge. This lesion may be related to idiopathic myocardial hypertrophy. As in the right ventricle, deviation of the outlet septum, in association with ventricular septal defect, is also a common cause of left ventricular outflow obstruction. In these cases, coarctation or interruption of the aortic arch are also frequently found.

10

Tetralogy of Fallot

Tetralogy of Fallot is one of the more common cyanotic heart defects. Although it had been described much earlier, it was Etienne-Louis Arthur Fallot who, in 1888, separated this malformation from other anatomical lesions responsible for the 'maladie bleu'. The characteristic malformation is composed of four constant features (Fig. 10.1), namely subpulmonary arterial stenosis, a ventricular septal defect, biventricular origin of the aortic valve and hypertrophy of the right ventricle. The precise anatomy can range from hearts with minimal aortic overriding and minimal pulmonary stenosis to the extreme, where the pulmonary obstruction is so severe as to represent the commonest form of pulmonary atresia with ventricular septal defect.

Morphological Hallmarks

In order to understand the morphology of the ventricular outlets in tetralogy of Fallot, the muscular components must be carefully defined. In normal hearts, a prominent fold of muscle separates the leaflets of the tricuspid from those of the pulmonary valves. This is the supraventricular crest ('crista supraventricularis'). Anatomically, it is mostly made up of the musculature of the inner heart curvature, which we call the ventriculo-infundibular fold separating the subpulmonary and subaortic outlets. In the normal heart, only a very small part of the supraventricular crest can justifiably be described as an outlet septum. This is because the leaflets of the pulmonary valve are supported by a sleeve of infundibular muscle that stands proud of the ventricular mass (Fig. 10.2). Another important muscular structure within the normal right ventricle, is the characteristic large trabeculation on the septum (Fig. 10.3). This structure, the septomarginal trabeculation, is made up of a body

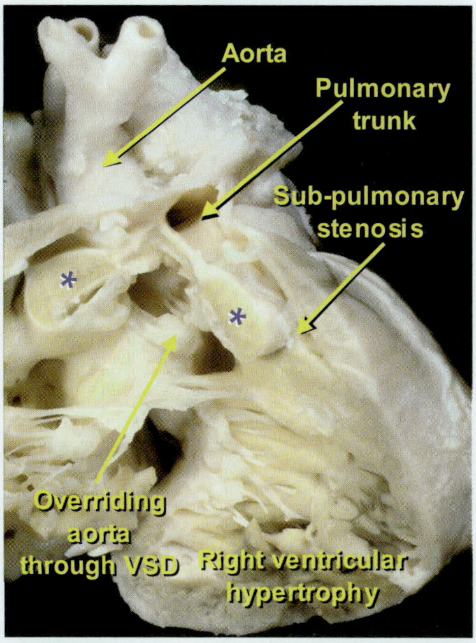

Figure 10.1 A specimen displayed in a fashion similar to the subcostal or right anterior oblique view. The outlet septum (**) has been transected to show the overriding of the aortic valve through the ventricular septal defect and muscular subpulmonary stenosis in Fallot's tetralogy.

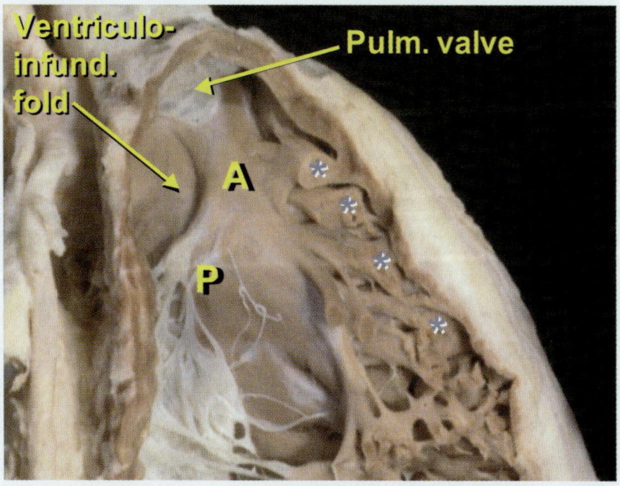

Figure 10.2 The right ventricular outflow tract is displayed in this normal heart. The ventriculo-infundibular fold is clasped between the anterior (A) and posterior (P) limbs of the septomarginal trabeculation. Smaller bundles of muscle, septo-parietal trabeculations (*), line the outflow.

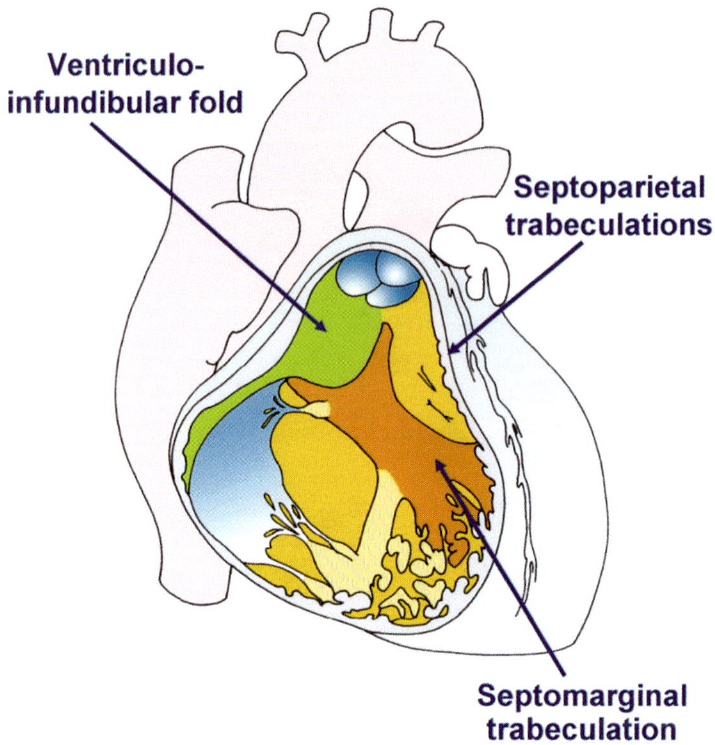

Figure 10.3 Schematic representation of the normal right ventricular outflow tract with naming of the muscular structures.

that divides superiorly into anterior and posterior limbs. In the normal heart, the supraventricular crest inserts into the ventricular septum between the limbs of the septomarginal trabeculation.

In hearts with Fallot's tetralogy, the normal architecture of the right ventricular outlet is distorted with the various muscular components achieving identity as discrete structures (Figs. 10.1 and 10.4). The outlet septum becomes a clearly defined right ventricular structure. It is inserted antero-cephalad to the anterior limb of the septomarginal trabeculation. In this location, it creates muscular obstruction of the subpulmonary outlet. Indeed, this antero-cephalad deviation of the outlet septum is the hallmark for diagnosis. Other smaller trabeculations, also present in the normal heart, contribute to the subpulmonary stenosis. These septoparietal trabeculations encircle the parietal wall of the subpulmonary infundibulum, extending from the anterior margin of the septomarginal trabeculation. They are prominent and hypertrophied in tetralogy (Fig. 10.5).

Because of its deviation into the right ventricular outflow tract, the outlet septum is malaligned relative to the rest of the muscular septum. This is a general feature of ventricular septal defects opening into the right ventricular outlet, with or without tetralogy of Fallot. The malalignment means that the aortic valve overrides the

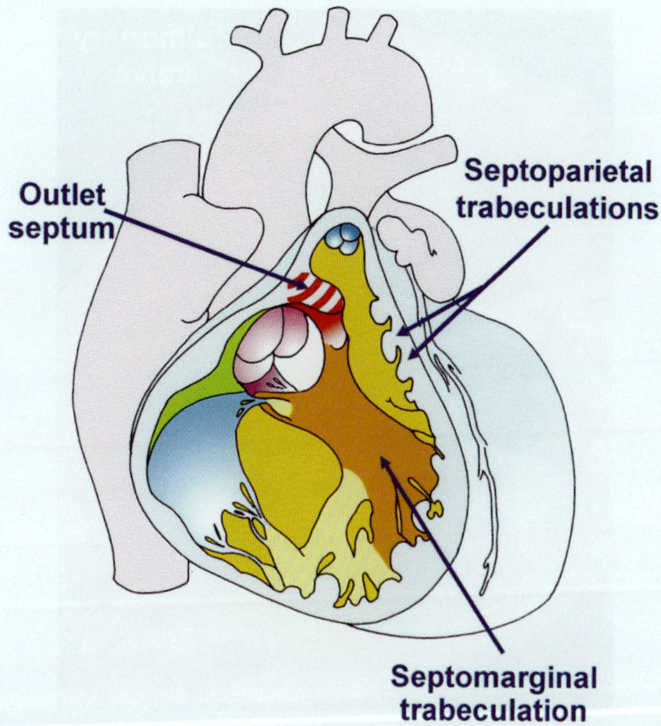

Figure 10.4 Schematic representation of the right ventricular outflow tract in Fallot's tetralogy. Note the insertion of the outlet septum to the anterior limb of the septomarginal trabeculation.

ventricular septum, being attached in part to right ventricular structures (Fig. 10.6). The outlet septum, therefore, is an exclusively right ventricular structure (Fig. 10.7).

Amongst hearts with these morphological hallmarks, there are variations in the anatomy of the ventricular septal defect, the nature of pulmonary infundibular stenosis, the degree of aortic override and the associated malformations.

The Ventricular Septal Defect

This is nearly always large and non-restrictive, except in rare cases where it is occluded by the leaflets of the tricuspid valve or tissue derived from them. When viewed from the right ventricle, the typical defect is cradled between the limbs of the septomarginal trabeculation and roofed by the leaflets of the overriding aortic valve. Its anterior border is formed by the fusion of the deviated outlet septum with the anterior limb of the septomarginal trabeculation (Fig. 10.8). The right ventricular margin of the roof is formed by the ventriculo-infundibular fold supporting the leaflets of the aortic valve.

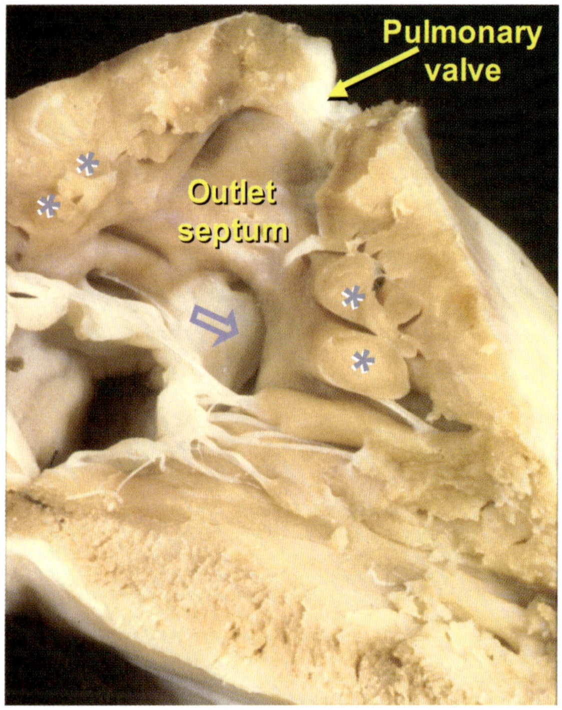

Figure 10.5 This heart with Fallot's tetralogy shows hypertrophy of septoparietal trabeculations (*) exacerbating subpulmonary stenosis. The aortic valve is visible through the perimembranous ventricular septal defect (arrow).

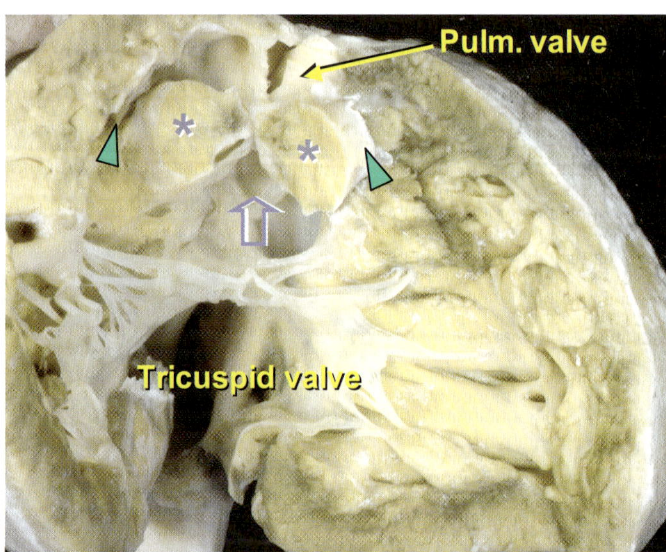

Figure 10.6 This right ventricular view shows the antero-cephalad deviation of the outlet septum (**) that causes narrowing of the subpulmonary outlet (ΔΔ). The aortic valve (open arrow) has attachments to both ventricles.

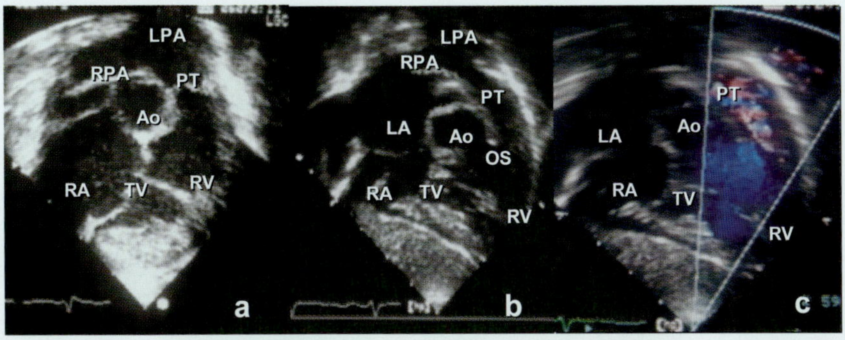

Figure 10.7 (a) Subcostal right anterior oblique view of a normal heart. (b) Subcostal right oblique section of Fallot's tetralogy showing aortic override and antero-cephalad insertion of the outlet septum (OS). (c) Colour flow Doppler emphasised infundibular pulmonary stenosis.

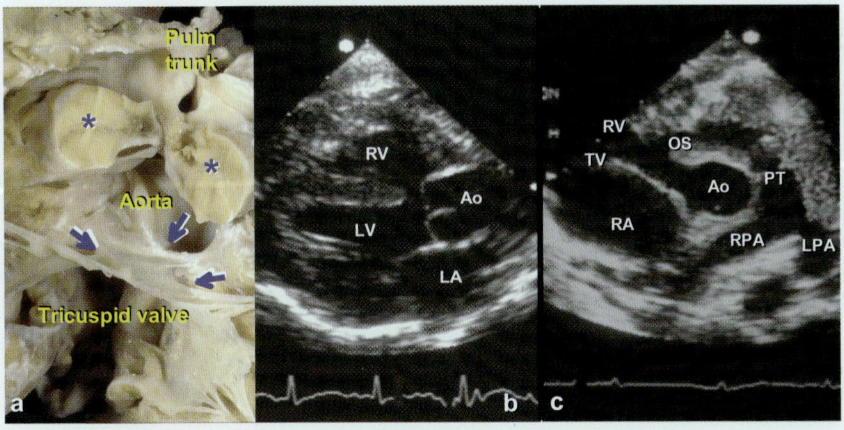

Figure 10.8 (a) This magnified view of Fig. 10.6 shows the borders of the ventricular septal defect. This defect is described as a perimembranous defect owing to fibrous continuity between tricuspid, aortic and mitral valves at its postero-inferior border (between arrows). The outlet septum (**) is confined to the right ventricle. (b) Parasternal long axis view shows overriding of the aorta. (c) Parasternal short axis view shows a perimembranous ventricular septal defect with tricuspid-aortic continuity, and anterior deviation of the outlet septum producing infundibular stenosis.

The area showing most variability is found postero-inferiorly. In about four-fifths of cases, this margin is made up of fibrous continuity between the leaflets of the aortic, mitral and tricuspid valves (Fig. 10.8). In these cases, the defect is perimembranous, and the atrioventricular conduction tissue penetrates through the area of fibrous continuity in the same way as in 'isolated' ventricular septal defects. The fibrous margin is duplicated in many of these cases to produce a so-called membranous flap. In the remaining fifth of cases, there is muscular separation between the aortic and tricuspid valves in the postero-inferior margin. This is produced by fusion of the

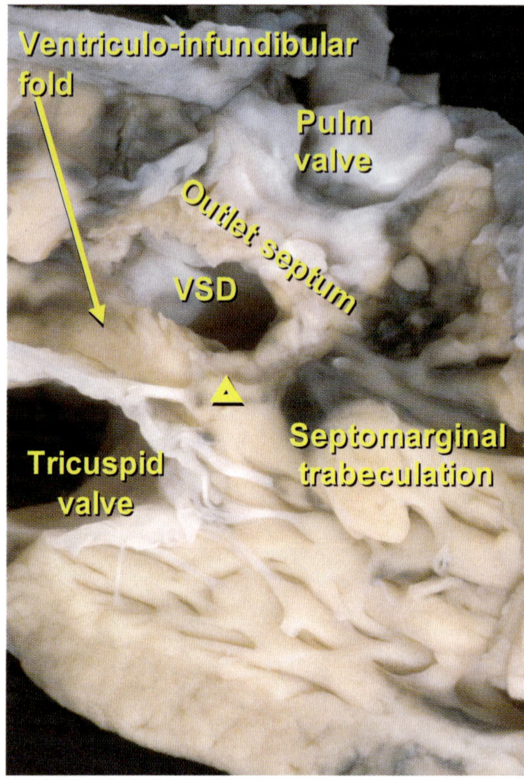

Figure 10.9 The borders of the ventricular septal defect in this heart are completely muscular. There is override of the aortic valve but owing to fusion of the ventriculo-infundibular fold to the posterior limb (Δ) of the septomarginal trabeculation the aortic valve is separated from the tricuspid valve.

ventriculo-infundibular fold with the posterior limb of the septomarginal trabeculation (Fig. 10.9). This muscle separating the leaflets of the aortic and tricuspid valves in the right ventricular margin of the defect also serves to protect the atrioventricular conduction tissues.

Some patients have hearts with an anatomical arrangement very similar to tetralogy, but the ventricular septal defect is both subaortic and subpulmonary because of complete absence of the muscular outlet septum. This anatomical variant is particularly frequent in patients from the Far East and South America. In these cases, the ventricular septal defect is doubly committed and juxta-arterial. Many include these cases in the diagnostic category of the tetralogy of Fallot.

Pulmonary Infundibular Stenosis

There is general agreement that pulmonary stenosis, in the form of narrowing of the infundibulum, is an integral part of tetralogy. The major part of the obstruction is

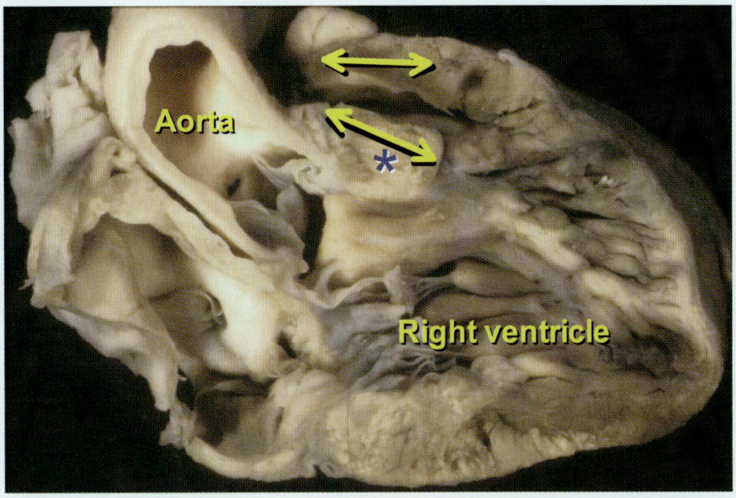

Figure 10.10 The subpulmonary infundibulum (arrows) is elongated in this heart. * = outlet septum.

due to deviation of the outlet septum. While occasional hearts exhibit a hypoplastic outlet septum, and, hence, a short subpulmonary infundibulum, most hearts have an extensive infundibulum that is longer than normal (Fig. 10.10). The proximal extent of the subpulmonary infundibulum is an orifice, the so-called 'os' to the infundibulum, which is surrounded by muscle. Further narrowing in this region is often due to superimposed accretions of fibrous tissue, and sometimes by hypertrophy of the anterior limb of the septomarginal trabeculation. Additional, but more proximal, stenosis may be caused by hypertrophy of the apical portion of the septomarginal trabeculation. This apical obstruction produces one variant of the so-called 'two chambered right ventricle', which can also exist without the infundibular morphology of tetralogy of Fallot. Additional obstruction is usually present at the level of the pulmonary valve. This is due either to fusion and doming of the valvar leaflets or stenosis of a valve with two or three leaflets.

Overriding of the Aorta

Biventricular connection of the aortic valve usually described as overriding, is an essential feature of tetralogy. There is, nonetheless, a marked variation in the degree of rightward deviation of the aorta. The degree of override can be minimal, with the aorta mostly connected to the left ventricle, in other words, with concordant ventriculo-arterial connections. In other hearts, in contrast, the aortic valve is attached almost entirely within the right ventricle, thus producing double outlet ventriculo-arterial connection.

Associated Malformations

An interatrial communication is a frequent additional finding. Additional ventricular septal defects can also occur. If a second muscular inlet ventricular septal defect is present, the conduction axis is in the muscle bar between the two defects. Alternatively, the subaortic defect may extend inferiorly to the crux, producing an extensive perimembranous defect though which the tricuspid valve may straddle and override. The essence of this lesion is malalignment between the atrial and ventricular septal structures and, because of this, the conduction axis will be grossly abnormal. In other hearts, there may be a common atrioventricular, valve with the subaortic defect confluent with the ventricular component of an atrioventricular septal defect.

Other important associations are non-confluent origin of the pulmonary arteries, stenosis of the pulmonary arteries themselves, variations in branching from the aortic arch and origin of the anterior interventricular artery from the right coronary artery (Fig. 10.11). A right aortic arch, while not of functional significance, is present in about a fifth of cases with tetralogy. The arterial duct may be patent, closed or absent. Absence of the duct is usually associated with another notable lesion, namely the so-called 'absence' of the leaflets of the pulmonary valve (Fig. 10.12). In reality, these usually form an annular array at the ventriculo-pulmonary junction, as rudimentary

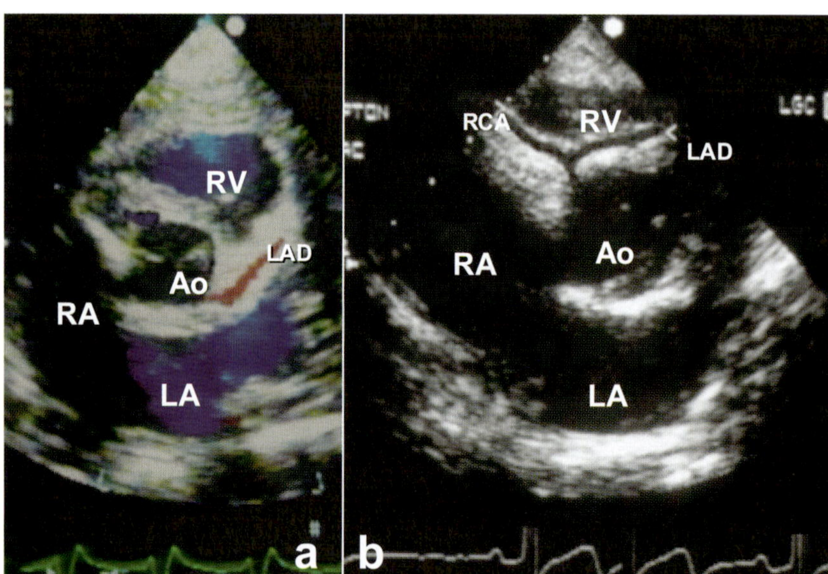

Figure 10.11 (a) Short axis section demonstrating origin of the anterior interventricular coronary artery (LAD) in the normal heart. (b) This case of Fallot's tetralogy has the origin of the anterior interventricular coronary artery (LAD) from the right coronary artery (RCA). The anterior interventricular artery courses along the anterior wall of the pulmonary infundibulum.

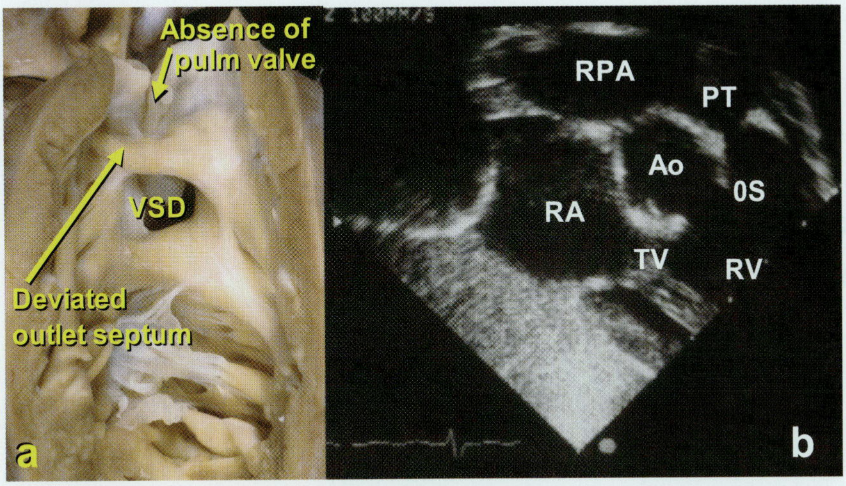

Figure 10.12 (a) This heart with Fallot's tetralogy is associated with under-development of the pulmonary valve. Instead of semilunar leaflets, the valve is represented by a ridge. (b) Subcostal right oblique section shows dilation of the right pulmonary artery in absent pulmonary valve syndrome. Dysplastic rudiments of the pulmonary and hypoplastic outlet septum are visible. There is a muscular postero-inferior rim to the ventricular septal defect, which separates the tricuspid and aortic valves.

leaflets, but the major feature is the marked dilation of the pulmonary trunk and arteries.

A very important subset of hearts with tetralogy have pulmonary atresia rather than pulmonary stenosis. These are part of the spectrum of pulmonary atresia with ventricular septal defect. They are of sufficient clinical import to warrant separate coverage.

11

Tetralogy of Fallot with Pulmonary Atresia

The spectrum of pulmonary atresia with ventricular septal defect includes many lesions. Thus, hearts with the segmental combinations producing transposition, namely concordant atrioventricular and discordant ventriculo-arterial connections, can have pulmonary atresia in the setting of a ventricular septal defect. So can those with the basic segmental arrangement of congenitally corrected transposition, or those with isomeric atrial appendages. Pulmonary atresia with a ventricular septal defect can also coexist with double inlet ventricle, or atrioventricular valvar atresia. In all these combinations, however, the blood supply to the lungs is almost always derived from the arterial duct with the pulmonary arteries themselves almost always being confluent, and supplying all the bronchopulmonary segments in normal fashion. There is a subset of hearts, nonetheless, in which the pulmonary arteries are fed by multiple systemic-to-pulmonary collateral arteries in the absence of the arterial duct. Almost always, these hearts have the intracardiac anatomy of tetralogy of Fallot, but with pulmonary atresia instead of stenosis. Hearts with tetralogy and pulmonary atresia can also be found when the pulmonary circulation is supplied by an arterial duct, or is fed from even rarer sources (Fig. 11.1). But, because this group includes the overwhelming majority of those with systemic-to-pulmonary collateral arteries, it is appropriate to describe them within the spectrum of tetralogy.

Intracardiac Anatomy

The ventricular septal defect, as in tetralogy, is perimembranous in the majority of cases, but can also be found with a muscular postero-inferior rim. In most of the hearts the antero-cephalad margin is the deviated outlet septum, which separates

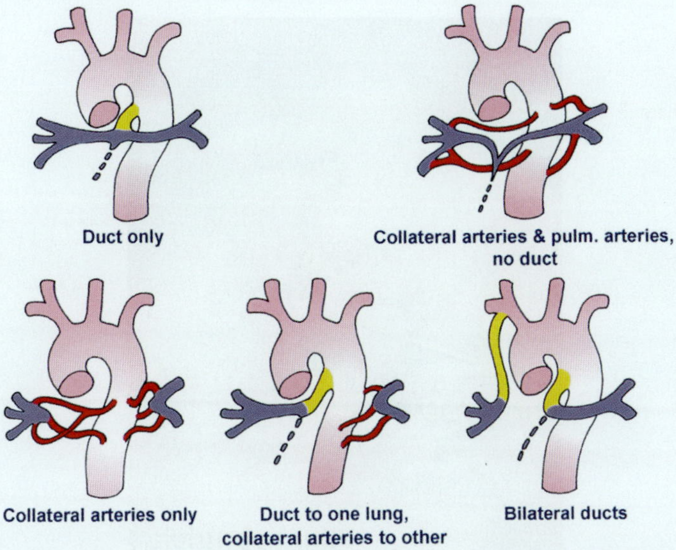

Figure 11.1 Diagram showing some of the variations in arterial supply to the lungs when there is atresia of the pulmonary valve, or right ventricular outlet, associated with a ventricular septal defect.

the overriding aorta from the atretic subpulmonary infundibulum (Fig. 11.2). In a minority of hearts, nonetheless, the outlet septum can be entirely lacking. The aortic valve leaflets can then be supported exclusively by the parietal wall of the right ventricle (Fig. 11.3), an arrangement reminiscent of common arterial trunk, or else be in fibrous continuity with an atretic pulmonary valve.

Infundibular Morphology

The majority of hearts have a blind-ending muscular subpulmonary infundibulum. Other arrangments are to be found, nonetheless, such as an imperforate pulmonary valve, or absence of the ventriculo-pulmonary connection. The imperforate pulmonary valve can be found either at the end of a patent subpulmonary infundibulum, producing atresia at valvar level (Fig. 11.4), or when the outlet septum is completely absent (Fig. 11.5). Atresia can also be found at the mouth of the subpulmonary infundibulum, and then the pulmonary valve itself can be patent.

Aortic Overriding

As with tetralogy of Fallot with pulmonary stenosis, the overriding aorta in the setting of pulmonary atresia can be predominantly connected with either the left or the right ventricle.

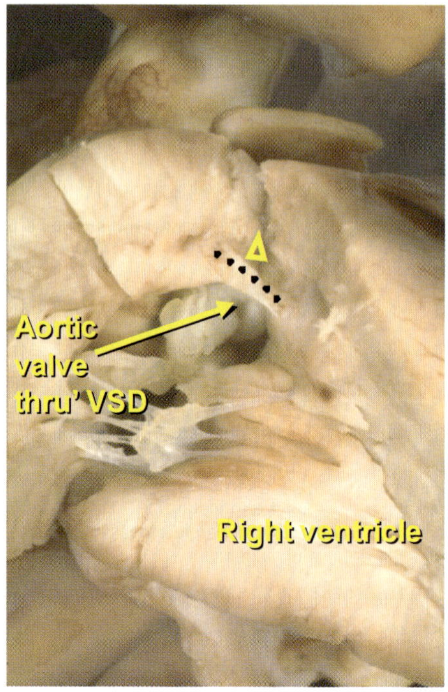

Figure 11.2 The right ventricular outlet in this heart shows extreme antero-cephalad deviation of the outlet septum (dotted line) markedly reducing the subpulmonary area to a blind ending muscular tunnel (Δ). There is a perimembranous ventricular septal defect with overriding of the aortic valve.

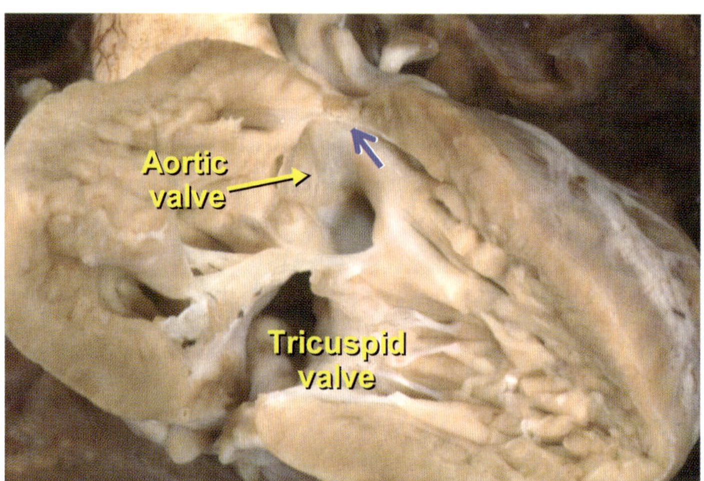

Figure 11.3 A discrete outlet septum cannot be identified in this heart. The anterior limb of the septomarginal trabeculation reaches to the parietal wall (arrow). The aortic valve is connected to both ventricles through the ventricular septal defect.

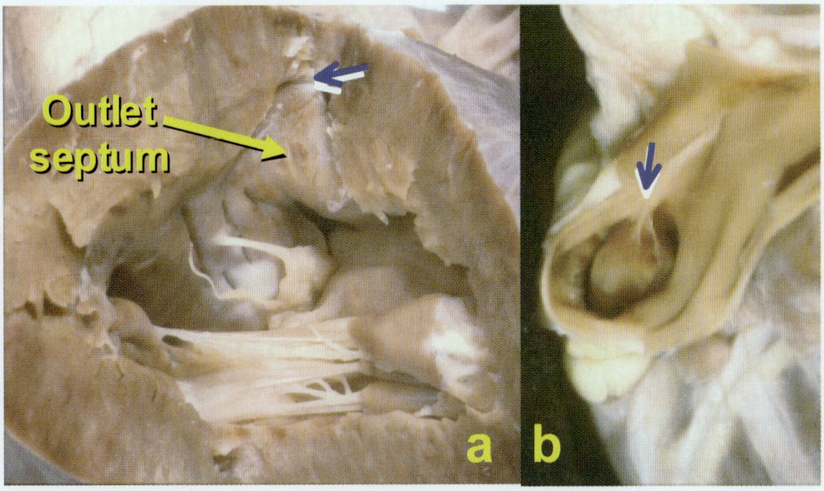

Figure 11.4 (a) A membrane (arrow) occludes the right ventricular outlet. The right ventricular wall is grossly hypertrophied. (b) The membrane is an imperforate valve that has only one rudimentary commissure (arrow).

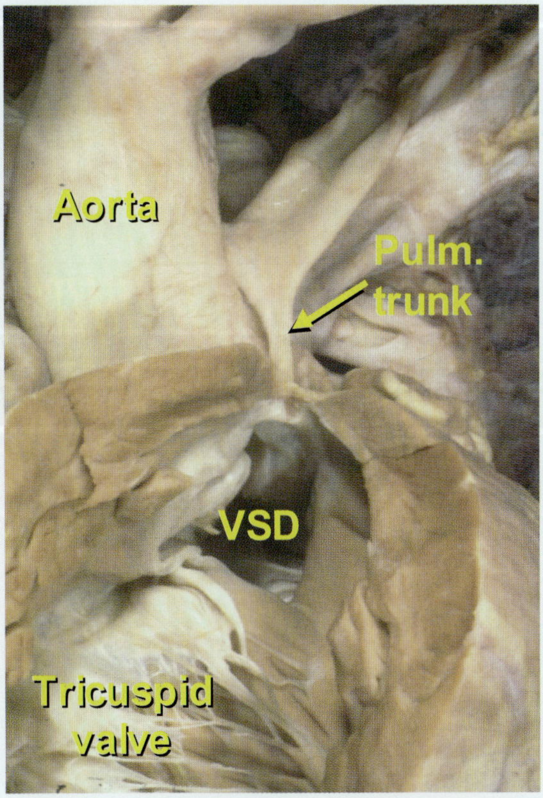

Figure 11.5 The aortic valve is in fibrous continuity with the atretic pulmonary valve. The outlet septum is absent.

The Pulmonary Arteries and their Supply

By far the most important feature in this group of hearts is the arrangement and supply of the pulmonary arteries. The pulmonary trunk itself can be patent to the level of an imperforate valve, can originate blindly above an area of muscular atresia (Figs. 11.6 and 11.7), or can be thread-like throughout its length (Fig. 11.8). The pulmonary trunk can also be completely absent, but then the trunk exiting from the ventricles is best described as a solitary arterial trunk (Fig. 11.9). This is because, when the intrapericardial pulmonary arteries are absent, there is no way of knowing whether had the trunk been present, it would have been an aorta or a common vessel (Fig. 3.10). The pulmonary arteries can themselves be confluent (Fig. 11.10), non-confluent (Fig. 11.11) or completely absent.

The supply to the pulmonary arteries also shows great variability (Fig. 11.1). When the supply is derived from a patent arterial duct, the pulmonary arteries are usually confluent, and branch to supply all the bronchopulmonary segments. Non-confluent pulmonary arteries, each with normal distribution, can be supplied by bilateral arterial ducts. Confluent arteries with normal distribution can also be fed by an aorto-pulmonary window, by a fifth aortic arch, or by a fistula from the coronary arteries.

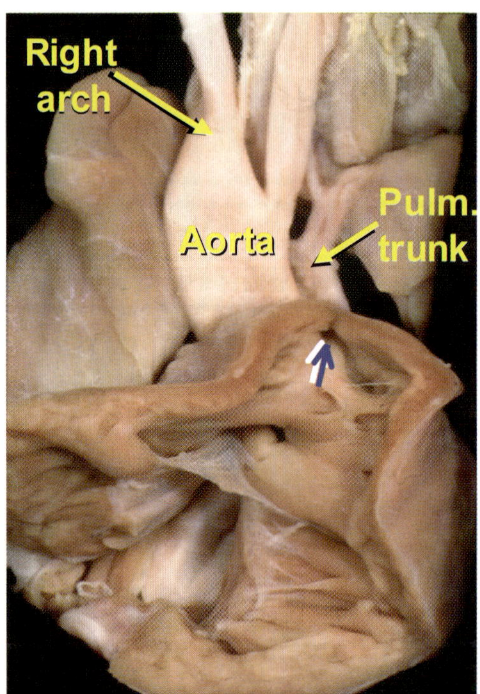

Figure 11.6 The right ventricular outflow tract terminated in muscular atresia. The pulmonary trunk is patent.

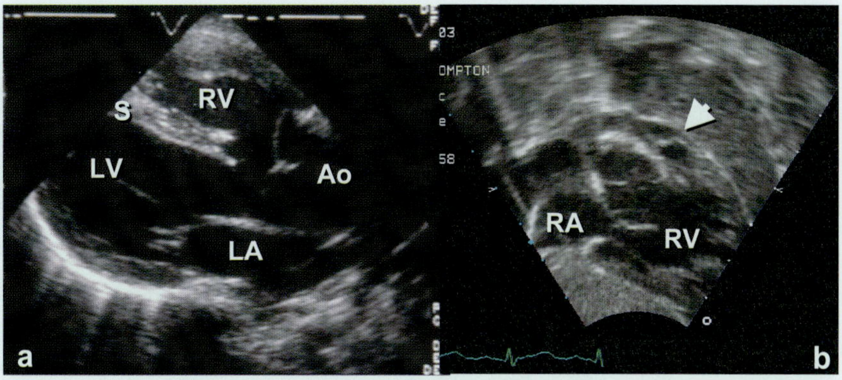

Figure 11.7 (a) Parasternal long axis section showing overriding of aorta. (b) Subcostal right oblique section showing muscular overgrowth of the subpulmonary infundibulum.

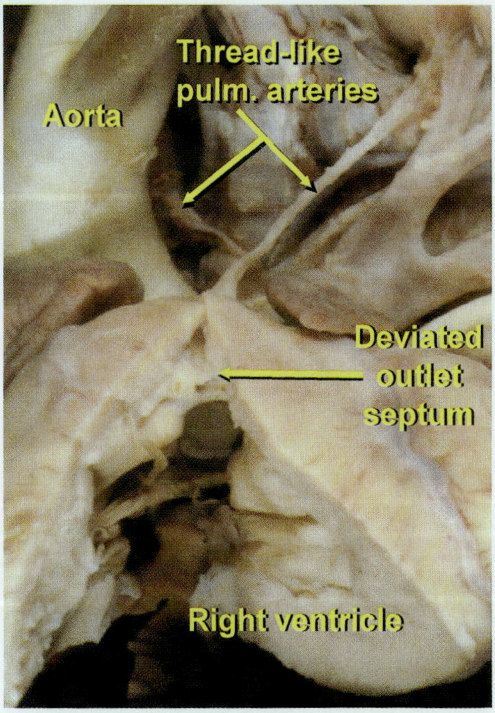

Figure 11.8 The pulmonary trunk and its bifurcation are thread-like.

The most interesting anatomical arrangements are to be found in the presence of systemic-to-pulmonary collateral arteries. These vessels, usually two or six in number, arise from the descending aorta or, more rarely, from the brachiocephalic, or even the coronary arteries. Usually, but not always, they coexist with confluent intrapericardial pulmonary arteries; hardly ever do they coexist with an arterial duct. The collateral arteries themselves can run into the hilums of the lung and become

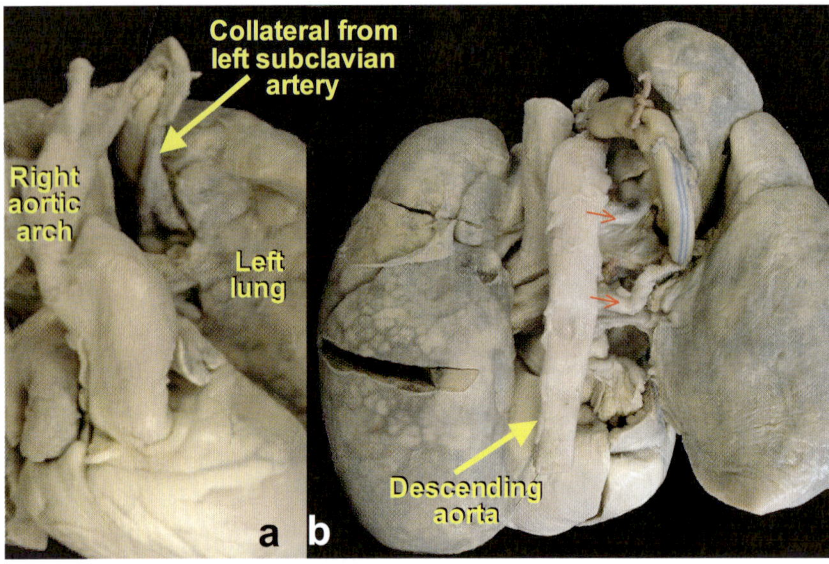

Figure 11.9 (a) Intrapericardial pulmonary arteries are not found in this case of solitary arterial trunk. (b) Posterior view shows the lungs supplied by collateral arteries (arrow) arising from the descending thoracic aorta.

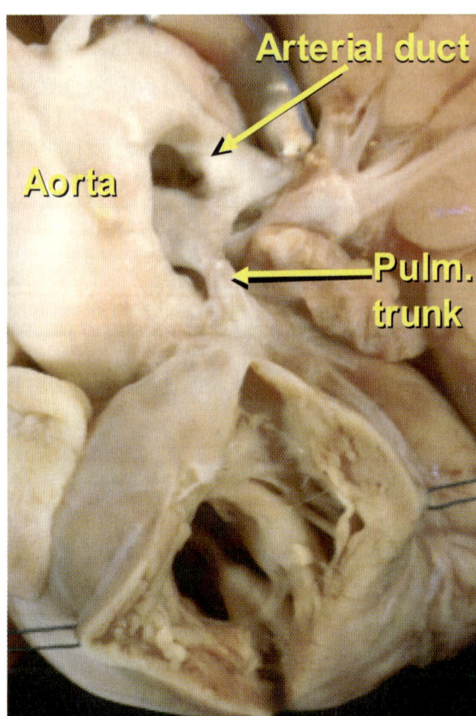

Figure 11.10 This case of pulmonary atresia has confluent pulmonary arteries supplied via a patent arterial duct.

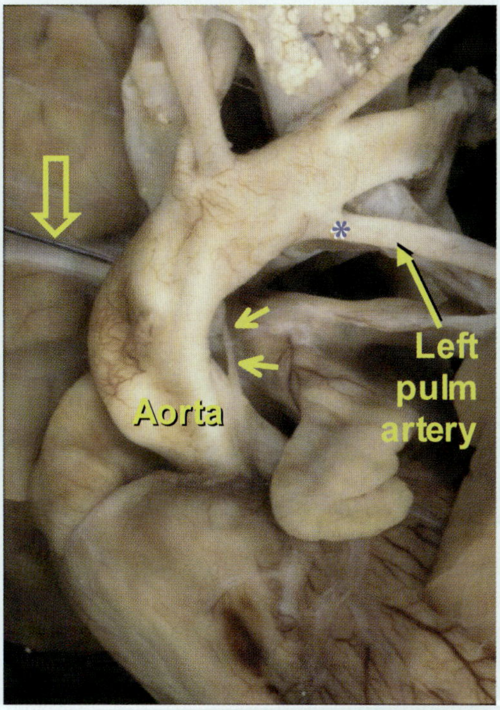

Figure 11.11 The pulmonary trunk is strand-like (small arrows) and continues into the right pulmonary artery (open arrow). The left pulmonary artery is not connected to the pulmonary trunk. Instead, it is connected to the arterial duct (*) that arises from the inner curvature of the aortic arch.

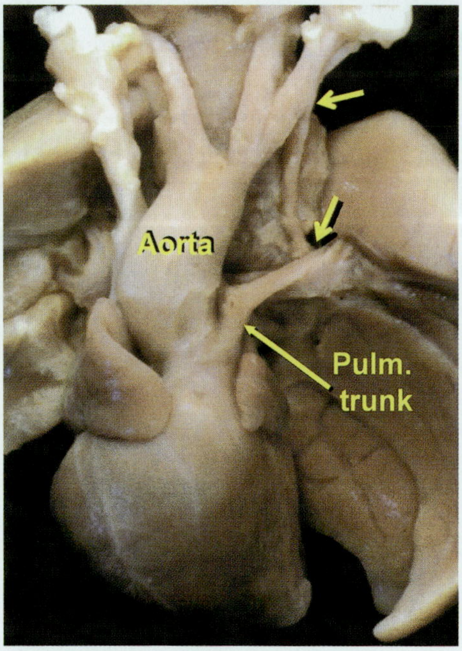

Figure 11.12 A collateral artery arising from the left subclavian artery anastomoses with the left pulmonary artery (short arrows).

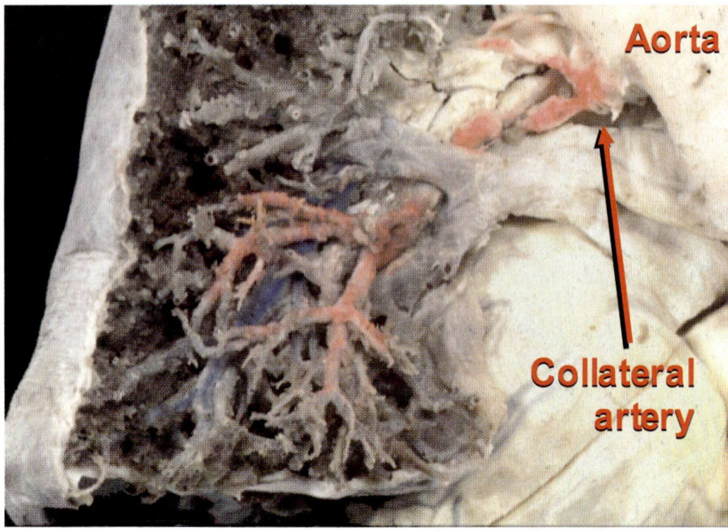

Figure 11.13 There is dual supply to this part of the lower lobe. Branches of systemic collateral arteries are coloured red. Arteries that can be traced to intrapericardial pulmonary arteries are coloured blue.

confluent with intraparenchymal pulmonary arteries. Alternatively, the collateral arteries can anastomose with intrapericardial pulmonary arteries at extrapulmonary, hilar, lobar or segmental levels (Fig. 11.12). They then supply the proportion of pulmonary parenchyma fed by the intrapericardial pulmonary arteries. Some bronchopulmonary segments receive a dual supply: a part directly through a collateral artery and a part through the branches of the intrapericardial pulmonary arteries (Fig. 11.13). The relationship between collateral arteries and bronchial arteries is unclear. Some of the collateral arteries have an origin and distribution that cannot be distinguished from bronchial arteries. Others seem to have a markedly different anatomical arrangement. Because of this, it is best to describe them simply as systemic-to-pulmonary collateral arteries, a term that is also accurate. Such arteries should be distinguished, nonetheless, from the acquired collateral arteries, which can develop from intercostal or similar systemic arteries.

12

Hypoplastic Right and Left Ventricles

Ventricles can be hypoplastic, but complete, in that each has inlet, trabecular and outlet portions. In such circumstances, one, two or all three of these components is underdeveloped. In most cases, the atrioventricular connections, as well as the ventriculo-arterial connections are concordant. Discordant ventriculo-arterial connections are rare. Hypoplastic but complete ventricles are to be distinguished from the rudimentary ventricles in hearts with univentricular atrioventricular connections. In the latter hearts, the ventricles are hypoplastic, but also incomplete or rudimentary in that they lack at least their inlet components.

Hypoplastic Right Ventricle

The most common setting for hypoplasia of the right ventricle is pulmonary atresia with intact ventricular septum (Fig. 12.1). Not all such hearts, however, have hypoplasia of the right ventricle. Indeed, there is a spectrum of ventricular cavity sizes. The majority have tiny or small right ventricular cavities, with a few having normal-sized or dilated ventricular chambers. In the hypoplastic forms, it is hypertrophy of the ventricular walls that squeezes out the cavity (Figs. 12.2 and 12.3). The apical trabeculations can be so overgrown as to totally obliterate the apical cavity, while overgrowth in the outlet component can produce muscular atresia, a feature to be contrasted with an imperforate valve. This distinction, between muscular and membranous atresia, is the single most important anatomical feature in classification.

A small right ventricle is also usually associated with a small orifice of the tricuspid valve. Anomalies of the tricuspid valve are frequent, although some valves

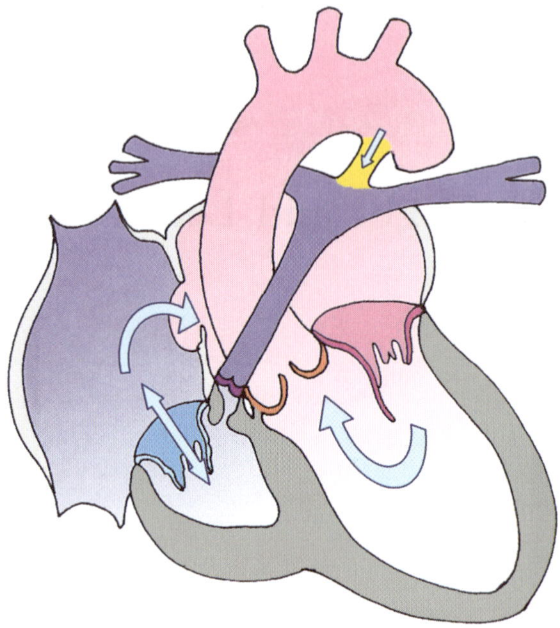

Figure 12.1 Diagram showing the circulatory pattern in pulmonary atresia with intact ventricular septum.

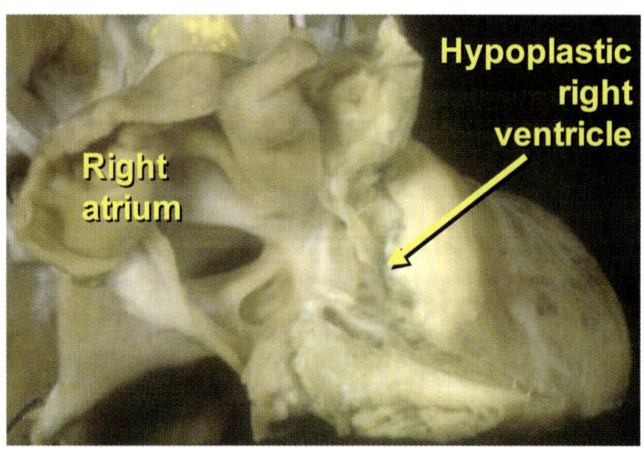

Figure 12.2 The cavity of the right ventricle is reduced in this heart with pulmonary atresia.

are normally formed but the valvar apparatus is miniaturised. Dysplasia of the valvar leaflets is common. Severely dysplastic tricuspid valves are sometimes seen in hearts with normal or near normal-sized ventricles (Fig. 12.4). Ebstein's malformation is another common malformation of the tricuspid valve seen in hearts with pulmonary atresia and intact ventricular septum, affecting about a quarter of cases. In the mildest

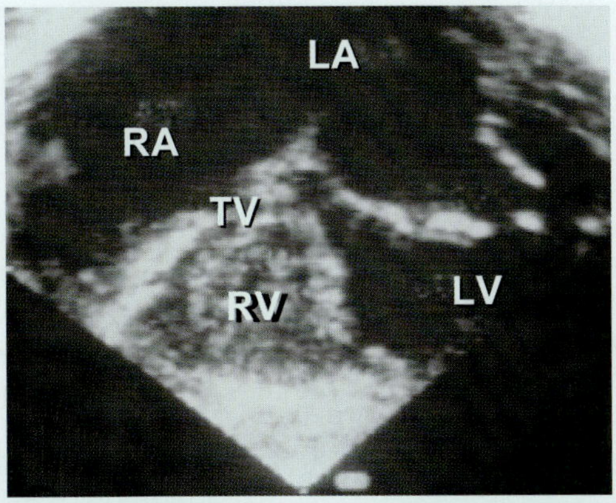

Figure 12.3 Parasternal four-chamber section showing hypoplasia of the right ventricle with severe muscular hypertrophy and minaturised tricuspid valve in a heart with pulmonary atresia and intact ventricular septum.

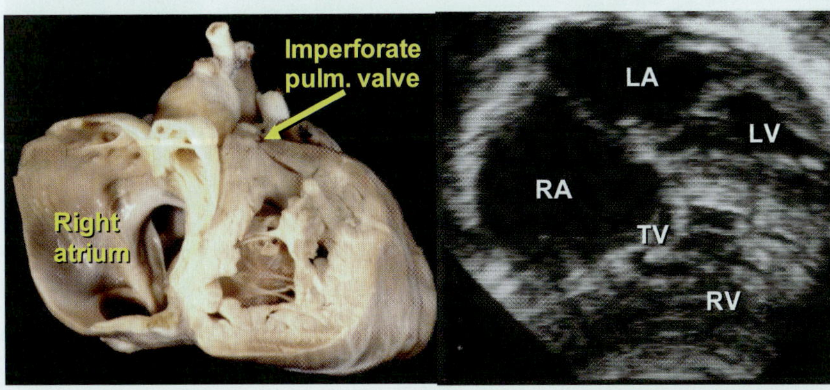

Figure 12.4 (a) This heart shows dilation of the right atrium caused by tricuspid incompetence. The right ventricle is a good size. (b) Subcostal four-chamber section with dysplastic tricuspid valve and severe right ventricular hypertrophy.

form, there is only apical displacement of the hinge of the septal leaflet. In others, the septal leaflet is almost absent and the antero-superior leaflet is curtain-like. Distortions producing severe tricuspid regurgitation are associated with the largest right ventricles (Fig. 12.5). Ebstein's malformation may also produce obstruction between inlet and outlet portions of the ventricle. The obstruction is caused by the insertion of the antero-superior leaflet.

The key to differentiation within the lesion is the recognition of the two forms of pulmonary atresia at the ventriculo-arterial junction. In one, the right ventricular infundibulum is patent to the undersurface of the valve, which is a dome-shaped imperforate membrane (Figs. 12.6 and 12.7). In the other, there is no evidence of the

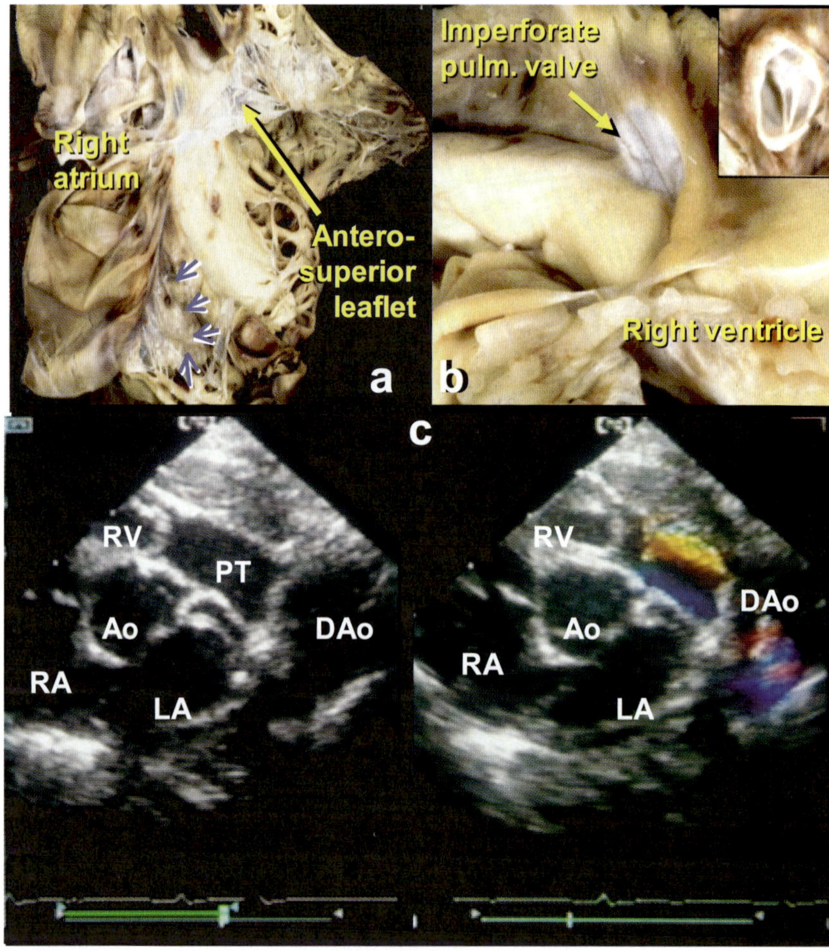

Figure 12.5 This heart has an imperforate pulmonary valve associated with dilation of the right atrium and right ventricle. (a) The right atrium and ventricle have been opened to show Ebstein malformation of the tricuspid valve. (b) The pulmonary outflow tract leads to an imperforate valvar membrane. The inset shows a fused commissure and two other rudimentary commissures on the arterial aspect. (c) Parasternal short axis view at the level of the aorta in pulmonary valve atresia. With colour flow Doppler, a small arterial duct is demonstrated.

valve because of muscular obliteration of the ventriculo-arterial junction (Figs. 12.8 and 12.9). The pulmonary trunk ends blindly in three sinuses and is separated from the ventricular cavity by the muscular wall of the infundibulum.

Despite the atresia at the ventriculo-arterial junction, the pulmonary trunk is usually of good size. The pulmonary circulation is fed through an arterial duct, which is long and tortuous, joining the aorta at a more acute angle than normal. The oval foramen also tends to be widely patent. The left atrium and left ventricle are

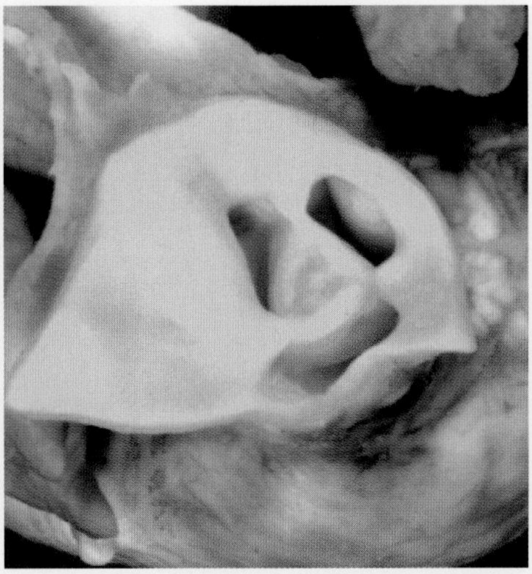

Figure 12.6 This is the more commonly seen dome-shaped and imperforate pulmonary valve.

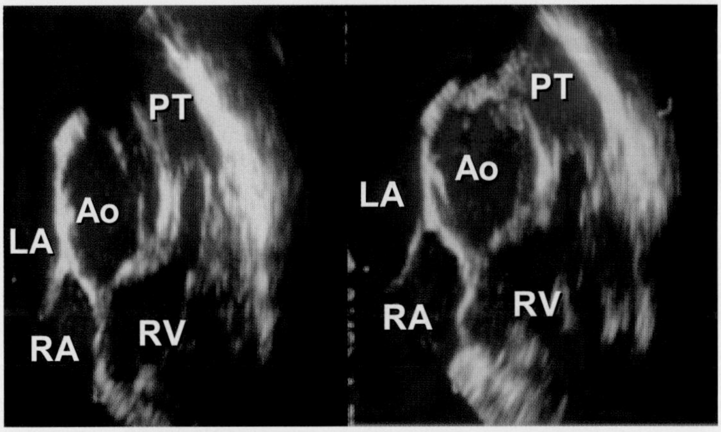

Figure 12.7 Echocardiographic sections showing doming of an imperforate pulmonary valve. The right panel fails to demonstrate forward flow with colour flow Doppler.

usually well developed. High pressures in the right ventricle can result in a convex bulging of the septum into the left ventricle.

Abnormalities of the coronary arteries are common. When the right ventricle is small, almost always with muscular atresia as opposed to an imperforate pulmonary valve, fistulous communications between the right ventricle and the coronary arterial system are frequently found (Fig. 12.10). Atresia or complete absence of the proximal portion of one or both main coronary arteries occurs rarely. In these hearts, it is the fistulous communications which provide the coronary arterial flow, which is therefore right ventricular dependent.

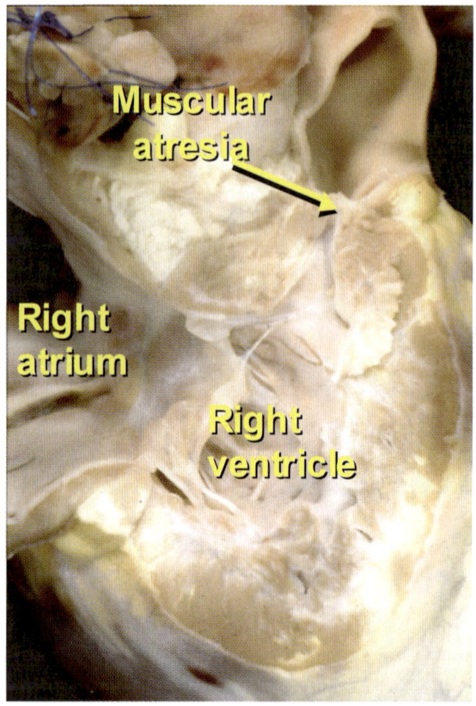

Figure 12.8 A heart showing muscular atresia of the right ventricular outflow tract. The pulmonary trunk ends blindly, without formation of a membrane or valvar elements. Note the areas of scarring in the right ventricular wall.

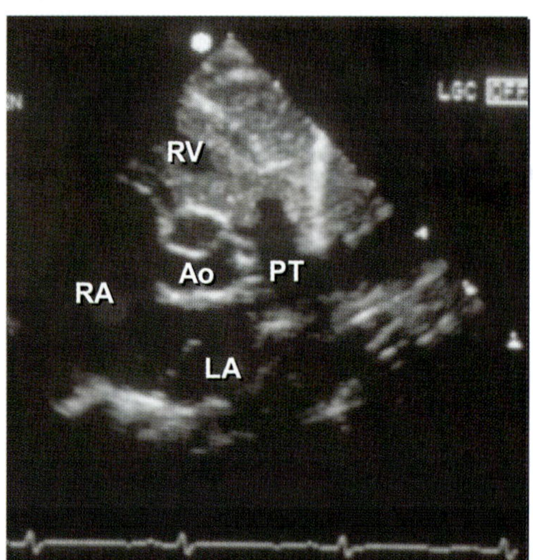

Figure 12.9 Parasternal short axis view at the level of the aorta showing muscular atresia of the infundibulum.

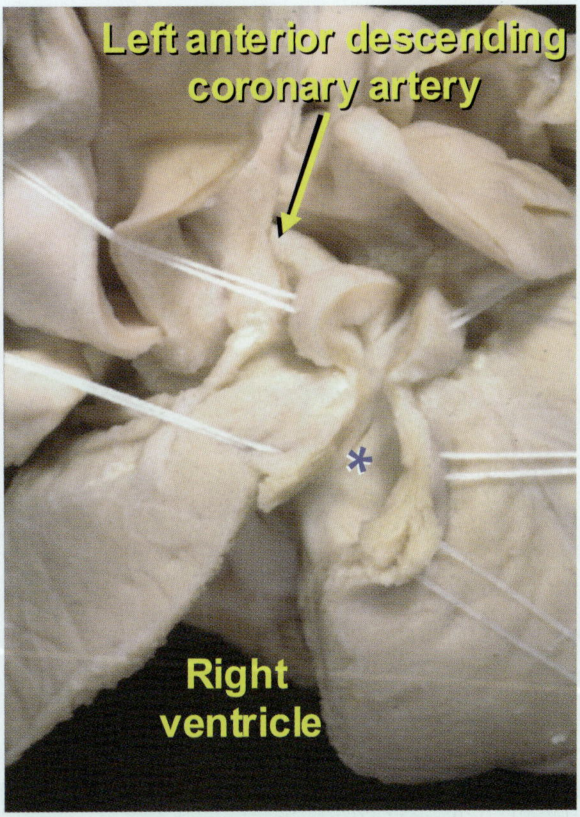

Figure 12.10 There is fistulous communication between the right ventricle and the anterior descending coronary artery in this heart with hypoplastic right ventricle.

Hypoplastic Left Ventricle

In 1952, Lev described a group of congenital heart anomalies, which he collectively termed 'hypoplasia of the aortic tract complex'. Infants with these lesions presented with a typical clinical picture, which Noonan and Nadas named the 'hypoplastic left heart syndrome', synonymous with 'hypoplasia of the left ventricle'. The hypoplasia involving the left ventricle, however, is variable, but usually associated with aortic atresia or critical anomalous (Fig. 12.11). Aortic atresia occasionally exists with a near-normal or normal-sized left ventricle, especially when there is a large ventricular septal defect. Hearts with hypoplastic left ventricle, however, generally have mitral stenosis or atresia together with aortic stenosis or atresia. There are two anatomical forms of mitral atresia, namely absence of the left atrioventricular connection or an imperforate mitral valve.

When perforate, the mitral valve is usually severely stenotic. The leaflets are thickened, the tendinous cords are short, and intercordal spaces are reduced (Fig. 12.12). The papillary muscles are diminished, with some cords inserting directly into the

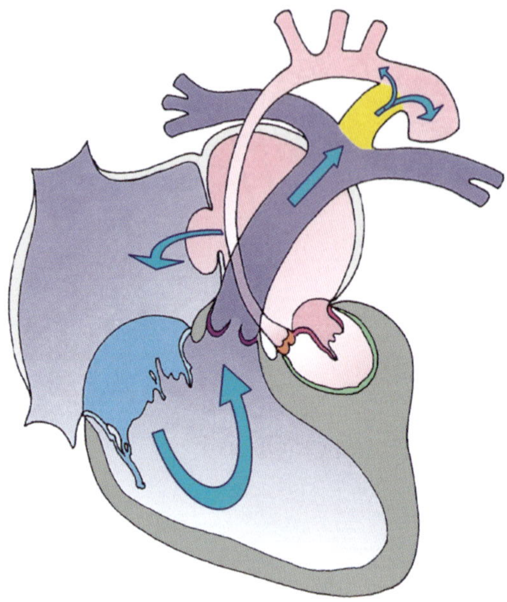

Figure 12.11 Diagram showing the flow pathways in a hypoplastic left heart with aortic atresia.

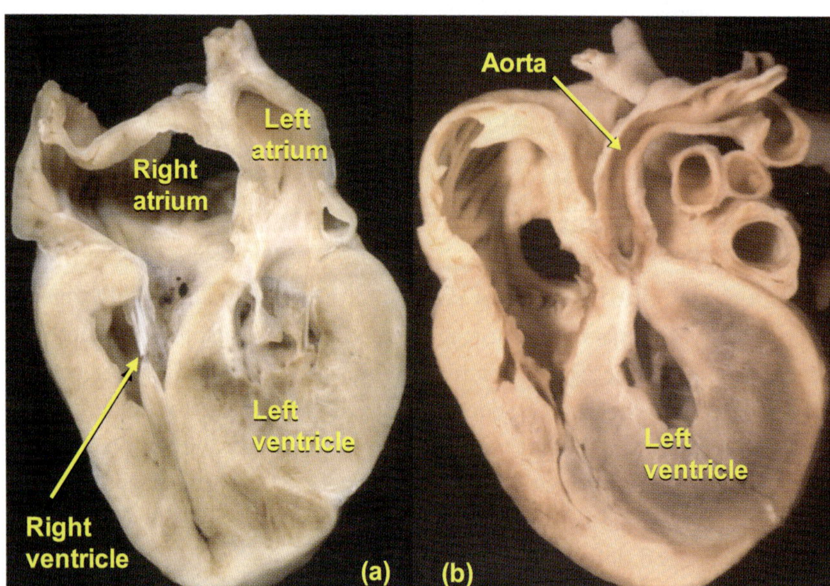

Figure 12.12 (a) Four-chamber section through a heart with mitral stenosis and hypoplastic left ventricle. Endocardial fibroelastosis lines the left ventricle. (b) This section of the same heart shows aortic atresia with muscular obliteration of the left ventricular outlet.

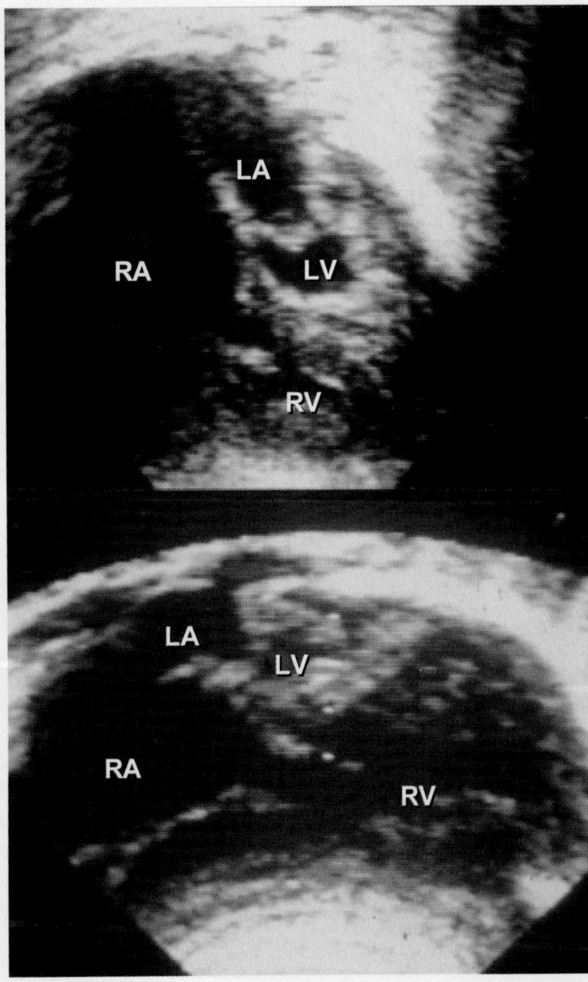

Figure 12.13 The upper panel is a parasternal four-chamber section and the lower panel is a subcostal four-chamber section showing miniaturised and dysplastic mitral valve. Echocardiograms of a case with a spherical hypoplastic left ventricle.

endocardium. The endocardial surface is covered by a layer of endocardial fibroelastosis, but only when the mitral valve is patent. The left ventricular wall is usually hypertrophied, producing a small, spherical cavity (Figs. 12.12 and 12.13). Fistulous communications between the ventricular chamber and the coronary arterial system are common in these cases.

At the ventriculo-arterial junction, the root of the aorta is usually blind and terminates in three sinuses. The coronary arteries arise from the blind end. The epicardial distribution of the coronary arteries is helpful in assessing the size of the left ventricle. The aorta widens as it ascends to continue into the arch (Figs. 12.14 and 12.15). Discrete coarctation occurs in 50–75% of cases. It is located in either the preductal or

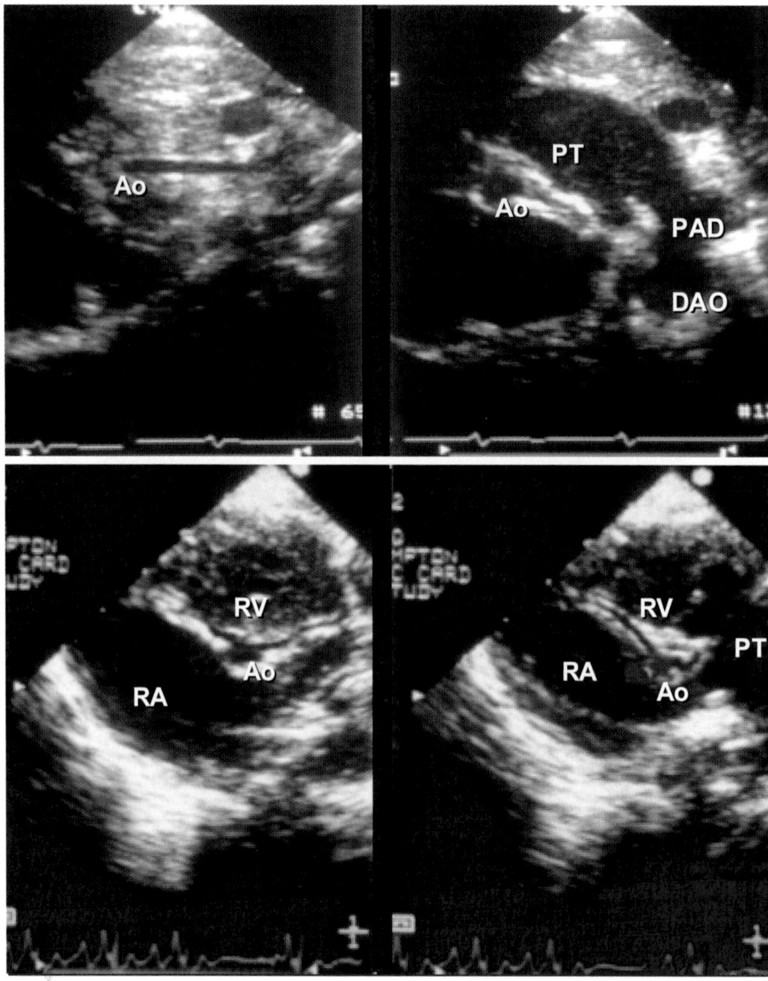

Figure 12.14 The upper panels show high parasternal long axis sections of the tiny aorta and large pulmonary trunk and arterial duct. The patent arterial duct (PAD) supplies the coronary arteries retrogradely. The lower panels are parasternal short axis sections through the aorta to show the origins of the coronary arteries.

paraductal position. When the aortic valve is an imperforate membrane, the ascending aorta can be near-normal in size. The major flow pathway to the descending aorta is from the pulmonary trunk through a patent arterial duct.

The left atrium is usually small, although the left appendage can be disproportionately large. Often, the atrial wall is muscular and has thickened white endocardial lining. When the outlet of the left atrium is restricted, the pulmonary veins tend to be thick-walled. The veins usually connect to the left atrium but may occasionally terminate elsewhere, sometimes via a laevoatrial cardinal vein (Fig. 12.16). The right side of the heart is usually enlarged. The floor of the oval foramen bulges aneurysmally into the right atrium when the atrial septal defect is inadequate. In a few hearts,

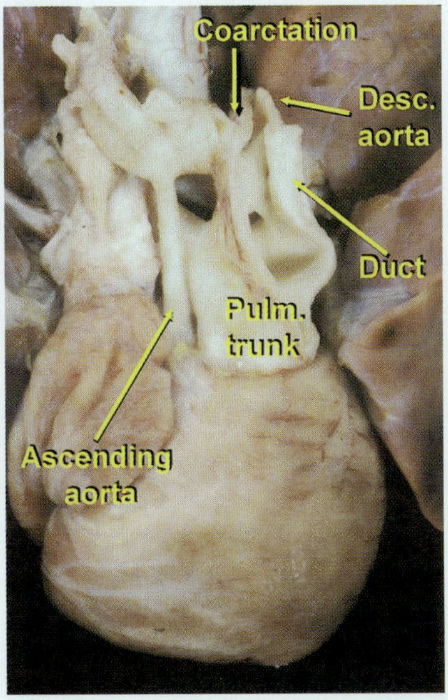

Figure 12.15 This case of hypoplastic left heart has aortic atresia. The ascending aorta is very narrow and there is a coarctation lesion opposite the entrance of the arterial duct.

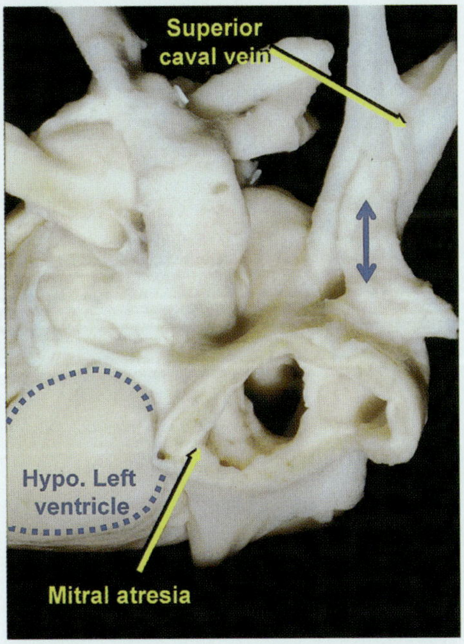

Figure 12.16 The left atrioventricular connection is absent (so-called mitral atresia). The left atrium is small and has a thick wall. The atrial septum was intact. Surgical excision leaves a large atrial communication. With an intact atrial septum, pulmonary venous return exited the heart via a laevoatrial cardinal vein (double headed arrow) that connected with the superior caval vein.

the atrial septum is intact due to premature closure of the oval foramen. Malalignment between the flap valve and the anterocephalad margin of it muscular rim is present in some hearts. Although the right ventricle is usually well formed, it may be associated with other malformations such as anomalous muscle bands, dysplastic tricuspid valve and division of the ventricular chamber.

13

Double Outlet Right Ventricle

There have been many arguments concerning the essential morphological features needed to make the diagnosis of double outlet from the morphologically right ventricle. Some authorities have insisted that there should be bilateral infundibular muscle supporting the entire circumference of both arterial valves. If this criterion is used, it is hardly ever appropriate to diagnose examples of tetralogy of Fallot as having a double outlet right ventricle. Far fewer patients will then be diagnosed as having a double outlet right ventricle than if the diagnosis is regarded solely as a description of ventriculo-arterial connection. Our preference is to define a double outlet as one specific ventriculo-arterial connection. We make the diagnosis whenever more than half of the circumference of both arterial valves, irrespective of the nature of their supporting structures, is connected to the morphologically right ventricle (Fig. 13.1). We have no problem, therefore, in classifying some examples of tetralogy of Fallot, in which more than half of the circumference of the aortic valve is supported by the right ventricle, as also having a double outlet right ventricle (Fig. 13.2).

Defined in this way, a double outlet right ventricle encompasses a huge variety of hearts. For example, it can include patients with isomerism of the atrial appendages. In these patients, the picture will be dominated by the anomalous venoatrial connections. It also includes patients with abnormal atrioventricular connections, such as discordant connections, double inlet ventricle or atrioventricular valvar atresia. It is possible, nonetheless, to focus on a subgroup of patients with usual or, rarely, mirror-imaged, atrial arrangement and with concordant atrioventricular connections. It is the morphology of these patients that we will illustrate. Even amongst this smaller group, there is marked variety of morphology, most importantly with the location of the interventricular communication.

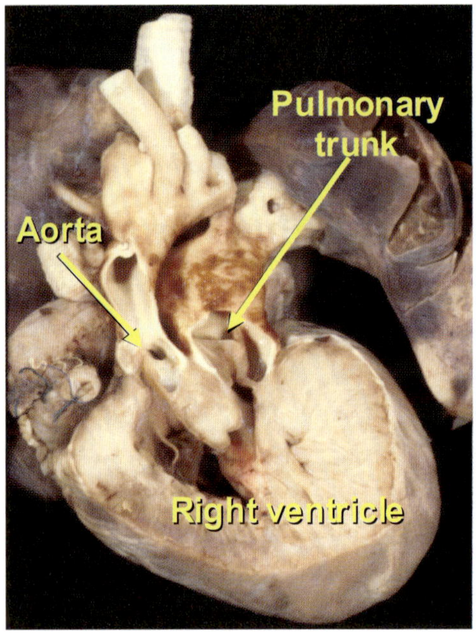

Figure 13.1 A section showing both great arteries arising from the right ventricle. Both sets of arterial valves are supported by muscular infundibulums.

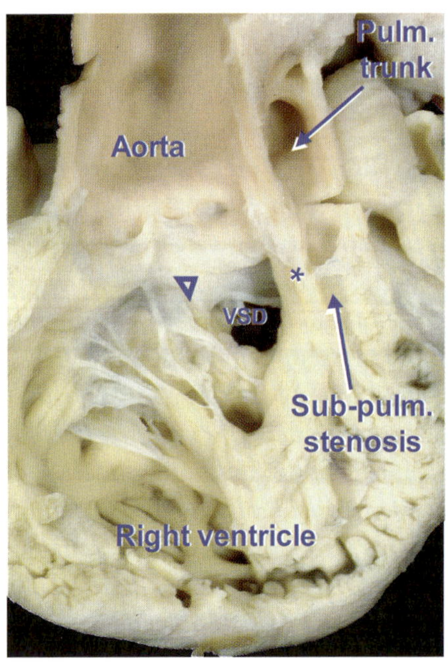

Figure 13.2 This heart clearly has both great arteries arising from the right ventricle but the aortic outlet lacks a complete muscular infundibulum. The ventricular septal defect is perimembranous with the postero-inferior margin (∇) of the defect abutting the area of fibrous continuity between tricuspid, aortic and mitral valves. The subpulmonary outflow tract is obstructed by antero-cephalad deviation of the outlet septum (*) typical of Fallot's tetralogy.

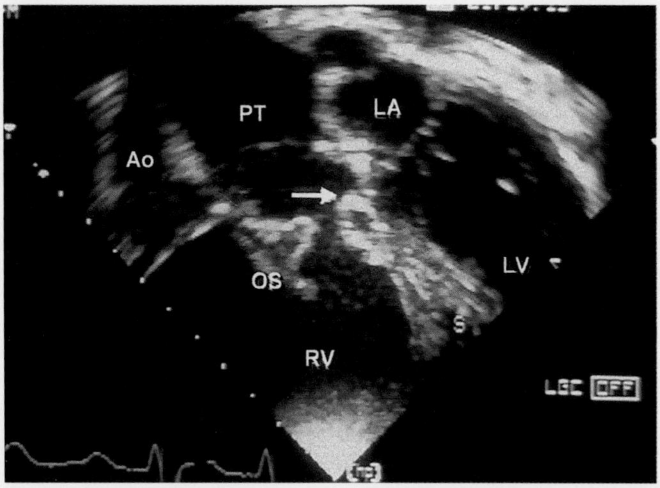

Figure 13.3 Subcostal long axis section in a double outlet right ventricle with restrictive subpulmonary ventricular septal defect, aneurysm of membranous septum (arrow) and severe subpulmonary stenosis.

Although it is a relatively straightforward procedure to identify the nature and relationships of the great arteries, it is much harder to diagnose the presence of a double outlet ventriculo-arterial connection with certainty by cross-sectional echocardiography. This is because the angulation of the ventricular septum makes it difficult to profile both great arteries at the same time. The diagnosis must be made by integrating the information obtained from several planes. One essential feature, nonetheless, is to find the outlet septum as an exclusively right ventricular structure, malaligned relative to the rest of the ventricular septum (Fig. 13.3).

The Interventricular Communication

In hearts with a double outlet right ventricle, the morphology of the interventricular communication is markedly different from the arrangement where each ventricle supports its own arterial trunk (Fig. 13.4). When there is a double outlet, closure of the communication would be incompatible with life of the patient. This is because the hole between the ventricles is, in effect, the outlet from the morphologically left ventricle. To 'correct' the circulations, ignoring any other factors, the surgeon must connect the hole to one or the other arterial trunk. The most popular convention for describing the variability in the interventricular communication, therefore, is to relate its position to the subarterial outlets. Very rarely, hearts will be found in which the ventricular septum is intact (Fig. 13.5). These rare examples almost certainly represent spontaneous closure of a pre-existing defect.

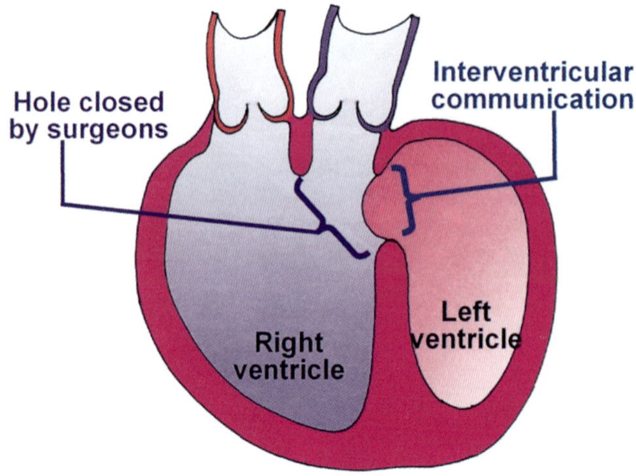

Figure 13.4 Diagram showing the ventricular septal defect as the exit from the left ventricle. To restore a one-to-one ventriculo-arterial connection, the patch needs to include one of the arterial outlets.

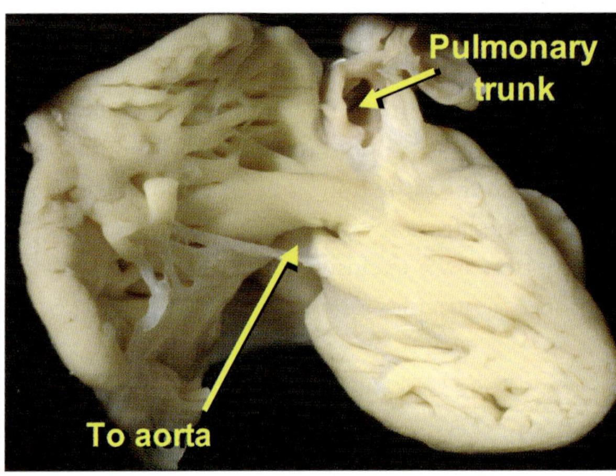

Figure 13.5 A rare case of a double outlet right ventricle with intact ventricular septum.

When, as in the majority of cases, the septal deficiency is the outlet from the left ventricle, its position can be described as subaortic, subpulmonary, doubly committed (opening beneath both arterial trunks) or non-committed (Fig. 13.6). The position of the hole between the ventricles has a major influence on the haemodynamics and presentation of patients with a double outlet right ventricle. Those with the defect in the subaortic position (Figs. 13.7 and 13.8) have a relatively normal pattern of circulation. In contrast, the presence of the defect in the subpulmonary position (Figs. 13.9 and 13.10) creates a circulation comparable to that seen in transposition.

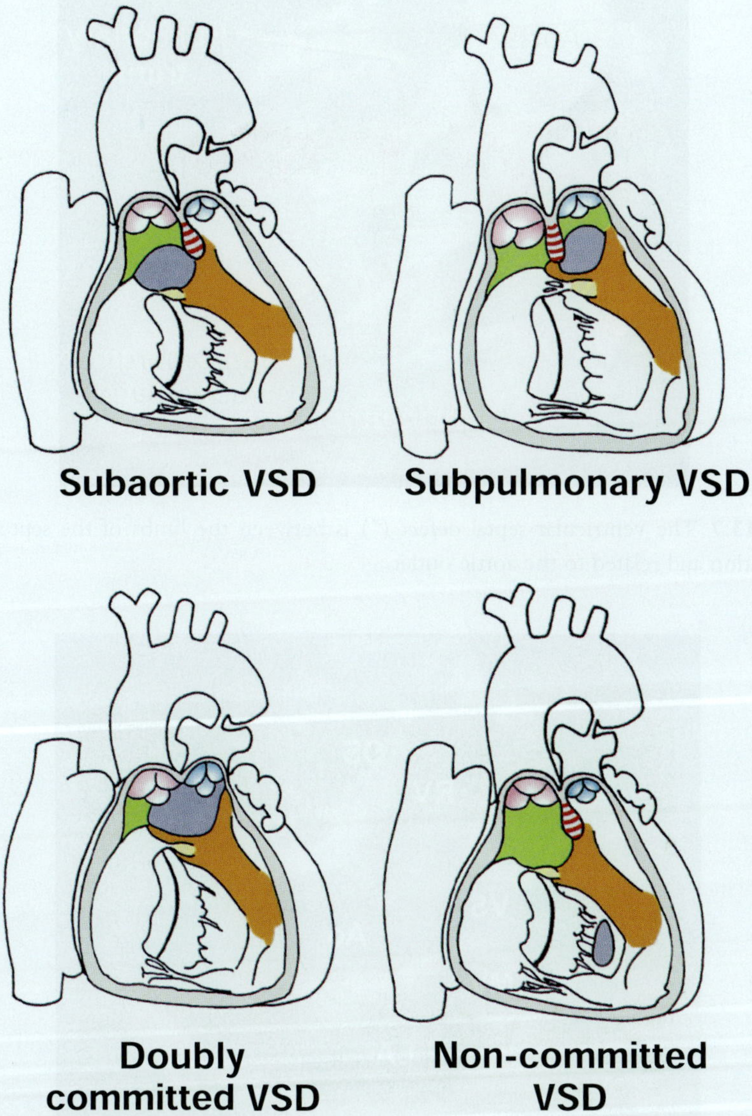

Figure 13.6 Diagram showing the variability in locations of the ventricular septal defect (VSD-dark grey). Red stripes indicate outlet septum.

The key anatomical feature determining these patterns is the ventricular attachments of the outlet septum (Fig. 13.6). The outlet septum is, by necessity, an entirely right ventricular structure. Most defects lie between the limbs of the septomarginal trabeculation. When the outlet septum is firmly attached to the anterior limb of the trabeculation, the defect will be in subaortic position. In contrast, when the outlet septum is attached to the posterior limb of the trabeculation, and to the ventriculo-infundibular fold, the defect is subpulmonary. Complete absence, or marked attenuation, of the outlet septum allows the defect to open beneath both arterial valves

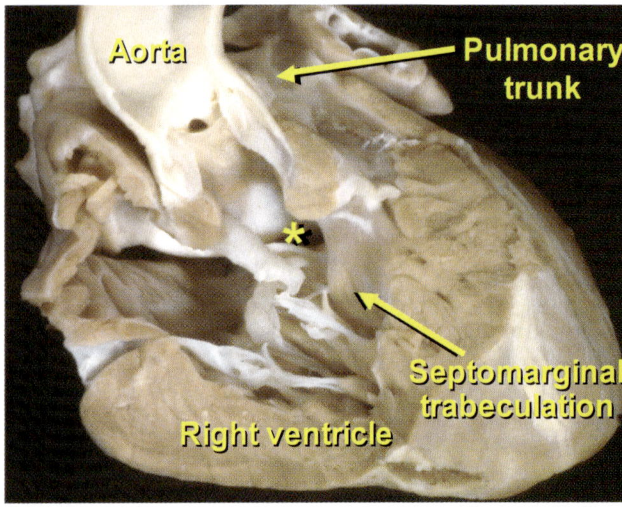

Figure 13.7 The ventricular septal defect (*) is between the limbs of the septomarginal trabeculation and related to the aortic outlet.

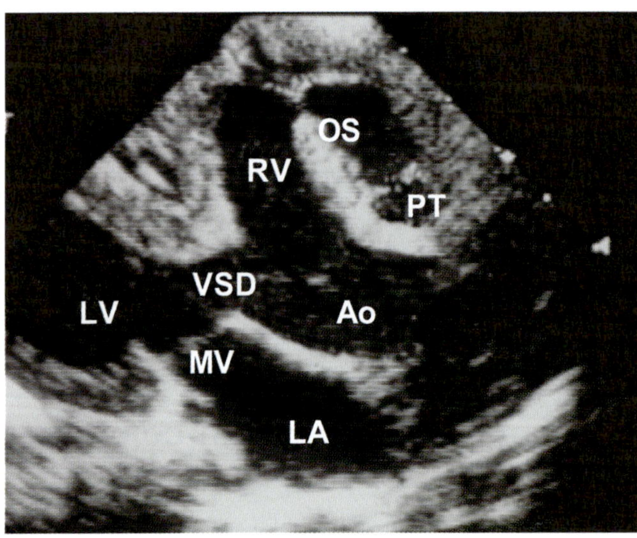

Figure 13.8 Parasternal long axis section showing a subaortic ventricular septal defect and infundibular and valvar pulmonary stenosis.

(Figs. 13.11 and 13.12). Non-committed defects are the exception to the rule that the defect is always between the limbs of the septomarginal trabeculation. Sometimes a defect in this position is non-committed because of an unusually long subarterial infundibulum (Fig. 13.13). How long the infundibulum has to be to make a defect non-committed is a matter of judgement, ultimately for the surgeon. In other instances, the defect is the ventricular component of an atrioventricular septal defect, or a muscular defect in the inlet or apical trabecular components of the septum.

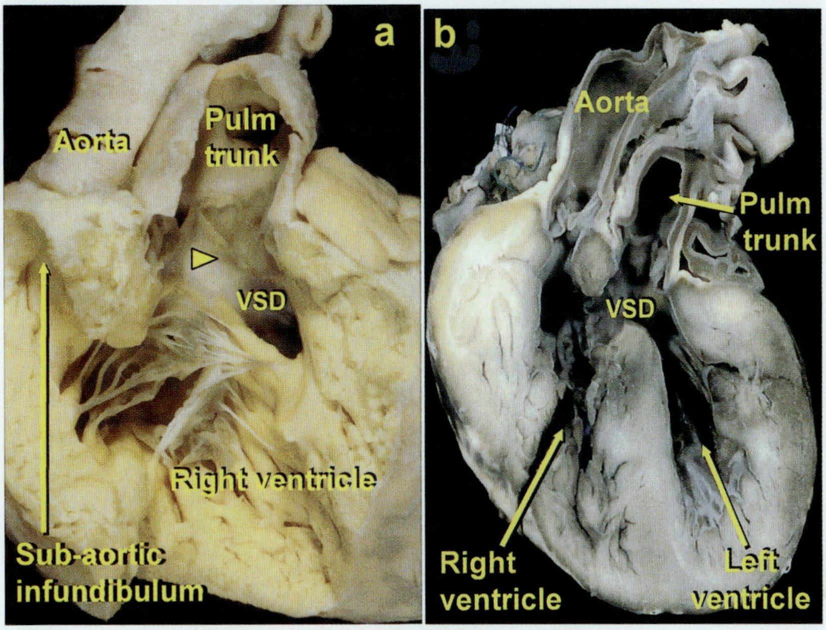

Figure 13.9 Two hearts with sub-pulmonary ventricular septal defect: (a) The pulmonary trunk arises almost entirely from the right ventricle. The ventricular septal defect between the limbs of the septomarginal trabeculation is perimembranous. Note its fibrous margin (Δ). The aortic valve is supported by a muscular infundibulum. (b) This heart shows overriding of the pulmonary valve with biventricular connections. The aorta arises entirely from the right ventricle.

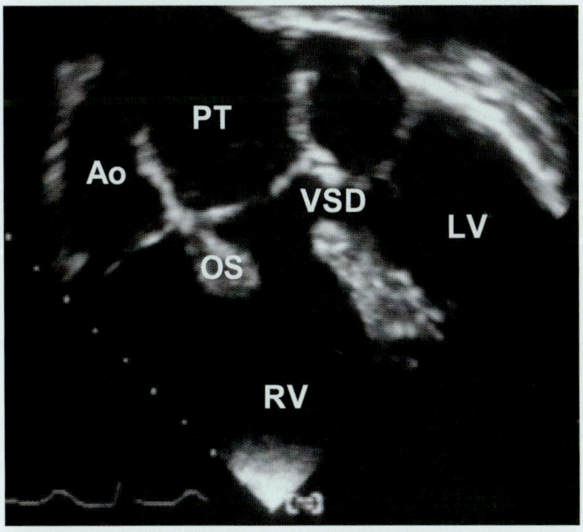

Figure 13.10 Parasternal long axis section showing a subpulmonary ventricular septal defect.

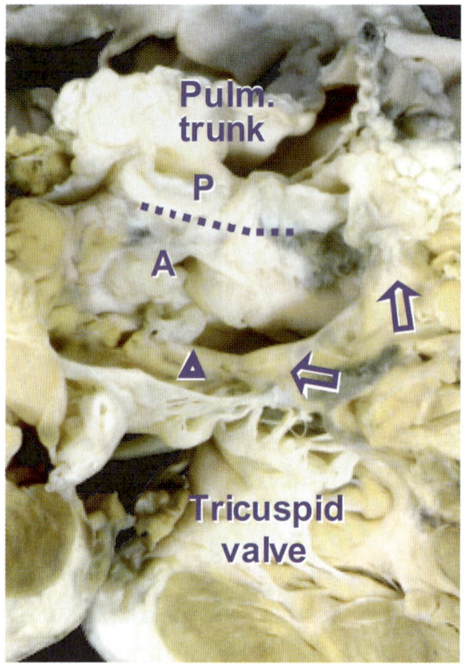

Figure 13.11 Double outlet right ventricle with a doubly committed and juxta-arterial ventricular septal defect. The defect is between the limbs of the septomarginal trabeculation (open arrows) but is roofed by the aortic (A) and pulmonary (P) valves. There is fibrous continuity between the arterial valves through a raphe (dotted line). The postero-inferior margin is muscular (Δ) owing to fusion between the ventriculo-infundibular fold and the posterior limb of the septomarginal trabeculation.

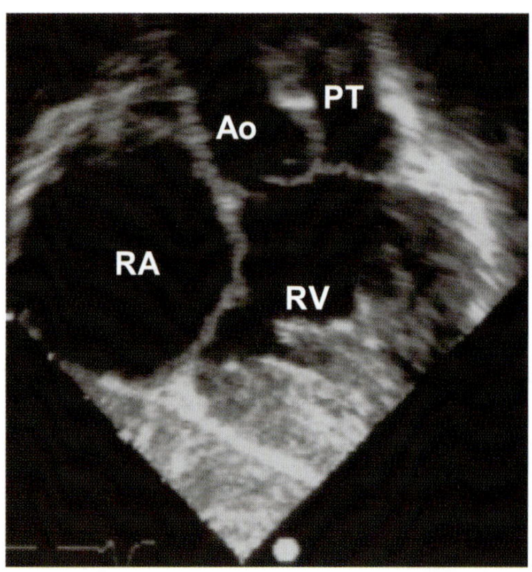

Figure 13.12 Echocardiogram showing a doubly committed and juxta-arterial and perimembranous ventricular septal defect (tricuspid-aortic continuity). The arterial valves are in fibrous continuity in this transgastric view (equivalent to the subcostal right oblique section).

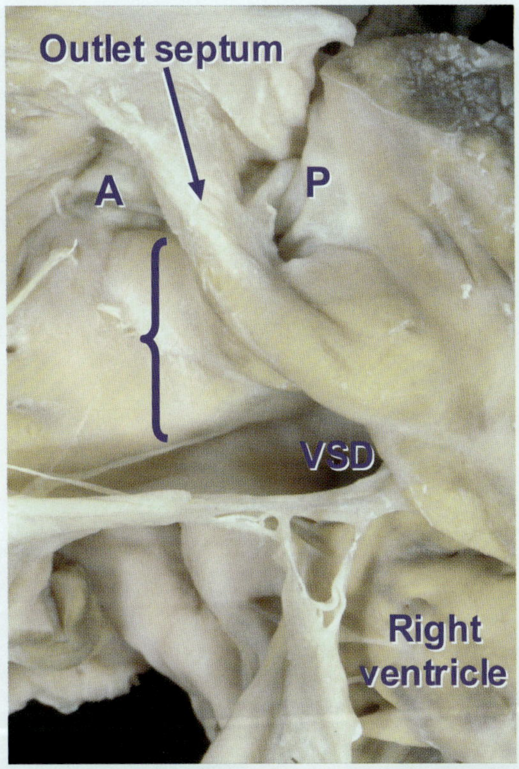

Figure 13.13 This double outlet right ventricle has bilatered infundibulums. Although the ventricular septal defect is subaortic, a long infundibulum ({) separates the aortic valve from the septal defect (VSD). There is a prominent outlet septum between the aortic (A) and pulmonary (P) valves.

In these circumstances, the defect is unequivocally distant from both sub-arterial outlets, and its non-committed nature is beyond question (Fig. 13.14).

One further factor is of importance when considering commitment of the defect. This is the interposition of anatomical structures between the defect and the subarterial outlets. Tension apparatus of atrioventricular valves, or straddling of the leaflets of such valves, can effectively, at least from a surgical point of view, transform a potentially subarterial defect into one that is non-committed.

Infundibular Morphology

As already disscussed, some authorities continue to insist upon the presence of an infundibulum supporting entirely the leaflets of both arterial valves before diagnosing a double outlet. In such circumstances, there is a complete muscular ring beneath both arterial valves, which separates the attachments of these valves from those of the atrioventricular valves. We do not agree with this definition, but we do take

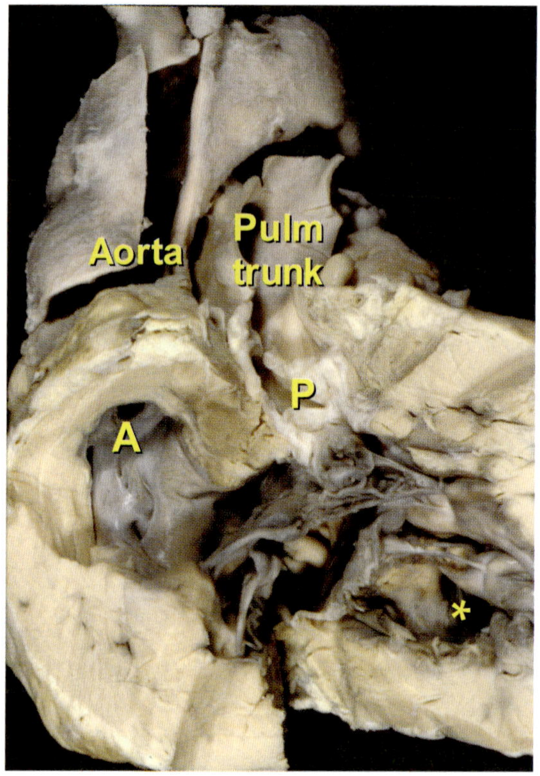

Figure 13.14 This ventricular septal defect is non-committed. The muscular inlet defect is distant from the outlets of both great arteries (A and P).

care to describe the infundibular morphology as it is one of the important variable features in hearts with double outlet. Fibrous continuity between the leaflets of the aortic and atrioventricular valves, or the pulmonary and the atrioventricular valves, is evidence of the lack of a complete infundibulum beneath the arterial valves. If the arterial valves are separated from the atrioventricular valves by muscle, it is always the ventriculo-infundibular fold that separates them. Where there is a complete infundibulum beneath both arterial valves, it is the presence of fibrous continuity between the mitral and tricuspid valves that determines whether the ventricular septal defect is perimembranous. If it is not, and there is a muscular postero-inferior rim, this muscle protects the atrioventricular conduction tissue (Fig. 13.15).

Arterial Relationships

The arterial trunks are often thought of as having a side-by-side relationship in hearts with a double outlet right ventricle. If the condition is defined in terms of a ventriculo-arterial connection, this is hardly ever the case. Usually, the arterial trunks spiral as they leave the base of the heart, in which case the interventricular

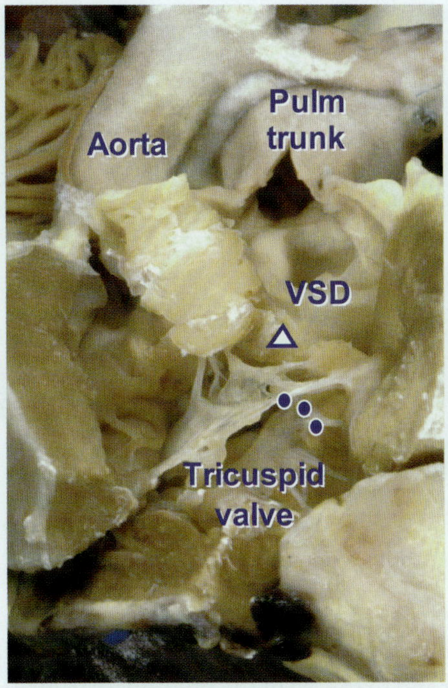

Figure 13.15 This subpulmonary ventricular septal defect has a muscular postero-inferior rim (Δ). The atrioventricular conduction bundle (●●●●) is some distance from the rim.

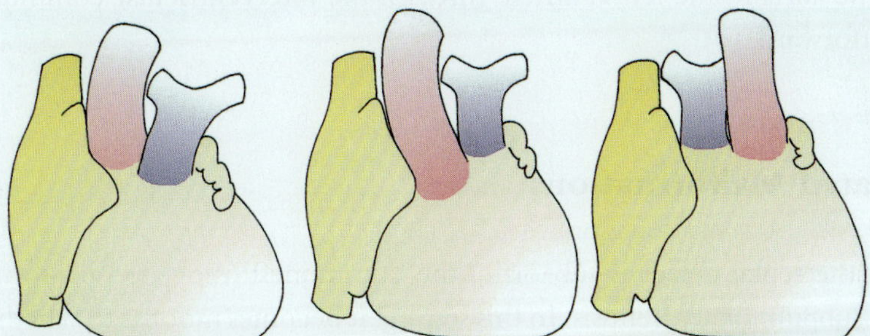

Figure 13.16 The spatial relationship between the aorta and pulmonary trunk is variable in the double outlet right ventricle but can provide a rough guide to the location of the ventricular septal defect.

communication is usually, but not always, subaortic (Fig. 13.16). If the trunks ascend in parallel fashion, with the aorta in anterior and rightward position, the defect is more frequently, but not always, subpulmonary. When the hole between its ventricles is sub-pulmonary, the heart is often called the Taussig–Bing anomaly.

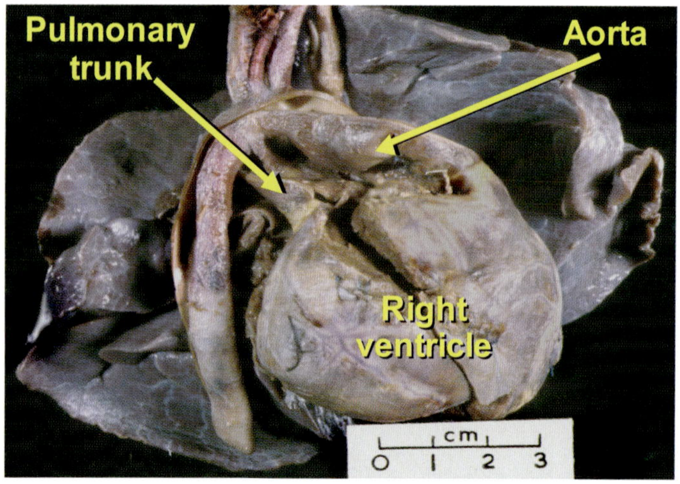

Figure 13.17 This case with left and anterior position of the aorta has a subaortic ventricular septal defect.

There is one small, but important, group in which the arterial trunks are in parallel but the aorta is anterior and to the *left* of the pulmonary trunk (Fig. 13.17). This group is important, first, because the atrioventricular connections are usually concordant, and not discordant as in congenitally corrected transposition, the typical anomaly in which the aorta is leftward and anterior, and second, because, almost always, the hole between the ventricles is subaortic. Surgical correction of these hearts, connecting the aorta to the left ventricle through the interventricular communication, is straightforward.

Associated Malformations

When the septal defect is subaortic, the commonest associated malformation is probably subpulmonary stenosis. In this setting, it becomes moot as to whether hearts are described as tetralogy of Fallot or a double outlet connection. The hearts with fibrous continuity between the aortic and mitral valves are often distinguished from those with a bilateral infundibulum and a subaortic defect. In reality, if there is subpulmonary stenosis due to deviation of the muscular outlet septum, the anatomical differences are minimal, although the presence of bilateral infundibulums should be noted when analysing surgical results. With the defect in subpulmonary position, the subaortic infundibulum is frequently narrowed and obstructed. Subaortic obstruction is often accompanied by either severe coarctation or interruption of the aortic arch. Straddling and overriding of the mitral valve is often present with this combination. Another important feature is the course of the left coronary artery across the subpulmonary infundibulum. Atrioventricular septal defects, when present, usually produce a non-committed defect. The defect can, however, extend antero-superiorly to reach the outflow tract of either, or both, great arteries. A straddling tricuspid valve can rarely occur with a non-committed defect. Other associated lesions, such as defects of the atrial septum, patency of the arterial duct or juxtaposition of the atrial appendages can occur with the interventricular communication defect in any location.

14

Common Arterial Trunk

In segmental analysis of the heart, a common arterial trunk is one variant of a single outlet from the heart. The other types of single outlets include pulmonary atresia with solitary aorta, and aortic atresia with solitary pulmonary trunk. In both of these, there is a second atretic trunk, but it cannot be traced to the ventricle. The final variant is the solitary arterial trunk, in which there is no second atretic trunk (Fig. 14.1). The distinction between a pulmonary trunk and an aorta is straightforward when one vessel is patent and the other atretic. When the atretic vessel is strand-like, and closely adherent to the wall of the patent vessel, it may be impossible to identify by cross-sectional echocardiography. To demonstrate such an arrangement anatomically, the prosector may need to dissect very carefully. Care must also be taken not to mistake a hypoplastic ascending aorta in the setting of aortic atresia as an anomalous origin of the coronary artery from the brachiocephalic artery in the setting of a common arterial trunk.

The common arterial trunk is characterised by a single arterial vessel arising from the base of the heart, through a common arterial valve, from which the systemic, pulmonary and coronary arteries directly originate. This situation should be distinguished from the aorto-pulmonary window, which describes a communication between the arterial trunk, in the setting of separate pulmonary and aortic valves. Collett and Edwards described four main anatomical types of common arterial trunk on the basis of the origin of the pulmonary arteries (Fig. 14.2). Their 'Type IV', however, is better described as a solitary arterial trunk (Fig. 14.2). Most commonly, the right and left pulmonary arteries arise close together from the leftward and posterior aspect of the trunk (Type II — Fig. 14.2). A common pulmonary trunk, which then divides into left and right pulmonary arteries, arises from the trunk in some cases (Type I — Fig. 14.2). Rarely, the pulmonary arteries arise separately

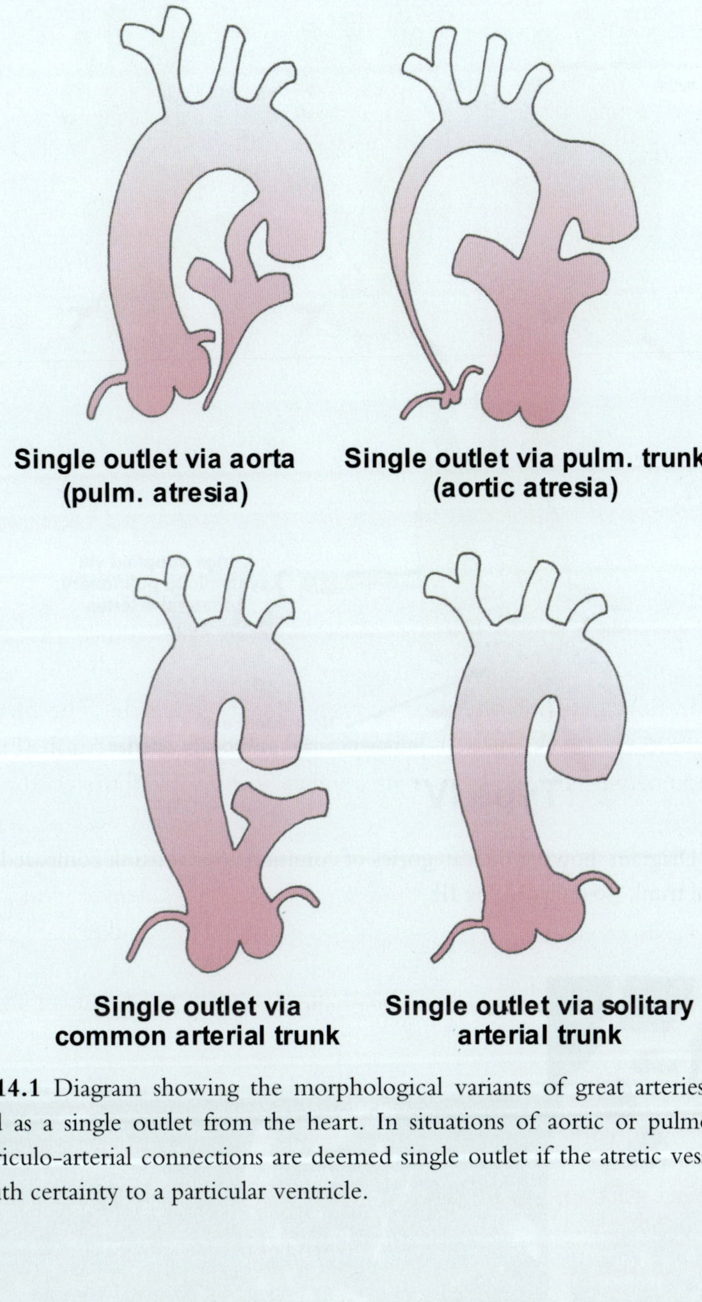

Figure 14.1 Diagram showing the morphological variants of great arteries that can be described as a single outlet from the heart. In situations of aortic or pulmonary atresia, the ventriculo-arterial connections are deemed single outlet if the atretic vessel cannot be traced with certainty to a particular ventricle.

from the right and left lateral aspects of the trunk (Type III). Other variations can occur, including cases in which only one pulmonary artery arises from the trunk with the other arising via an arterial duct. The pulmonary arteries can also arise within one of the common truncal sinuses. On echocardiography, it is visualisation of the origins of the pulmonary arteries directly from the truncal root which differentiates the common trunk from Fallot with pulmonary atresia (Fig. 14.3).

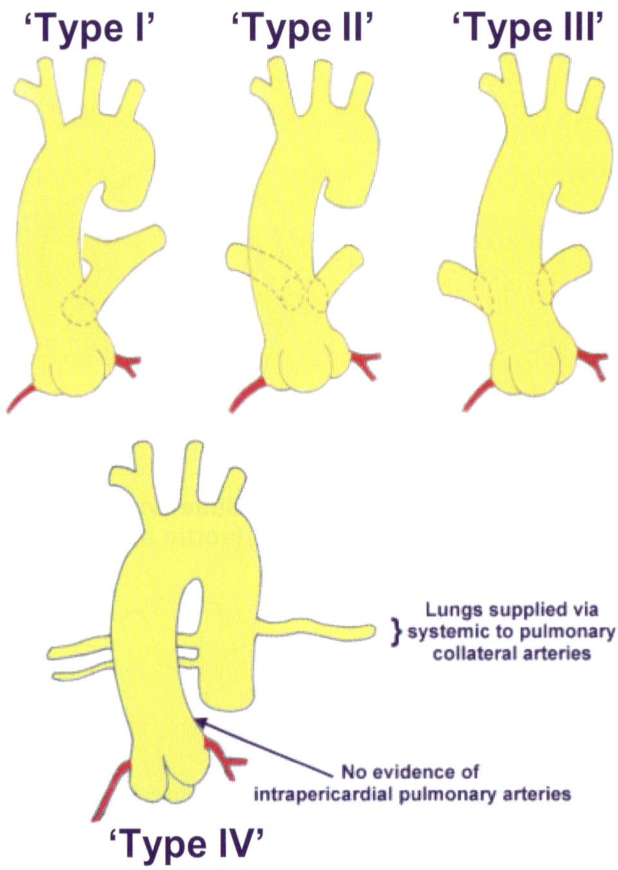

Figure 14.2 Diagram showing the categories of common arterial trunk compared with the solitary arterial trunk (so-called Type II).

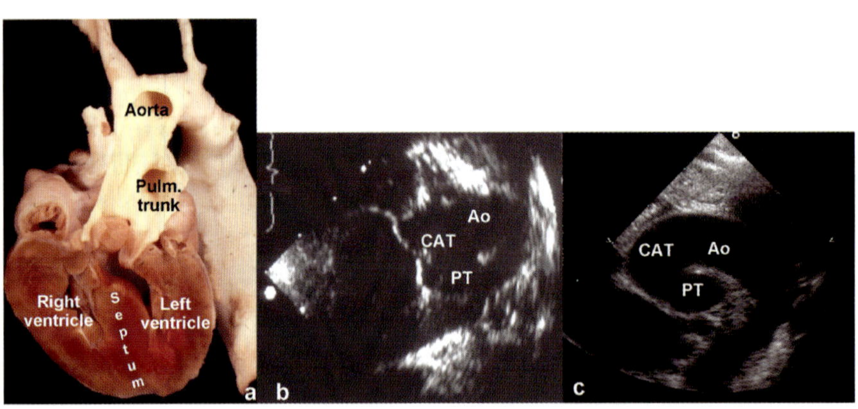

Figure 14.3 (a) Specimen showing a common arterial trunk with dysplastic valvar leaflets. (b) Subcostal long axis section of a common arterial trunk (CAT) dividing into ascending aorta and pulmonary trunk. (c) Suprasternal parasagittal section clearly shows the aorta and pulmonary trunk arising from the common trunk.

Since a common arterial trunk is a type of ventriculo-arterial connection, it can exist with any atrioventricular connections and with any atrial arrangement. Most frequently, atrioventricular connections are concordant and the ventricular septum is well formed apart from a subtruncal ventricular septal defect. Rarely, the common trunk can be associated with an atrioventricular septal defect, or other malformations of ventricular inlets.

A key feature of a common arterial trunk is the presence of a ventricular septal defect. The typical defect is large, is located between the limbs of the septomarginal trabeculation and is roofed by the truncal valve (Figs. 14.3 and 14.4). In most hearts, fusion between the ventriculo-infundibular fold and the posterior limb of the septomarginal trabeculation produces a muscular postero-inferior margin to the defect, which separates the attachments of the tricuspid and truncal valves. This muscular border protects the conduction tissues. In other hearts, there is fibrous continuity between the leaflets of the tricuspid, truncal and mitral valves, and the defect is consequently perimembranous in position. In these, the conduction tissues are more closely related to the postero-inferior margin of the defect. Rarely, the defect is small, and may be closed by the leaflets of the truncal valve during diastole (Fig. 14.5). In exceedingly rare circumstances, the ventricular septum may be intact,with the trunk arising exclusively from one or the other ventricle.

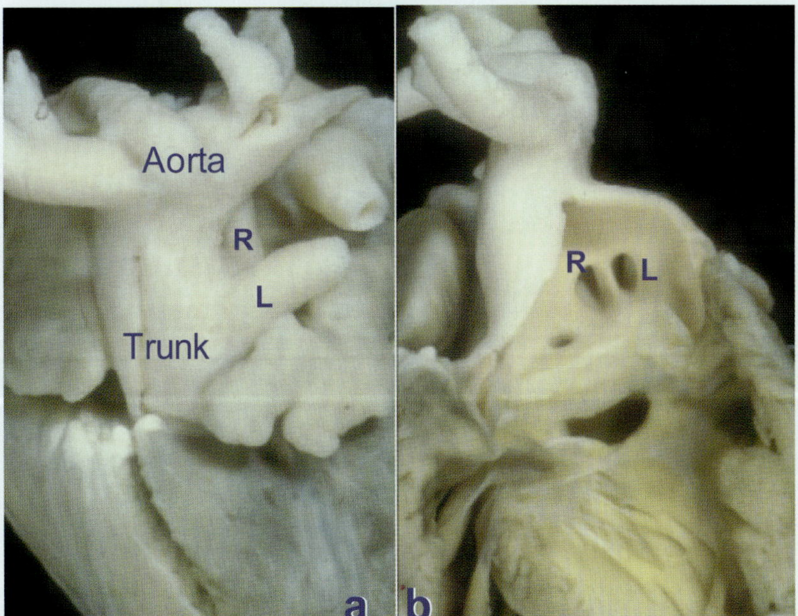

Figure 14.4 (a) External aspect showing separate pulmonary arteries (R and L) arising from the common trunk. (b) Internal aspect of the same heart shows the right (R) and left (L) pulmonary arteries.

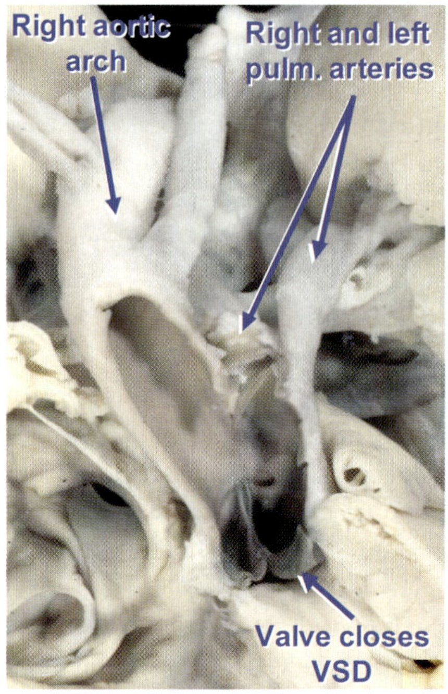

Figure 14.5 The ventricular septal defect is obliterated by leaflets of the aortic valve when the valve closes.

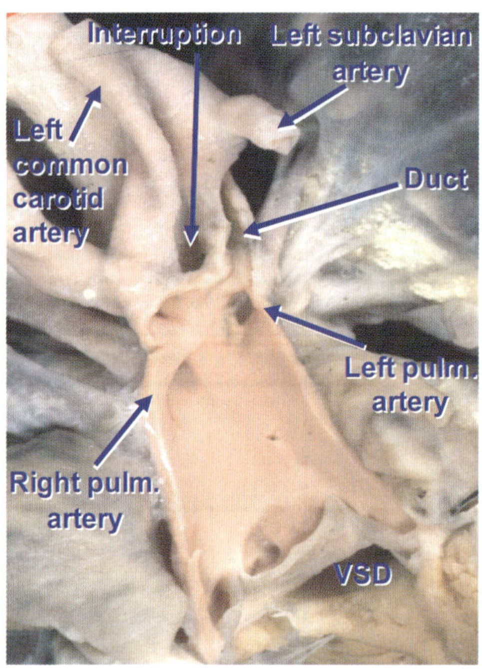

Figure 14.6 This common arterial trunk arises entirely from the right ventricle. The ventricular septal defect is small. Note the separate origins of the pulmonary arteries from either side of the common trunk. There is interruption of the aortic arch between the left common carotid artery and the left subclavian artery.

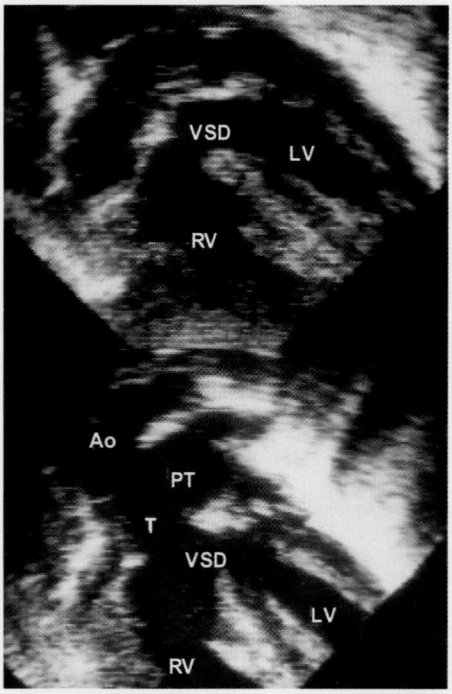

Figure 14.7 Subcostal sections showing the ventricular septal defect and the common arterial trunk committed entirely to the right ventricle.

The truncal valve usually overrides the ventricular septum so as to arise approximately equally from right and left ventricles. Alternatively, the trunk may be committed predominantly, or even exclusively, to one or the other ventricle, usually with a ventricular septal defect (Figs. 14.6 and 14.7) but very rarely with an intact septum as discussed above. The common arterial trunk may be associated with an atrioventricular septal defect (Fig. 14.8).

The truncal valve most frequently has three leaflets, but may have two or four leaflets. Valves with five or even six leaflets have also been reported. Insufficiency of the truncal valve is common, and can be caused by thickened and dysplastic leaflets. Valvar stenosis is less common.

The arrangement of the truncal sinuses relative to the area of fibrous continuity with the mitral valve is unlike that of the normal aortic valve. In some cases, there is a complete subtruncal infundibulum. There is also considerable variability in the origins of the coronary arteries. Even in those hearts with three sinuses, the majority of the orifices of the coronary arteries are situated above the sinutubular junction, or are found close to the margins of the sinuses (Fig. 14.9). A single coronary artery and variations in the epicardial distribution are common. Associations found frequently with the common arterial trunk include the right aortic arch, interrupted aortic arch, aberrant subclavian artery, defects within the oval fossa and persistent left superior

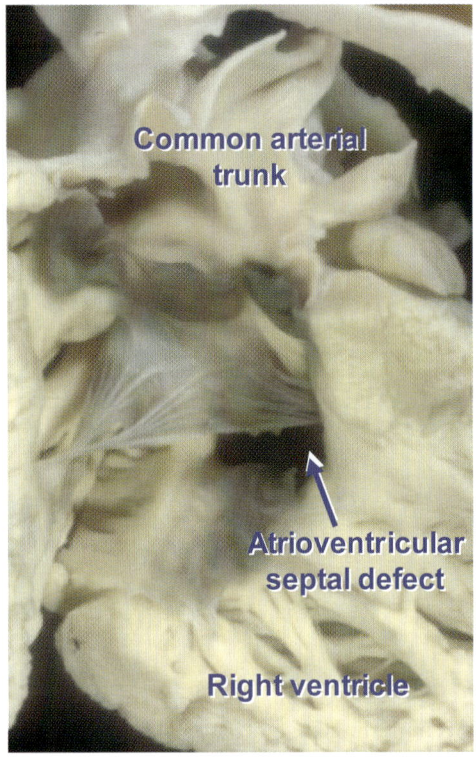

Figure 14.8 This common arterial trunk is associated with an atrioventricular septal defect.

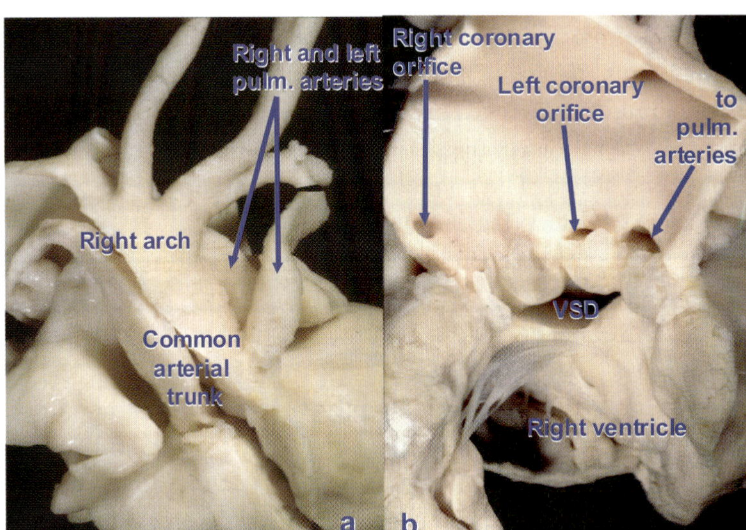

Figure 14.9 (a) The external aspect of this case shows the pulmonary arteries arising from close to the base of the common arterial trunk. (b) This internal view shows a common orifice to the pulmonary arteries. This orifice is located at the sinutubular junction and opens in part to the truncal sinus. Note the slit-like left coronary orifice and the high take-off of the right coronary artery.

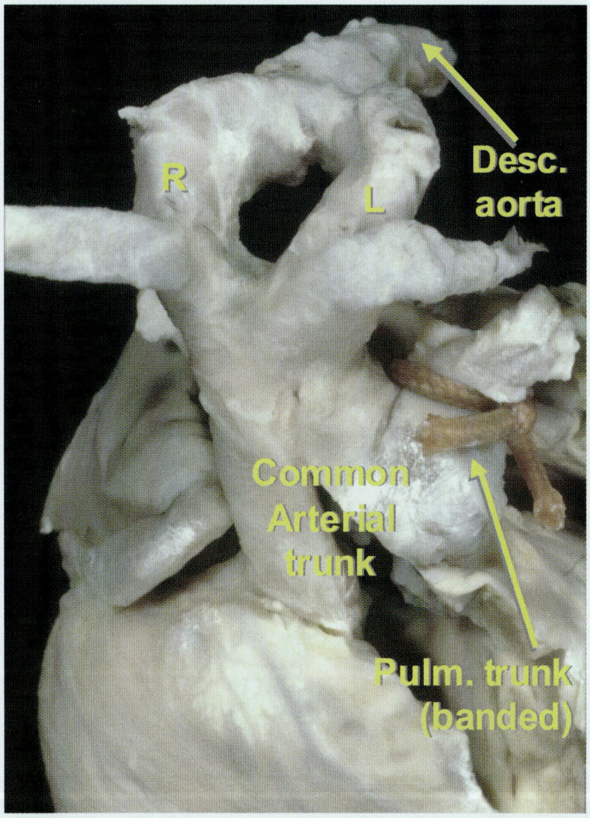

Figure 14.10 This common arterial trunk is associated with a double aortic arch. The right (R) and left (L) arches form a vascular ring that surrounds the trachea and oesophagus. The pulmonary trunk has been banded.

caval vein draining to the coronary sinus. Occasionally, there may be a double aortic arch forming a vascular ring (Fig. 14.10). The arterial duct is usually absent, other than in cases with coarctation or interruption of the aortic arch (Fig. 14.11). When present in those with normal arches, it may remain patent postnatally.

Other Arterial Lesions

There are other arterial lesions that can be confused with the common arterial trunk. One of these, the solitary arterial trunk, is an important variant of the single outlet of the heart. The solitary trunk leaves the heart to supply the aorta and its branches and the coronary arteries, while the lungs are supplied by systemic-to-pulmonary collateral arteries arising from the descending aorta (Fig. 14.2). The intrapericardial pulmonary arteries are either absent, or discontinuous pulmonary

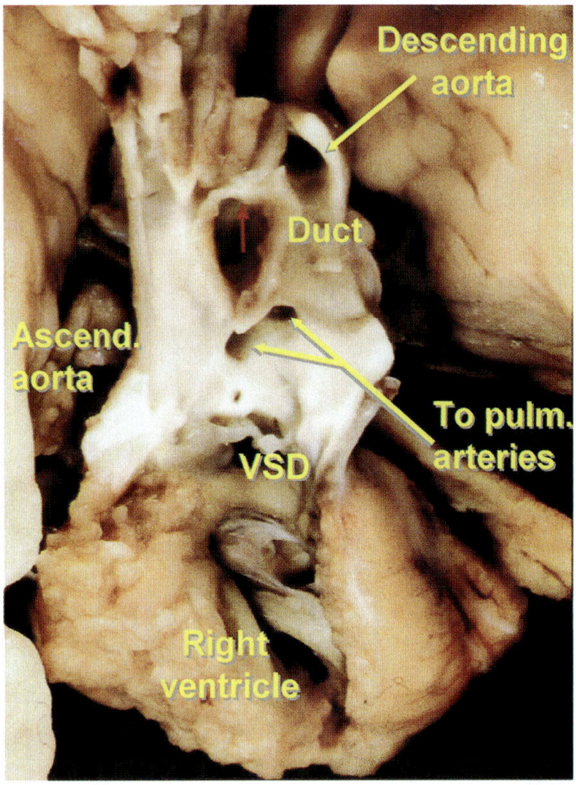

Figure 14.11 This foetal heart shows a common arterial trunk associated with atresia of the aortic isthmus. The arrow indicates the fibrous strand. The descending aorta is supplied via a widely patent arterial duct. There are separate origins of the pulmonary arteries.

arteries are each fed by an arterial duct. As already discussed, this arrangement was originally described by Collett and Edwards as a variant of the common arterial trunk ('Type IV'). Careful dissection by other investigators has demonstrated remnants of the pulmonary trunk and its main branches in many cases previously thought to be examples of this lesion. There is, however, no doubt that cases do exist with absence of intrapericardial pulmonary arteries. In these, there is no way of defining whether the single trunk is an aorta or a common arterial trunk. Because of this, it is best to describe it simply as a solitary arterial trunk.

Other lesions with potential for confusion are the aorto-pulmonary window, and the so-called 'hemitruncus'. In contrast to the common arterial trunk, separate aortic and pulmonary valves are present in hearts with an aorto-pulmonary window (Figs. 14.12 and 14.13). The malformation is characterised by a communication between the great arteries, usually involving the left side of the aorta and the right wall of the pulmonary trunk. The size of the defect varies from a few millimetres in diameter to virtual absence of the walls between the great arteries. In the latter situation, the pathophysiology is similar to the common arterial trunk. The defect can

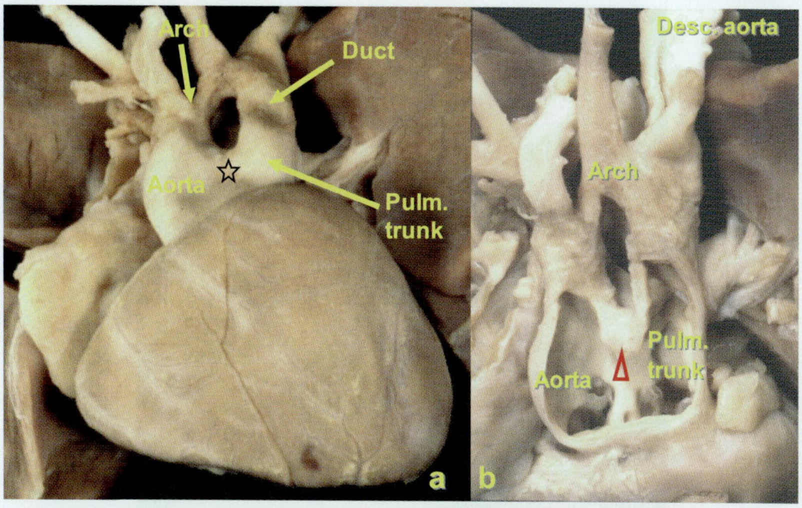

Figure 14.12 (a) The aorta and pulmonary trunk are joined at the base through an aorto-pulmonary window (⋆). (b) This dissection shows the aorto-pulmonary window (Δ). There are separate aortic and pulmonary valves.

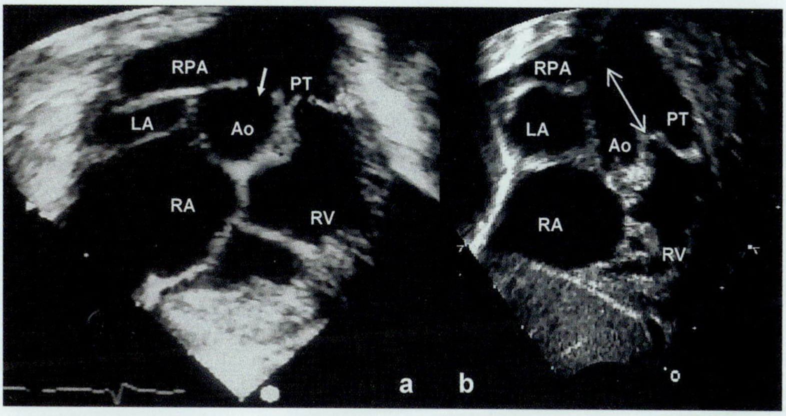

Figure 14.13 Echocardiograms of two cases with aorto-pulmonary window. (a) Subcostal right oblique section showing a fenestration between the pulmonary trunk and the aorta. (b) Subcostal right oblique section showing a large communication (double headed arrow) between the pulmonary trunk and the aorta. Note the right pulmonary artery arising from the aorta.

be located near the insertion of the arterial valves or more distally, confluent with the origin of the right pulmonary artery. In contrast to hearts with the common arterial trunk, the ventricular septum is usually intact in hearts with the aorto-pulmonary window.

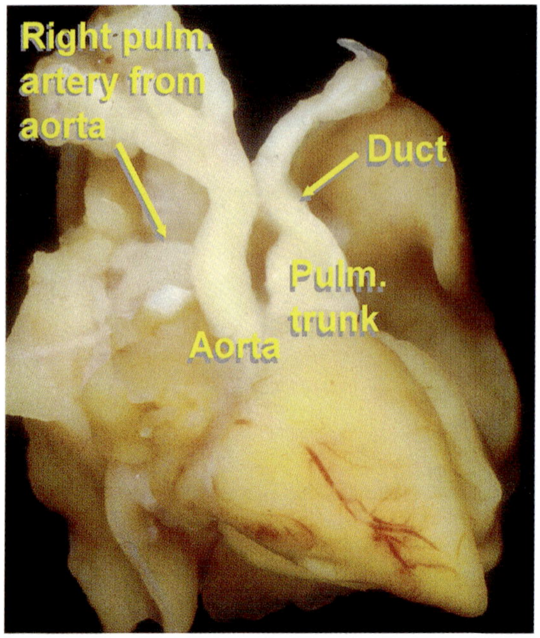

Figure 14.14 The right pulmonary artery arises from the ascending aorta while the left pulmonary artery arises from the pulmonary trunk.

'Hemitruncus', a term best avoided, is the arrangement in which one pulmonary artery arises from the ascending aorta, while the other pulmonary artery arises directly from the heart via a second arterial valve (Fig. 14.14). The arrangement is far better described simply as the anomalous origin of one pulmonary artery from the ascending aorta.

15

Complete Transposition

The lesion most frequently described as 'transposition' is a specific combination of abnormal arrangement of the chambers of the heart. The morphologically right atrium is connected to a morphologically right ventricle which, in turn, gives rise to the aorta. The morphologically left atrium is connected to a morphologically left ventricle that supports the pulmonary trunk (Fig. 15.1). In segmental terms, therefore, the connections are concordant at the atrioventricular junctions, but discordant at the ventriculo-arterial junctions. Defined in this manner, transposition can exist in patients with either usual (solitus) or mirror-imaged (inversus) arrangement of the atriums, but not in hearts with isomerism of the atrial appendages.

Previous definitions of 'transposition' emphasised the abnormal position of the great arteries, either relative to each other or to the ventricles. This led to the inclusion within the definition of 'transposition' of a variety of other malformations, such as double outlet right ventricle. Restricting the phrase 'transposition' to the specific segmental combination described above, we believe, avoids many, if not all, of the numerous previous problems of description.

Basic Anatomy

Clinicians recognise 'simple' and 'complex' forms of transposition. In the 'simple form' are those patients with an intact, or virtually intact, ventricular septum, and absence of obstruction of the left ventricular outflow tract. They may have coexisting lesions, such as patency of the arterial duct. Presence of other associated malformations, such as a large ventricular septal defect, pulmonary stenosis or aortic coarctation, represents the so-called 'complex' lesion.

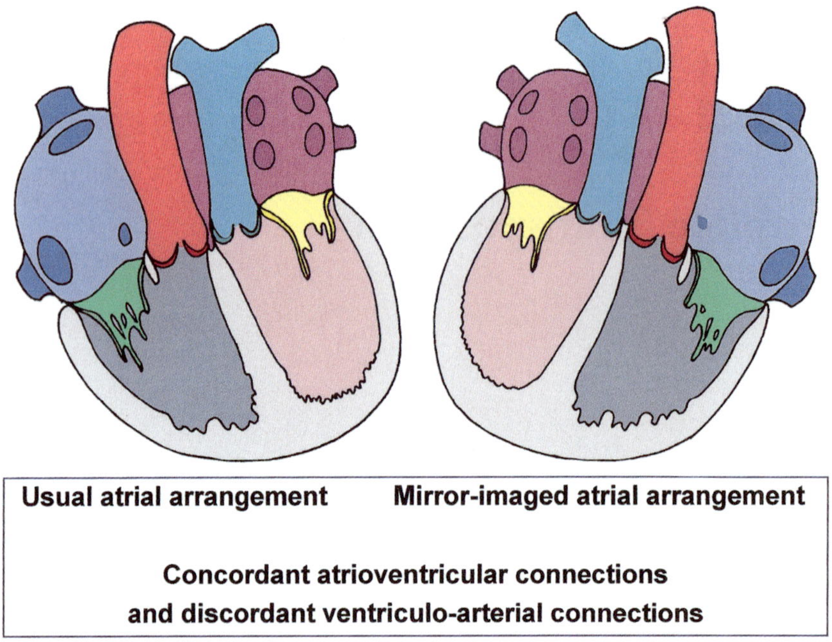

Figure 15.1 Diagram showing the segmental arrangement of complete transposition.

The atrial chambers are essentially normal, even when arranged in mirror image fashion. The sinus node is in its anticipated position and, in keeping with normal atrial anatomy, the atrioventricular node is also in its usual position. Almost always the oval foramen is probe patent, or else its floor is defective. The atriums are connected to the appropriate ventricles, but subtle differences exist in the anatomy of the atrioventricular junctions because of the abnormal ventriculo-arterial connections. The membranous component of the septum is often small, or even absent in hearts with an intact ventricular septum. The ventricular septum in the majority of hearts is straight, without the curvature so typical of the normal heart (Figs. 15.2 and 15.3). This reflects the fact that the outflow tracts from the left and right ventricles usually run in parallel, instead of having the normal cross-over arrangement. Apart from these minor anomalies, the ventricles are structurally normal. The mural thicknesses, however, may be very different from normal. Although more-or-less the same at birth, the thickness of the right ventricular wall rapidly exceeds that of the left ventricle in the immediate postnatal period in those with transposition and intact verticular septrum. This is important for surgical correction at the arterial level, because the left ventricle will be required to support the systemic circulation. This will not be possible if the left ventricle has undergone too much regression.

The coronary arteries always arise from the aortic sinuses that are nearest the pulmonary trunk, irrespective of the position of the aorta relative to the pulmonary trunk. This is important, since it means that, almost always, the surgeon can transfer these arteries satisfactorily during the arterial switch procedure. There are, however,

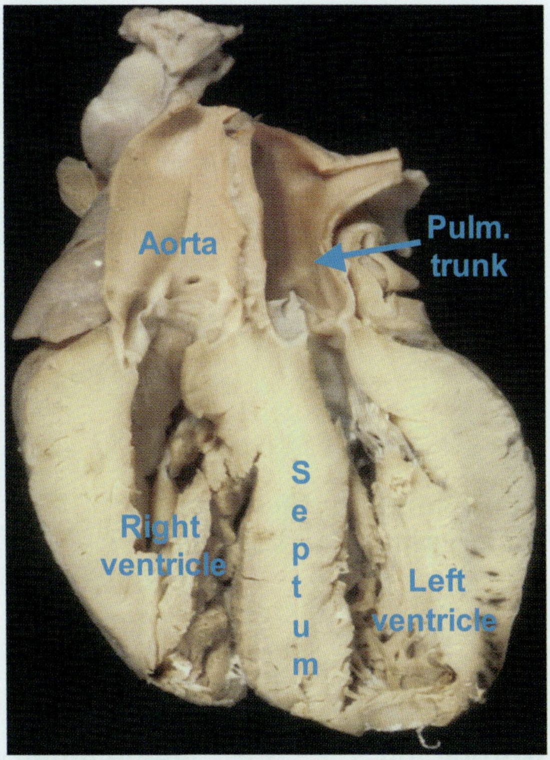

Figure 15.2 This longitudinal section shows the straight ventricular septum in a heart with complete transposition.

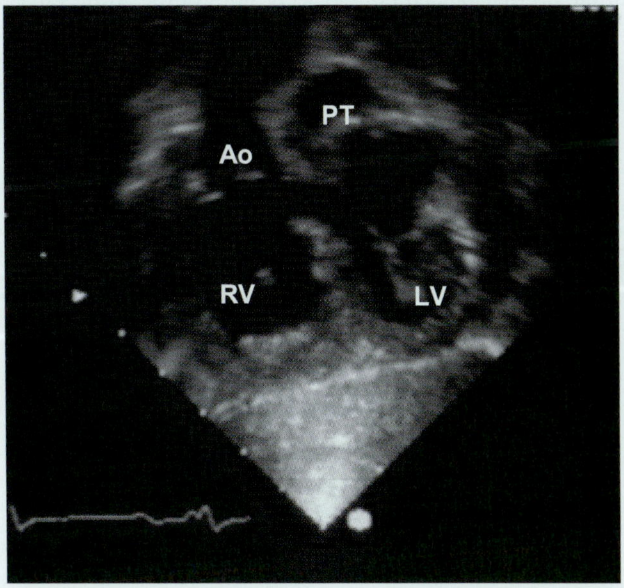

Figure 15.3 Subcostal long axis view in complete transposition showing straight ventricular septum.

significant variations in the epicardial distribution of the coronary arteries that are of surgical significance. Several patterns have been described, often using alpha-numeric codifications. We find such classifications confusing, and difficult to remember. Description can be facilitated by imagining an observer to be in the non-facing sinus of either the aorta (Fig. 15.4) or the pulmonary trunk (Fig. 15.5). By looking straight towards the middle of the adjacent arterial valve, the observer will then see the two facing or adjacent aortic sinuses, those being the ones closest to the pulmonary valve.

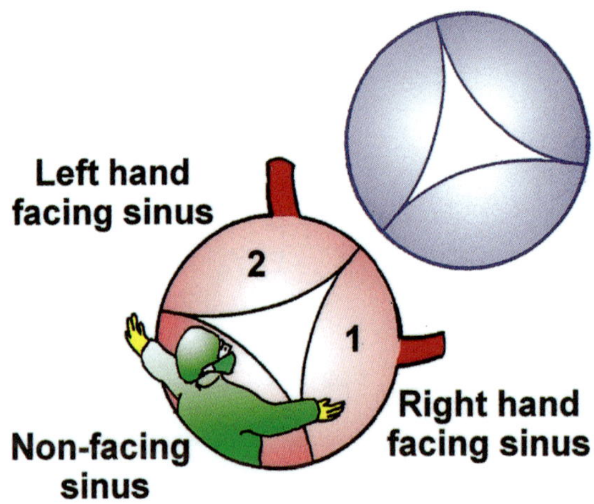

Figure 15.4 Diagram showing the convention of naming the aortic sinuses with the imaginary observer in the non-facing and non-adjacent sinus of the aortic valve.

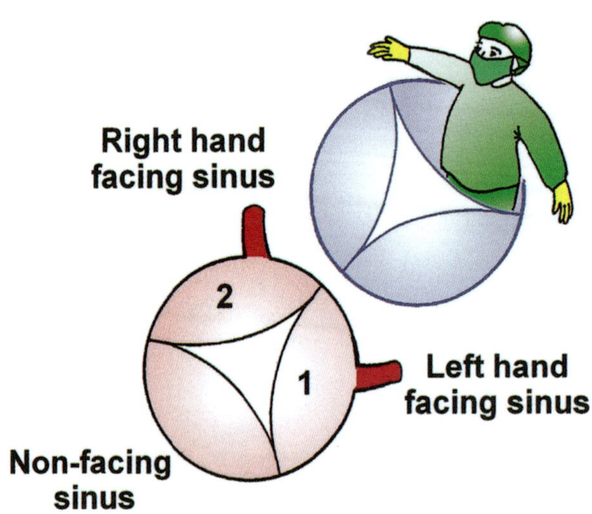

Figure 15.5 Diagram showing the convention of naming the aortic sinuses with the imaginary observer in the pulmonary valve.

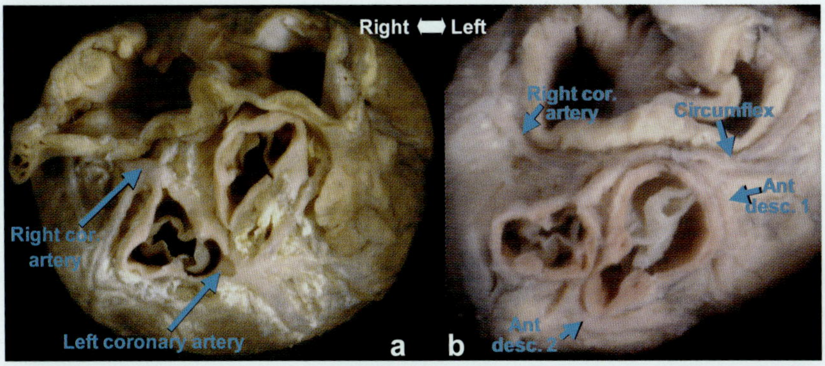

Figure 15.6 (a) The coronary arteries arise from the facing aortic sinuses. Note the malalignment of the facing commissures in this heart. (b) Dissection of a heart with the aorta arising to the right of the pulmonary trunk. This shows the coronary arteries arising from the facing sinuses of the aorta. There are dual anterior descending coronary arteries. Note the intramural course at the origin of the anterior descending coronary artery 2.

One aortic sinus will be to the right hand, and the other sinus to the left hand. This description holds good irrespective of the relationships of the aortic and pulmonary trunks. The coronary arteries virtually always arise from both, or one, of these facing sinuses (Fig. 15.6). Whether the sinuses are to the right or the left hand then varies according to whether the observer is stationed in the aorta or the pulmonary trunk. The convention of naming the two sinuses #1 and #2, however, does not change, and this is the system of description we now recommend. Use of this convention, combining it with an account of epicardial course, permits all patterns of the coronary arteries to be described without ambiguity.

Relationship of the Great Arteries

The most obvious external abnormality of hearts with transposition is that the aorta is abnormally positioned relative to the pulmonary trunk. An aorta anterior and right sided relative to the pulmonary trunk is the commonest relationship. The aorta may also be either directly anterior, or even anterior and left sided, in hearts with usual arrangement of the atriums. There are also rare cases in which the aorta is posterior and right sided, the so-called 'normal' relationship. In hearts with mirror-imaged atrial arrangement, the aorta is most often left sided and anterior. Whilst it is important to describe arterial relationships, they are only one of the variables in patients with transposition. The relationships are not sufficiently constant to be used as a criterion for definition. In a similar way, although most hearts have a subaortic infundibulum together with fibrous continuity between the leaflets of the pulmonary and mitral valves, infundibular morphology is not a hallmark of transposition. A few patients have bilateral infundibulums, while those rare hearts with 'normal' arterial relationships tend also to exhibit fibrous continuity between the leaflets of the aortic and mitral valves through the roof of a ventricular septal defect.

Ventricular Septal Defect

This is probably the most significant and frequently associated lesion. Its location and size can vary as in otherwise normal hearts, and the defects can be multiple. The same system for description is used as for isolated ventricular septal defects (Fig. 15.7). The most frequent defects are those associated with malalignment of the outlet septum with respect to the muscular ventricular septum. These defects open into the outlet portion of the right ventricle (Fig. 15.8). They may have entirely muscular right ventricular margins, or may extend posteriorly to be bordered by fibrous continuity between the leaflets of the pulmonary and tricuspid valves. The latter variant is perimembranous. The outlet septum is usually deviated into the right ventricle, allowing the pulmonary valve to override the crest of the ventricular septum (Figs. 15.8 and 15.9). With greater degrees of overriding, the malformation merges

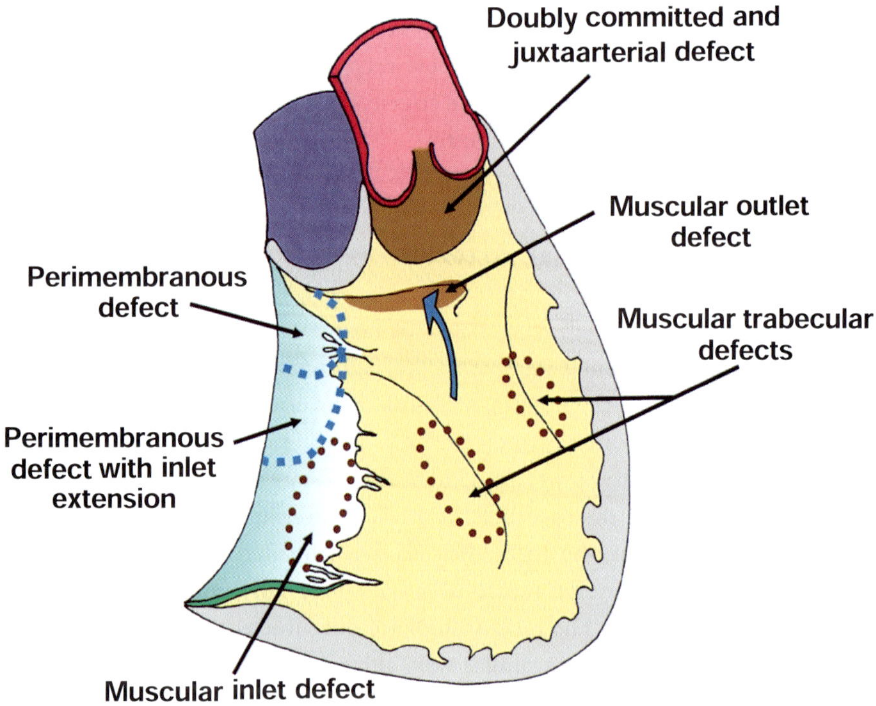

Figure 15.7 Diagram showing variations in locations and margins of ventricular septal defects.

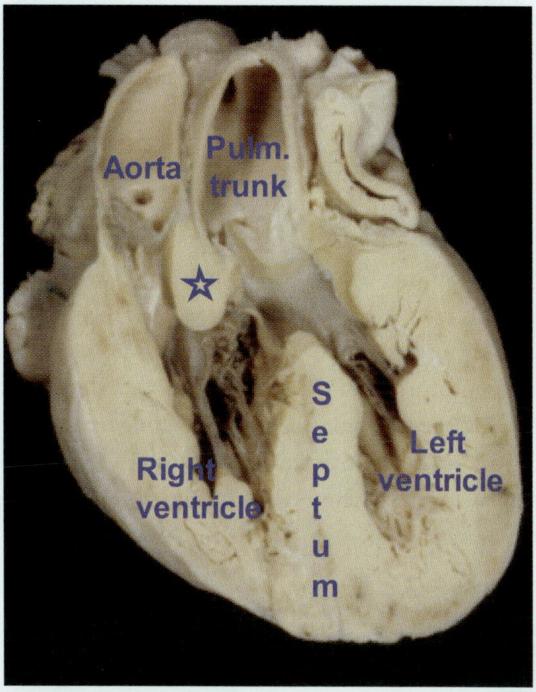

Figure 15.8 The outlet septum (☆) is deviated into the right ventricle, allowing the pulmonary valve to override the ventricular septum through the septal defect.

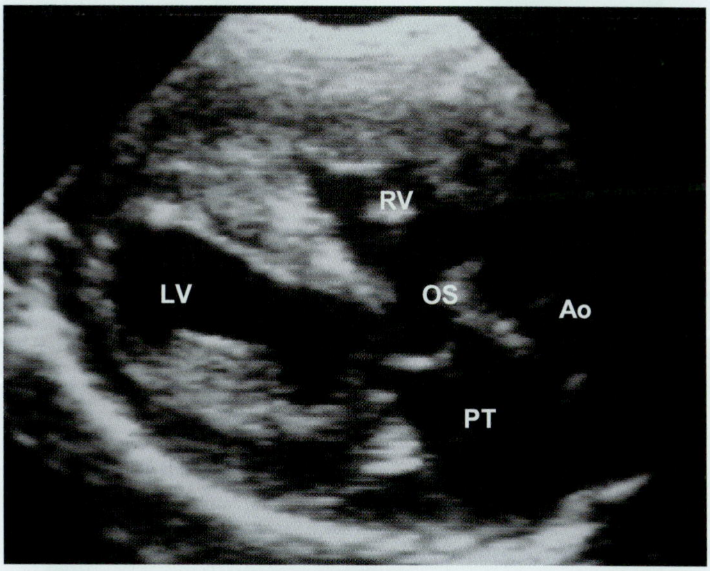

Figure 15.9 Parasternal long axis view shows ventricular septal defect with override of the pulmonary valve and deviation of the outlet septum.

into the spectrum of hearts with double outlet right ventricle with subpulmonary defect — the so-called Taussig–Bing anomaly. We divide this spectrum of override halfway, and use the description 'transposition' only for those hearts with less than half the circumference of the orifice of the pulmonary valve attached within the right ventricle. When viewed from the right ventricle, cords of the tricuspid valve may be seen crossing the defect to insert into papillary muscles arising from the outlet septum. This is of obvious significance for surgical repair.

Equally significant are those defects that extend so as to open into the inlet of the right ventricle. Such defects may be hidden by the septal leaflet of the tricuspid valve, complicating their surgical repair. In others, there is malalignment between the atrial and ventricular septums, with overriding and straddling of the tricuspid valve (Fig. 15.10). In these, since the inlet septum no longer reaches the cardiac crux, the penetrating portion of the atrioventricular conduction axis is displaced, and the atrioventricular node is formed where the muscular ventricular septum meets the right atrioventricular junction.

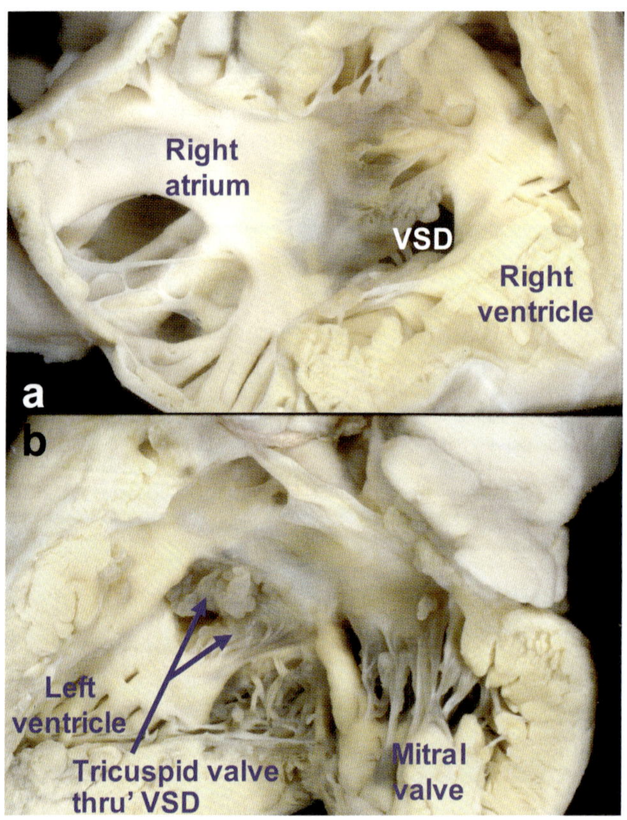

Figure 15.10 This case of complete transposition is associated with straddling of the tricuspid valve. (a) The septal leaflet of the tricuspid valve has insertions through the ventricular septal defect (VSD). (b) This view shows the straddle of the tricuspid valve into the left ventricle.

Other types of defect, such as muscular trabecular defects, multiple muscular defects, or doubly committed and juxta-arterial defects, are seen in some hearts. Hearts with a doubly committed and juxta-arterial defect in the setting of usual atrial arrangement tend to have a left-sided, or anterior and left-sided, aortas, making it much easier surgically to connect the aorta to the left ventricle. Generally, the conduction axis is where it would be expected to be in 'isolated' ventricular septal defects.

Obstruction of the Left Ventricular Outflow Tract

Obstruction of the left ventricular outlet produces pulmonary stenosis in hearts with transposition (Fig. 15.11). Subvalvar obstruction is more common than isolated valvar obstruction. When the ventricular septum is intact, dynamic obstruction produced by bulging of the septum is common, but its effect is difficult to quantify. In severely affected cases, the septum itself is thickened, rather like in hypertrophic cardiomyopathy. There may be a superimposed fibrous shelf, or an elongation of the fibrous area to produce a tunnel. Other causes of obstruction include anomalous attachments of the mitral valve, or its tension apparatus, across the outflow tract (Fig. 15.12). All these forms of obstruction can be found either with or without a ventricular septal defect. Where there is a ventricular septal defect, the outlet

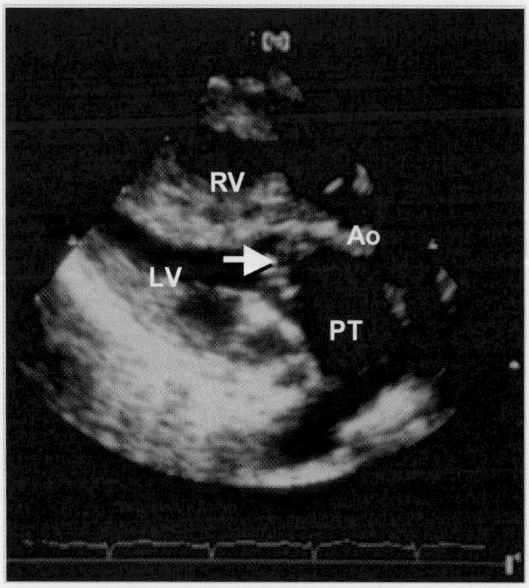

Figure 15.11 Parasternal long axis section in complete transposition showing dysplastic pulmonary valve (arrow), dilated pulmonary trunk and parallel great arteries.

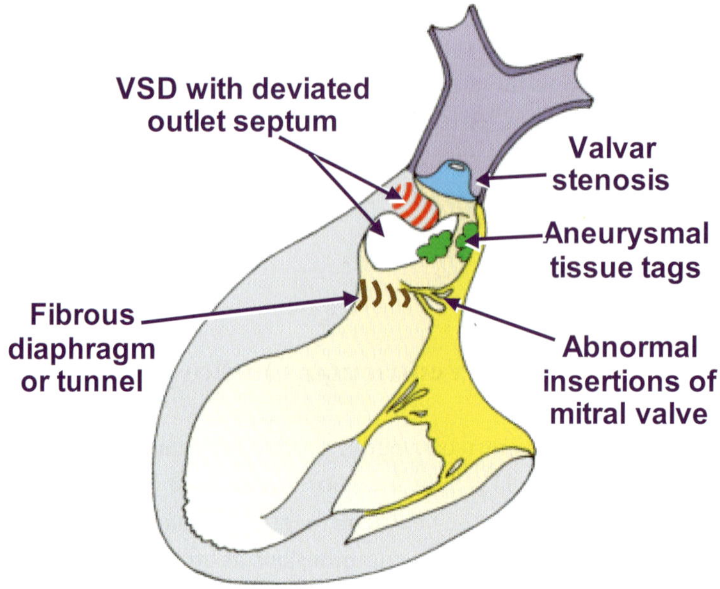

Figure 15.12 Diagram showing potential substrates for left ventricular outlet obstruction.

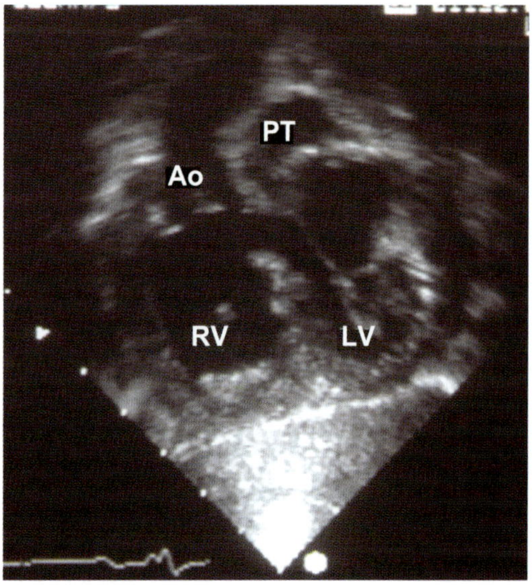

Figure 15.13 Echocardiogram showing deviation of the outlet septum into the left ventricle, compromising the outflow tract.

septum, instead of being deviated into the right ventricle, is occasionally deviated into the left ventricle (Figs. 15.13 and 15.14). This produces subpulmonary stenosis with overriding of the aortic valve. Tissue tags from either the tricuspid valve or the membranous septum may also cause subpulmonary obstruction.

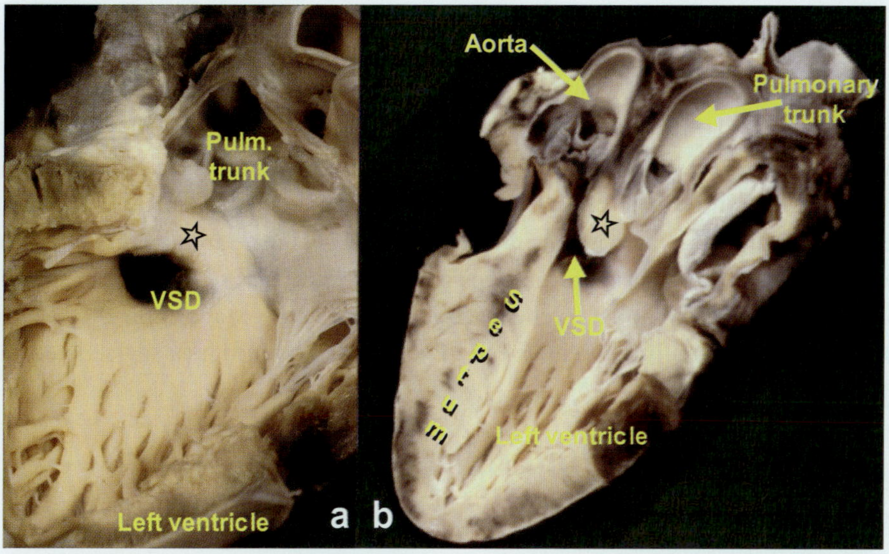

Figure 15.14 (a) The outlet septum (★) is deviated into the left ventricle in this heart. (b) A long axis section through the same heart shows the malalignment between the outlet septum (★) and the rest of the ventricular septum. Due to the deviated outlet septum, there is subpulmonary stenosis.

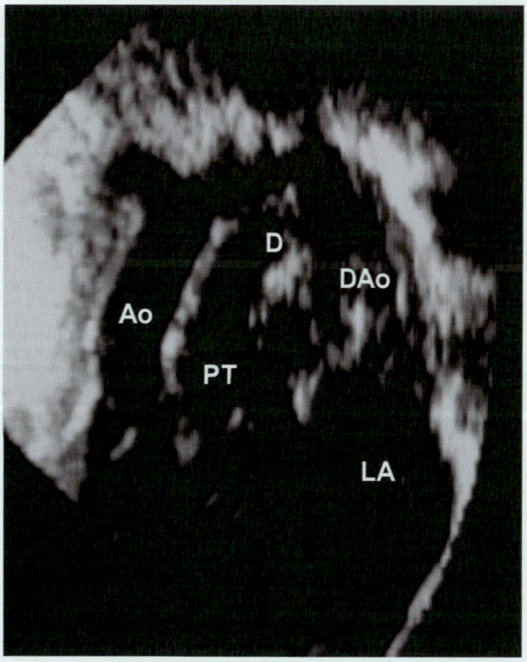

Figure 15.15 Suprasternal parasagittal section showing the parallel aorta and pulmonary trunk in a case of complete transposition with patent arterial duct (D).

Other Associated Malformations

A patent arterial duct may lead to a significant systemic-to-pulmonary shunt, overload of the left ventricle and congestive cardiac failure unless the pulmonary vascular resistance remains high. Patency of the arterial duct (Fig. 15.15) can also complicate the clinical picture where there are anomalies of the aortic arch, such as coarctation, tubular hypoplasia or interruption. A right aortic arch is fairly common. Other notable associated malformations are atrioventricular septal defects, anomalous systemic and pulmonary venous connections, and juxtaposition of the atrial appendage. The latter is frequently seen in hearts with a ventricular septal defect and left-sided aorta.

16

Congenitally Corrected Transposition

Congenitally corrected transposition describes hearts with discordant connections at *both* atrioventricular and ventriculo-arterial junctions. In such hearts, the morphologically right atrium is connected to the morphologically left ventricle, which supports the pulmonary trunk, while the left atrium is connected to the right ventricle, which gives rise to the aorta (Fig. 16.1). This should be contrasted with transposition, in which discordant connections are present only at the ventriculo-arterial junctions. Hearts with discordant atrioventricular connections can also exist, albeit more rarely, with any of the other possible ventriculo-arterial connections. When they are analysed in sequential fashion, identifying both the connections and relationships, all combinations can be fully described.

The Discordant Atrioventricular Connections

Discordant connections at the atrioventricular junction exist when both morphologically right and morphologically left atriums are connected to morphologically inappropriate ventricles. Discordant connections cannot exist, therefore, in hearts with isomerism of the atrial appendages, or with univentricular atrioventricular connections, such as double inlet left ventricle. Hearts with double inlet left ventricle can, in fact, have many similarities to those with discordant atrioventricular connections, such as left-sided rudimentary right ventricles and left-sided and anterior aortas. There are, nonetheless, also important differences between the two. To avoid confusion, therefore, it is best to use the description 'discordant atrioventricular connections' only for hearts with usual or mirror-imaged arrangement of the atriums, and with each atrium connected to the morphologically inappropriate

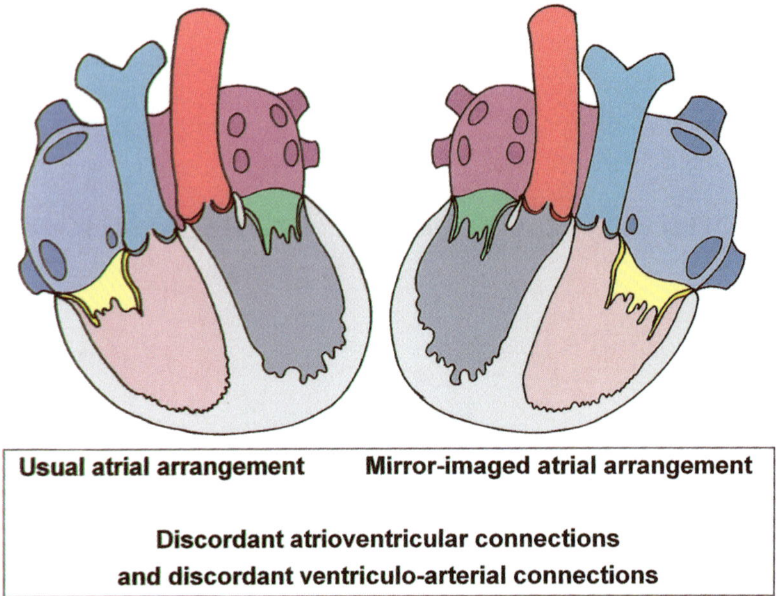

Figure 16.1 Diagram showing the segmental arrangement of congenitally corrected transposition.

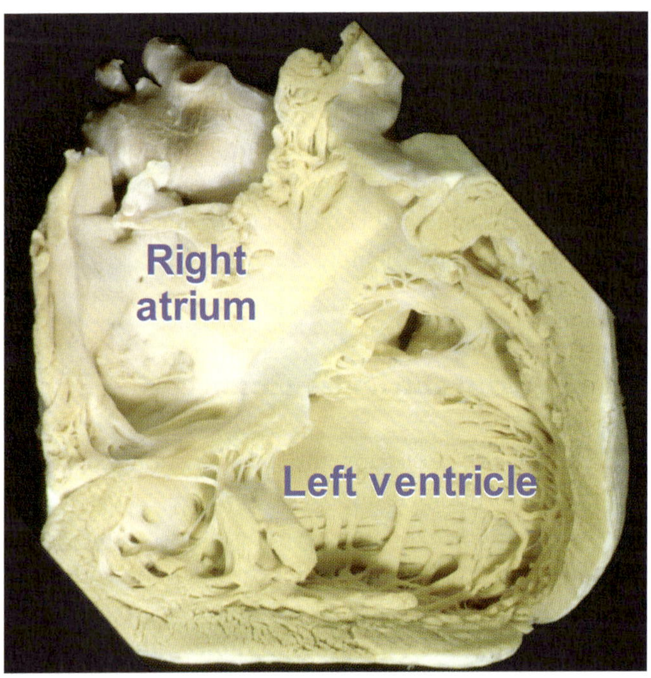

Figure 16.2 The morphologically right atrium opens through the mitral valve to a morphologically left ventricle. The left side of this heart is shown in Fig. 16.3.

ventricle (Fig. 16.1). In our experience, the morphologically right atrium is always connected to the left ventricle through a morphologically mitral valve, and the left atrium to the right ventricle through a tricuspid valve. Identification of two atriums, each supporting an inappropriate atrioventricular valve, therefore, is diagnostic of discordant atrioventricular connections (Figs. 16.2 and 16.3).

Discordant atrioventricular connections can exist regardless of the relationship of the ventricles to one another. Usually, with discordant atrioventricular connections and usual atrial arrangement, the morphologically left ventricle is right sided relative to the right ventricle, the two ventricles being side-by-side (Fig. 16.4). Similarly, with discordant atrioventricular connections and mirror-imaged atrial arrangement, the morphologically left ventricle tends to be left sided and side-by-side relative to the right ventricle. But these arrangements are not always present. Often there is a supero-inferior obliquity seen in the orientation of the ventricles, with the apex shifted rightwards with usual atrial arrangement, and leftwards with the mirror-imaged variant. The morphologically left ventricle then tends to be the superior ventricle (Figs. 16.5 and 16.6). Abnormalities of ventricular relationship can also be found because of rotation around the long axis of the ventricles. This means that all or part, of the morphologically right ventricle is right sided in hearts with the usual atrial arrangement, or left sided in those with mirror-imaged atrial arrangement. This rotational anomaly has been called a 'criss-cross heart'. Like the supero-inferior

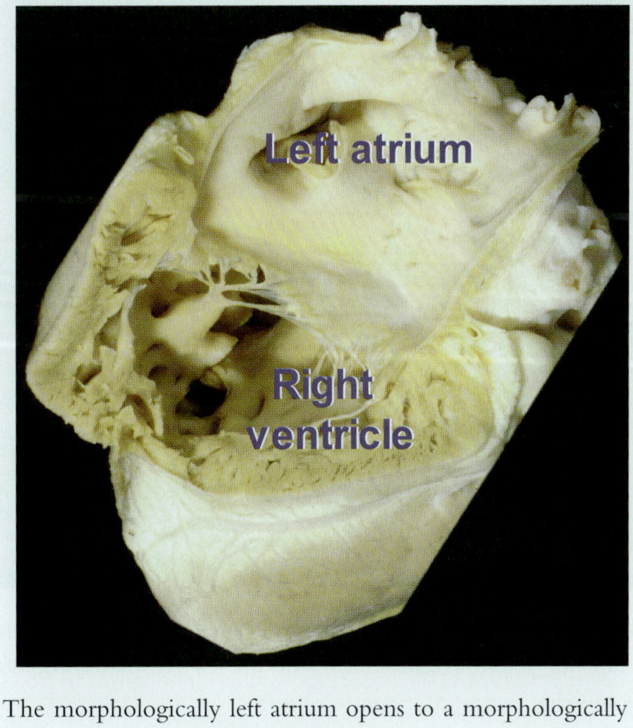

Figure 16.3 The morphologically left atrium opens to a morphologically right ventricle. The septal leaflet of the tricuspid valve is distinctive.

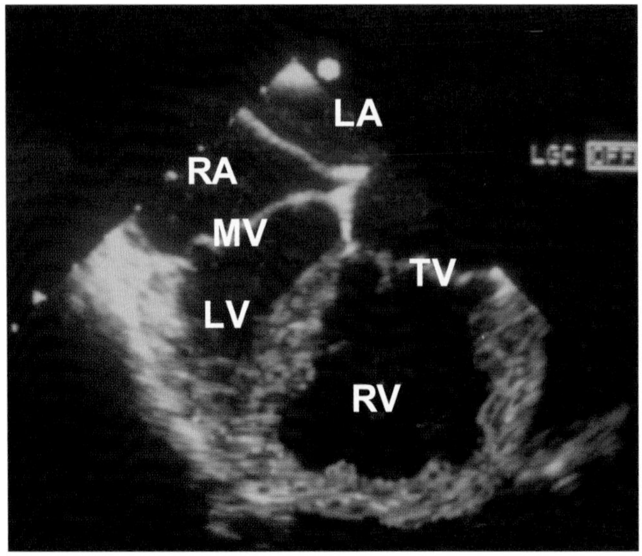

Figure 16.4 Parasternal of four-chamber view showing discordant atrioventricular connections with the lower hingepoint of the tricuspid valve on the left side offset from the higher hingepoint of the mitral valve on the right side.

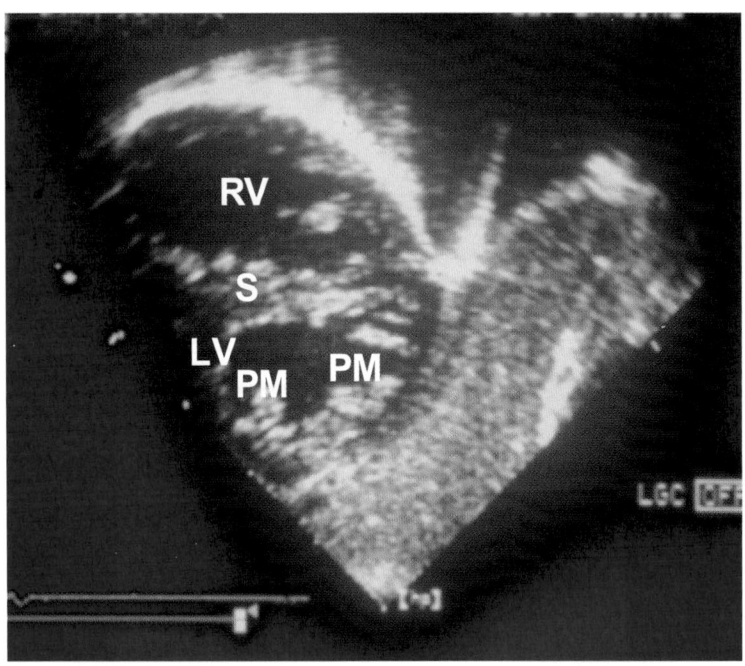

Figure 16.5 Subcostal short axis section. Instead of a side-by-side ventricular relationship, this case shows superior–inferior relationships with the left ventricle lying inferiorly defined by two papillary muscles.

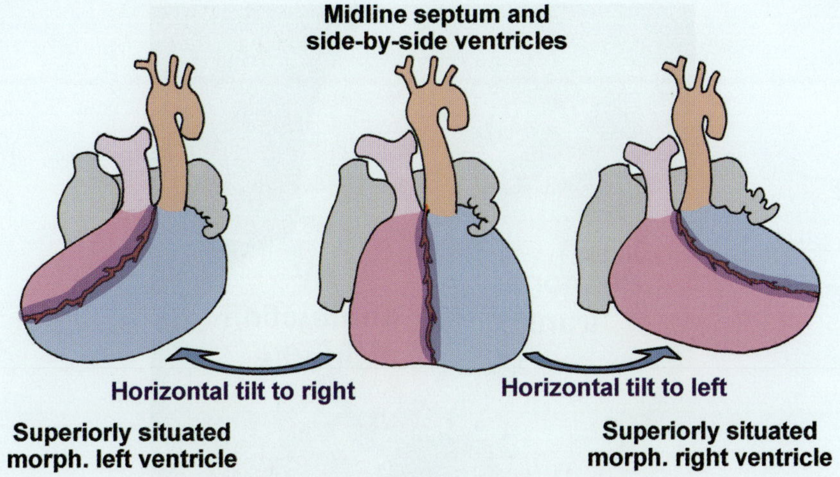

Figure 16.6 Diagram showing how tilting of the ventricular mass along the long axis can produce deviations in spatial relationships of the ventricles.

variant, with which it can coexist, it is found most frequently with discordant atrioventricular connections, but it can exist with any other type of atrioventricular connection. The important feature of these rotational and horizontal deviations in ventricular relationships is that they do not disturb the basic architecture of the two chambers within the ventricular mass.

Morphology of Congenitally Corrected Transposition

Congenitally corrected transposition exists when discordant atrioventricular connections are accompanied by discordant ventriculo-arterial connections. The two discordant connections, in terms of the circulation, cancel each other — hence the term 'congenitally corrected'. Anatomically, the arterial trunks arise from morphologically inappropriate ventricles. In other words, the pulmonary trunk arises from the morphologically left and the aorta from the morphologically right ventricle. Almost always, the leaflets of the pulmonary valve are in fibrous continuity with the mitral valve, while the aortic valve has a complete muscular infundibulum (Figs. 16.7 and 16.8). The aortic valve is usually found anterior and leftwards relative to the pulmonary trunk or anterior and rightwards in the mirror-imaged variant. Neither the infundibular anatomy, nor the arterial relationships, however, are always like this. Abnormalities in the arterial relationships, for instance, are often a feature of the so-called 'criss-cross' variants of congenitally corrected transposition.

When the pulmonary trunk originates from the left ventricle, its posterior position leads to an extensive anterior recess in the ventricle. The origin of the pulmonary trunk from the left ventricle also has a fundamental effect on septal morphology. As

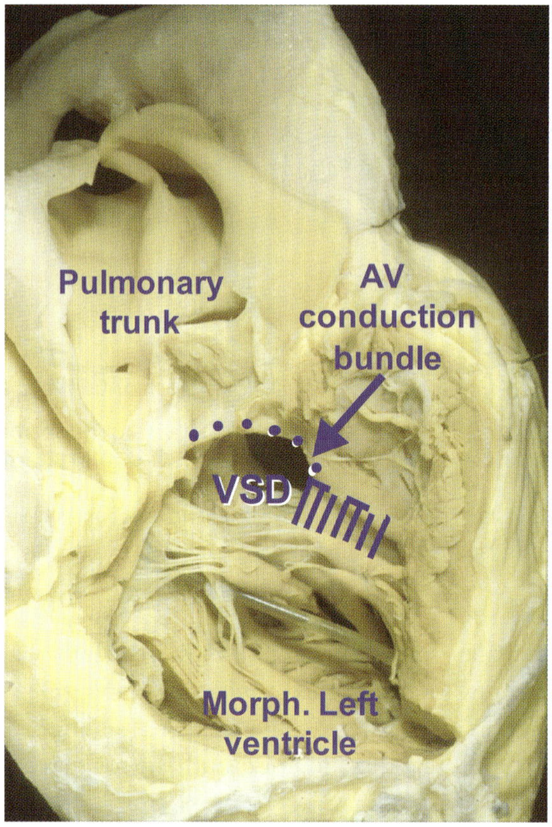

Figure 16.7 There is fibrous continuity between the pulmonary and mitral valves. The atrioventricular conduction bundle (●●●●) penetrates through the area of fibrous continuity to connect with an antero-superiorly located atrioventricular node. Note that the course of the conduction bundle is along the antero-superior margin of the ventricular septal defect (VSD). The hatched area depicts the left bundle branch on the septal aspect of the morphologically left ventricle.

in the normal heart, the outflow tract of the left ventricle has a deep posterior recess between the mitral valve and the septum. In the heart with discordant atrioventricular connections, this posterior recess produces malalignment between the atrial septum and the inlet ventricular septum (Fig. 16.9). The degree of atrioventricular malalignment has been reported to be greater in hearts with the usual atrial arrangement than in those with the mirror-imaged variant, but this reflects the coexistence in such hearts of severe pulmonary stenosis or atresia. This has important implications for the disposition of conduction tissues in the two types of corrected transpositions. When discordant atrioventricular connections occur with double outlet right ventricle or pulmonary atresia, the atrioventricular septal malalignment is less marked. This is because the pulmonary trunk no longer originates from the left ventricle, or else is atretic.

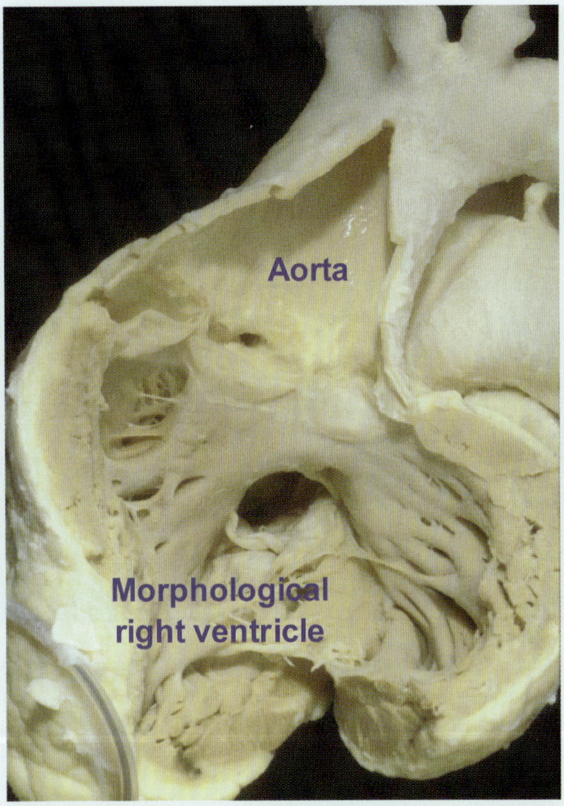

Figure 16.8 This right ventricular view of the same heart as shown in Fig. 16.7 shows the aortic valve supported by a complete muscular infundibulum.

The flow of blood in patients with congenitally corrected transposition is, potentially, entirely normal. In the absence of associated lesions, patients may be completely well. Cases are reported in which the segmental combination has been discovered incidentally as an autopsy finding in the eighth decade of life. Conventional wisdom, nonetheless, is that the morphologically right ventricle is unable to support the circulation for a full lifetime, even when the rest of the heart is normal. Some evidence supports this assertion. Other evidence suggests the morphologically right ventricle can function normally even when supporting a systemic load. Even so, it is most unusual to find patients with congenitally corrected transposition in which there is not some other lesion in the heart. Three of these lesions are sufficiently frequent to be considered part and parcel of the anomaly. These are a ventricular septal defect, obstruction to the left ventricular outflow tract and malformations of the morphologically tricuspid valve. Other important anomalies can also occur, such as subaortic obstruction and coarctation.

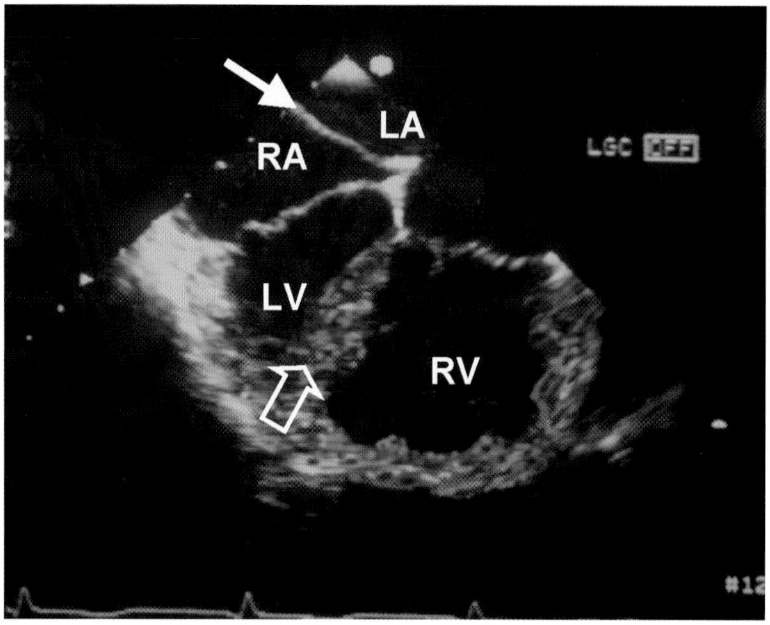

Figure 16.9 Echocardiogram showing a feature commonly seen in congenitally corrected transposition. The atrial septum (closed arrow) and ventricular septum (open arrow) are not aligned.

The Major Associated Lesions

A ventricular septal defect is found in about two-thirds of autopsied examples of corrected transposition. Most frequently, it is bordered by fibrous continuity between the leaflets of the pulmonary, mitral and tricuspid valves and is, therefore, described as perimembranous (Figs. 16.10 and 16.11). Usually, it opens mostly between the ventricular inlets. This is important for the echocardiographer, since the defect in the inlet septum removes the off-setting of the attachments of the mitral and tricuspid valves (Fig. 16.10). Although the perimembranous defect is seen most frequently, any type of defect can be found in the setting of discordant atrioventricular connections. As in other hearts, the doubly committed and juxta-arterial defect is found most frequently in occidental populations. Muscular defects are rare, and atrioventricular septal defects even rarer, but both lesions do exist.

Obstruction to the left ventricular outflow tract can be produced by various lesions, often coexisting with stenosis of the pulmonary valve (Figs. 16.12 and 16.13). Muscular subvalvar stenosis is particularly difficult to treat surgically because of the intimate relationship of the atrioventricular conduction tissue. A fibrous shelf is also difficult to remove for the same reason. Fibrous tissue tags, in contrast, are frequent and can often be resected safely. They can originate from any of the valves near the outflow tract, but most frequently arise from the tricuspid valve or from a remnant

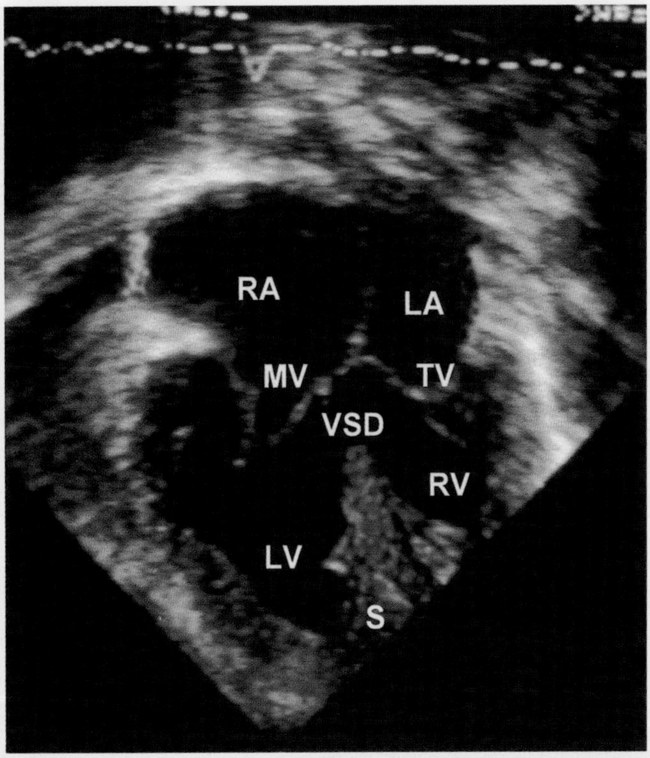

Figure 16.10 Parasternal four-chamber section shows a heart with perimembranous inlet ventricular septal defect. There is loss of off-set arrangement between tricuspid and mitral valves since these valves form the immediate border of the defect. Moderator band allows identification of the left-sided morphologically right ventricle.

of the interventricular component of the membranous septum. Usually, they coexist with a ventricular septal defect, but can be found with an intact ventricular septum.

Malformations of the morphologically tricuspid valve are the commonest associated lesions found in autopsied hearts, being observed in up to nine-tenths of all specimens. The anomalies are not always clinically identified. The most frequent lesion is Ebstein's malformation (Fig. 16.14). As in the setting of concordant atrioventricular connections, the valve is deformed by both anomalous attachment and dysplasia of its leaflets. Again, as with concordant connections, it is the mural and septal leaflets that show the greatest degree of distal displacement. The antero-superior leaflet is usually attached focally, but can exhibit a linear attachment. Although Ebstein's malformation is the commonest lesion of the tricuspid valve, straddling and/or overriding is probably the most significant abnormality. Certainly it produces the greatest problems with surgical correction. An overriding valve can be considered, depending on its attachments, as part of a spectrum of malformations between congenitally corrected transposition and double inlet left ventricle with left-sided rudimentary right ventricle. The mitral valve can also straddle and/or override in the setting of

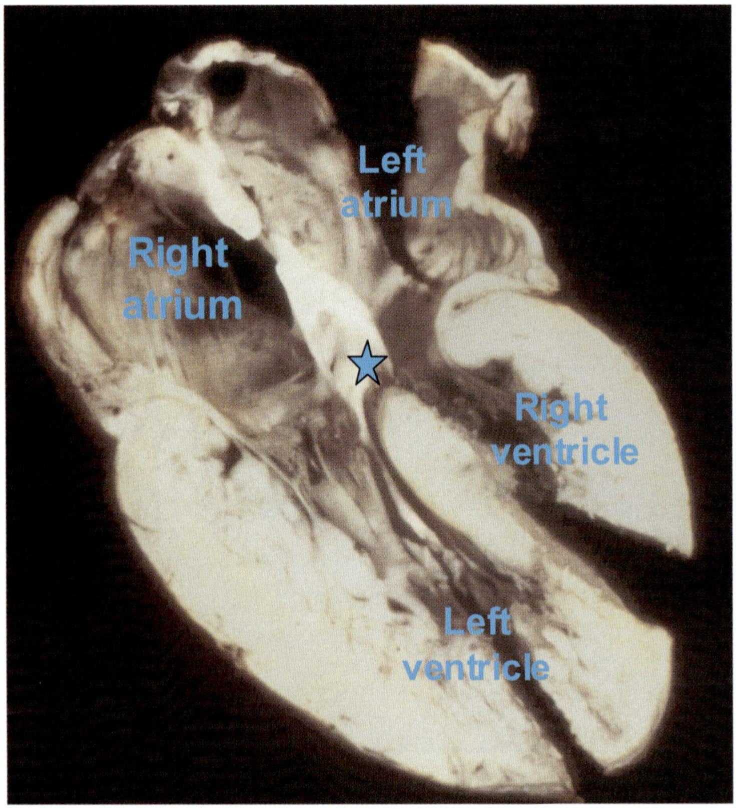

Figure 16.11 This heart shows a view corresponding to that shown in Fig. 16.10. Mitral and tricuspid valves 'roof' the ventricular septal defect (☆).

discordant atrioventricular connections. It straddles the outlet part of the septum, often in the presence of double outlet from the morphologically right ventricle. The straddling mitral valve is part of a series of lesions extending towards the double inlet right ventricle with right-sided rudimentary left ventricle.

Other lesions can occur in congenitally corrected transposition. Deficiencies of the atrial septum are frequent. Subaortic obstruction, when present, tends to coexist with coarctation. It is also well recognised that aortic atresia or interruption can be found. If aortic atresia is found in the setting of congenitally corrected transposition, it accompanies hypoplasia of the morphologically right ventricle. Likewise, pulmonary atresia (when found with an intact ventricular septum and a discordant atrioventricular connection) is part and parcel of hypoplasia of the morphologically left ventricle.

Although the majority of patients have discordant connections at the ventriculo-arterial junction, other ventriculo-arterial connections can occur. Double outlet right ventricle and single outlet coexisting with pulmonary atresia are the two most likely. As already discussed, with the double outlet right ventricle the malalignment

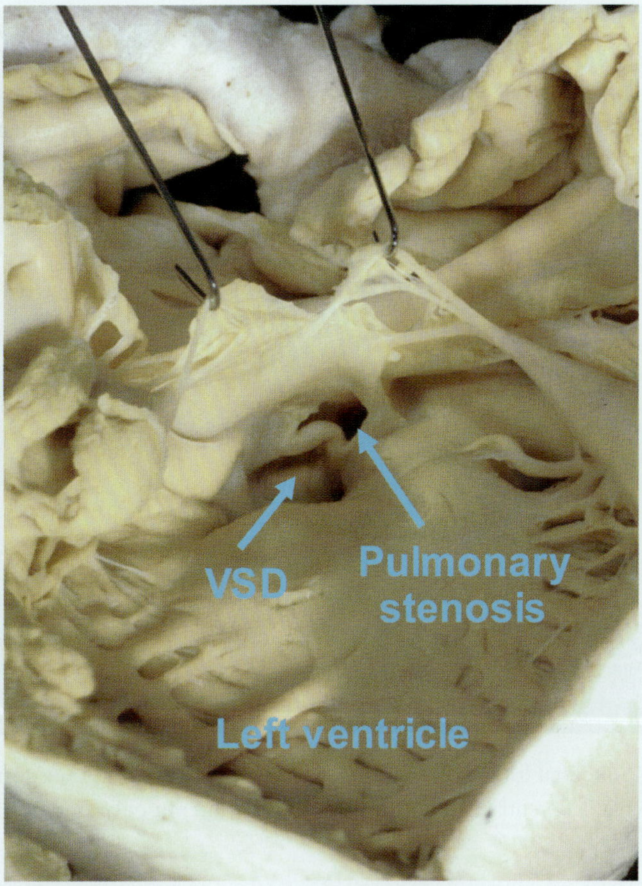

Figure 16.12 This left ventricular views shows the mitral valve retracted to reveal a fibrous diaphragm just beneath the pulmonary valve.

between the atrial and ventricular septums is much less. The ventricular septal defect with double outlet is almost always found in subpulmonary position. But there is no reason why it should not exist in other positions, such as subaortic, non-committed, or doubly committed.

Pulmonary atresia can be found with an intact ventricular septum and a hypoplastic left ventricle. More usually, it is found with a ventricular septal defect and with the aorta connected to the morphologically right ventricle. The remnant of the pulmonary trunk is then found posteriorly. It may be difficult to say whether it originated initially from the right or left ventricle. The pulmonary arterial supply in these circumstances has always, in our experience, been from the arterial duct, but cases are described with systemic-to-pulmonary collateral ateries.

Other ventriculo-arterial connections are much rarer. Concordant ventriculo-arterial connections are important because, when associated with discordant atrioventricular connections, they produce the circulatory pattern of transposition. Since

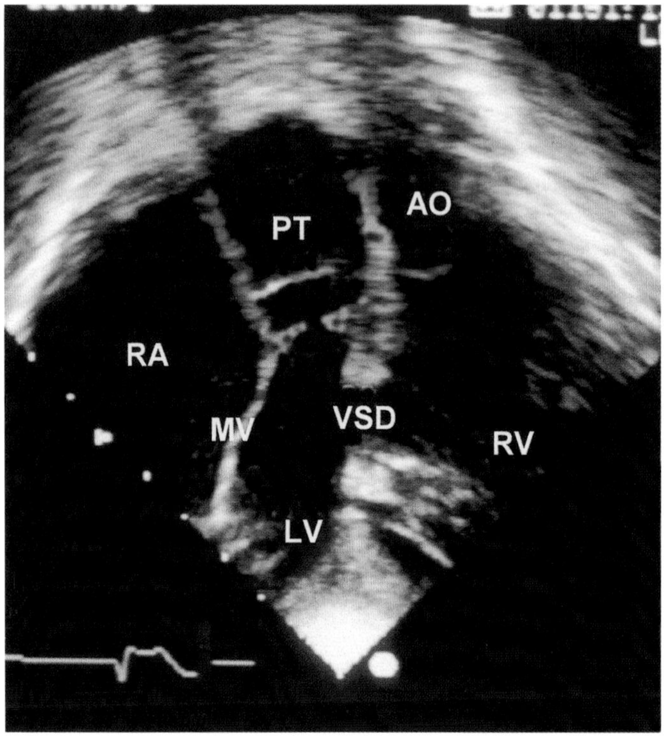

Figure 16.13 Subcostal long axis section in congenitally corrected transposition with discrete fibromuscular left ventricular outflow obstruction and muscular outlet ventricular septal defect.

the morphologically left ventricle supports the aorta, it can be corrected surgically by an atrial re-direction procedure (Mustard or Senning operation). The double outlet left ventricle, common arterial trunk, and single outlet with aortic atresia are all extremely rare, but do exist.

Discordant Atrioventricular Connections with Mirror-imaged Atriums

When discordant atrioventricular connections occur with mirror-imaged atrial arrangement, the pattern is not the same as the usual pattern 'in reverse'. Often, there is less atrioventricular septal malalignment, albeit typically in association with severe pulmonary stenosis or atresia. This means that, in most cases, the atrioventricular conduction axis originates from the regular atrioventricular node. Over and above this, there are differences in the frequency of associated lesions. A ventricular septal defect is less frequent, and subpulmonary stenosis or atresia more frequent than in the usual atrial arrangement.

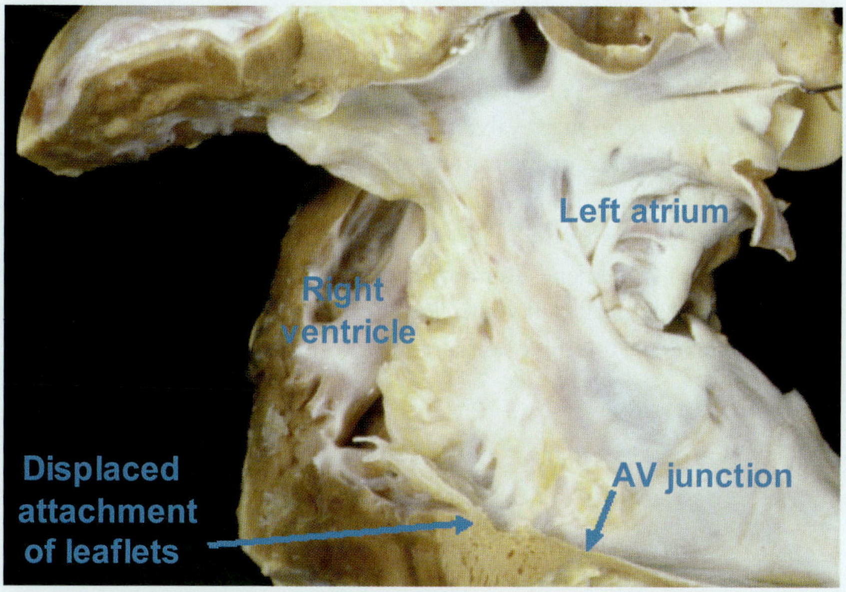

Figure 16.14 There is Ebstein malformation of the tricuspid valve in this heart with congenitally corrected transposition. Note that the right ventricular wall from the atrioventricular (AV) junction to the displaced hinge-line remains thick, without evidence of 'atrialisation'.

Anomalous Location of the Heart

An abnormal location of the heart is frequent in patients with discordant atrioventricular connections. The position of the heart within the chest, and the orientation of its apex, should be described separately. This avoids the need to create cryptic and confusing terms such as 'mixed laevocardia', or 'pivotal dextrocardia'.

The Conduction System

The sinus node is situated in its normal position in patients with the usual arrangement of the atrial appendages but is located in the left-sided morphologically right atrium in patients with mirror-imaged arrangement of the appendages.

In hearts with discordant atrioventricular and ventriculo-arterial connections, the left ventricular outflow tract is 'wedged' deeper than normal, extending posteriorly towards the crux. There is malalignment between the atrial septum and the inlet ventricular septum. This creates a considerable gap between the left atrium and the pulmonary outflow tract. In the absence of a ventricular septal defect in this region, the gap is filled by an extensive membranous septum. As a result of this distortion, the normal atrioventricular node, found in the atrioventricular septum at the apex of the triangle of Koch, is no longer in contact with the ventricular myocardium.

A connecting atrioventricular node, instead, is found in the right atrial wall at the right-hand limit of the area of fibrous continuity between the leaflets of the mitral and pulmonary valves. The conduction axis then penetrates through the fibrous area to pass in front of the pulmonary valve (Fig. 16.7). The course of the non-branching bundle is particularly relevant in hearts associated with a ventricular septal defect. The bundle runs anterior and cephalad to the pulmonary valve and then descends along the anterior margin of the defect before diverging into the bundle branches. The left bundle branch descends in immediate subendocardial position on the septal aspect of the morphologically left ventricle. The proximal portion of the right bundle branch usually takes an intramyocardial course to reach the morphologically right ventricle.

17

Hearts with Univentricular Atrioventricular Connections

There has been much argument about the description of hearts with a double inlet atrioventricular connection and those with atrioventricular valvar atresia. Although these two types of abnormality often have a remarkably similar morphology of their ventricular mass, there are distinct differences in their atrioventricular connections. All examples of hearts with double inlet ventricle, and the majority of those with atrioventricular valvar atresia, have both atriums connected to only one chamber within the ventricular mass (Fig. 17.1). They are distinguished from the majority of congenitally malformed hearts in which each atrium is connected to its own ventricle. It is simple and logical, therefore, to describe these hearts as having univentricular atrioventricular connections. The types of connection are double inlet ventricle and absence of the right and left atrioventricular connections. They always produce a functionally univentricular circulation. When analysing such patients, it helps to distinguish the type of atrioventricular connection from ventricular morphology, and from the morphology of the atrioventricular valves.

Morphology of Univentricular Atrioventricular Connections

Each atrioventricular junction consists of an atrial myocardium potentially connected to the adjacent ventricular mass. In most hearts, there are two atrioventricular junctions, the morphology of which is independent of the nature of the valve they contain. In a heart with a common valve, the atrioventricular junction is deficient at the septum, but the two parietal atrioventricular junctions connecting to the atrial mass are connected to the ventricular myocardium through the common valve (Fig. 17.2). The double inlet ventricle, therefore, is best defined as the connection

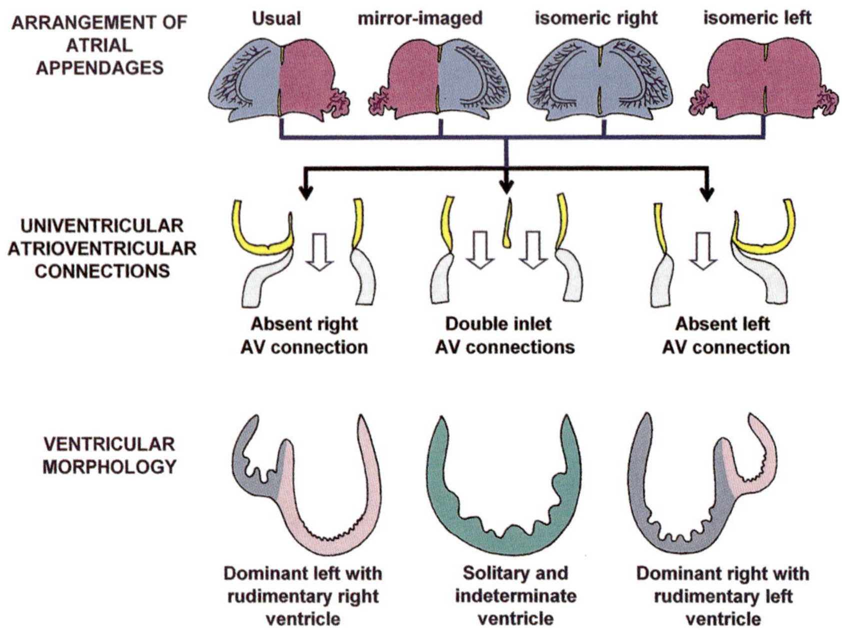

Figure 17.1 Diagram illustrating the concept of univentricular atrioventricular connections. As discussed in Chapter 3, most hearts thus categorised have two ventricular chambers, one large and dominant and the other smaller and rudimentary.

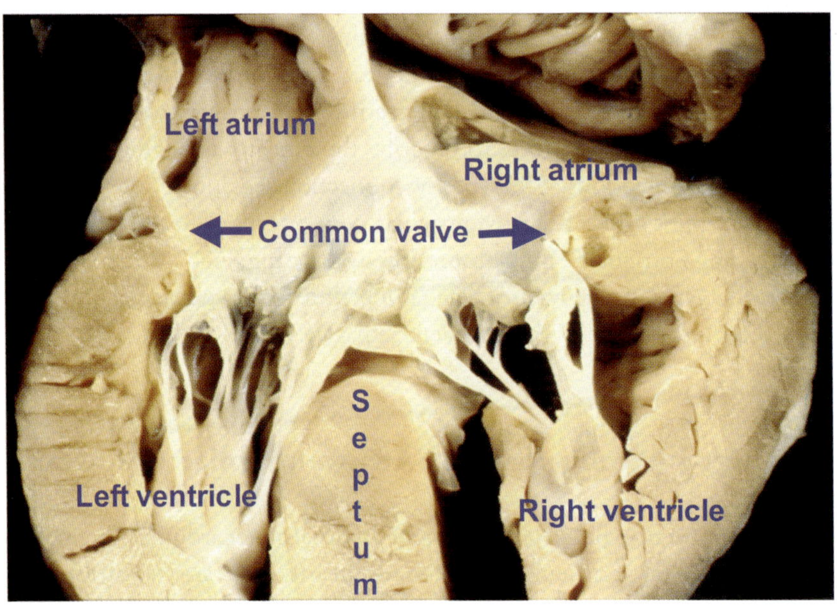

Figure 17.2 This heart has biventricular atrioventricular connections through a common atrioventricular valve and atrioventricular septal defect. Each atrium is connected to a ventricular chamber, hence the term biventricular connections.

of both atrioventricular junctions to the same ventricle. There may be two atrioventricular valves or a common valve guarding these junctions (Fig. 17.3).

It is often assumed that atrioventricular valvar atresia is caused by an imperforate atrioventricular valve that blocks a potential communciation between an atrium and a ventricle. Such variants of valvar atresia do exist (Fig. 17.4), but they are rare. In these, the imperforate membrane typically balloons into the ventricle during atrial systole. In some instances, a hypoplastic tension apparatus may be detected on the ventricular aspect of the membrane. Much more frequently, there is complete absence of the atrioventricular connection (Fig. 17.5). The atrial floor is entirely muscular, and is separated from the ventricular mass by the fibrofatty tissue of the atrioventricular groove. Either the right or the left atrioventricular connection can be absent in this way. The other atrium connects, in most cases, with only one ventricle. So, like the double inlet ventricle, this arrangement is accurately described as producing a univentricular atrioventricular connection, and supporting a functionally univentricular circulation.

Some hearts with atrioventricular valvar atresia do not have univentricular atrioventricular connections. For instance, those with imperforate Ebstein's malformation of the tricuspid valve have atrioventricular valvar atresia with concordant, and biventricular, atrioventricular connections.

The Ventricular Mass with Univentricular Atrioventricular Connections

Most hearts with univentricular atrioventricular connections are not, in any sense of the words, 'univentricular hearts' or 'single ventricles'. They have one big and one small ventricle. The only feature that is truly univentricular is the atrioventricular

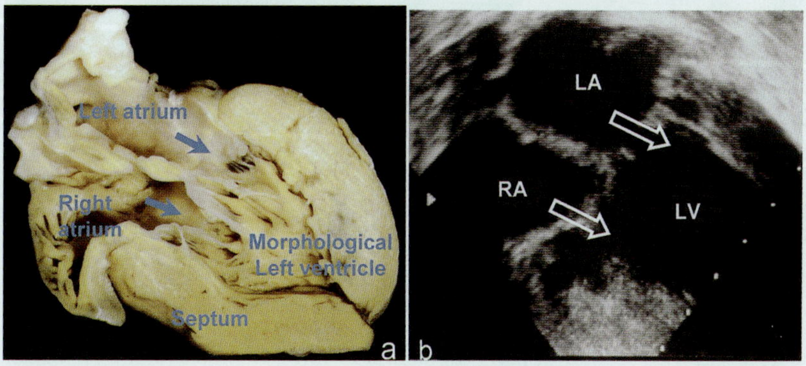

Figure 17.3 (a) Both atrial chambers are connected (arrows) to the same ventricular chamber, which is recognised as a morphologically left ventricle. Very little of the morphologically right ventricle is visible since this plane of section is inferior to it. This univentricular atrioventricular connection is the double inlet left ventricle. Two discrete valves guard the junction. (b) Subcostal four-chamber sections in the double inlet left ventricle with two atrioventricular valves.

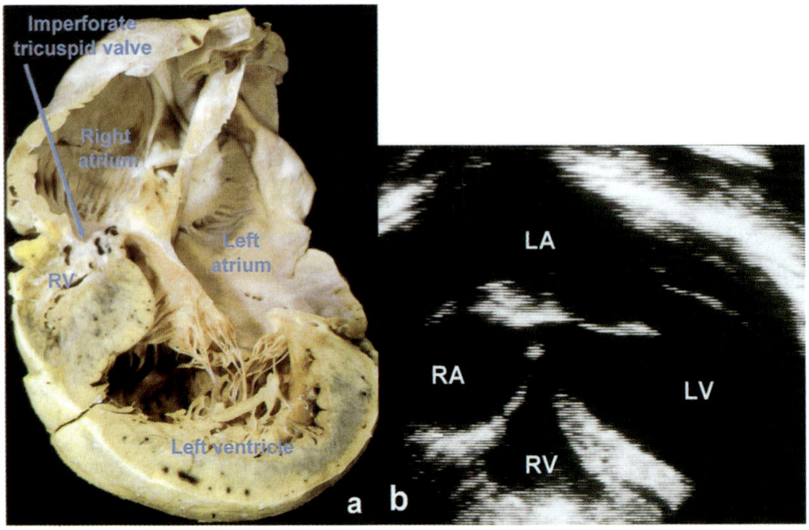

Figure 17.4 (a) This four-chamber section shows concordant biventricular atrioventricular connections. An imperforate valve blocks the outlet from the right atrium. (b) A corresponding subcostal four-chamber view demonstrates an imperforate tricuspid valve and perimembranous inlet ventricular septal defect.

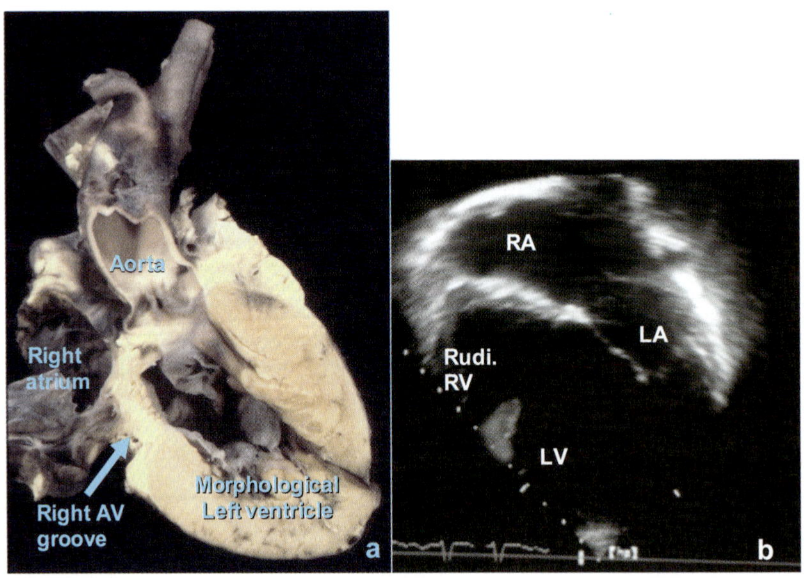

Figure 17.5 (a) This section displays the common form of tricuspid atresia, which is due to absence of the right atrioventricular connections. The right atrium has a muscular floor, which is separated from the ventricular mass by fibro-fatty tissue of the right atrioventricular groove. (b) This parasternal four-chamber section shows the deep right atrioventricular groove indicative of absence of the atrioventricular connection. There is a large ventricular septal defect.

connection. The circulation, nonetheless, is functionally univentricular. Whether there is a double inlet ventricle, or absence of one atrioventricular connection, the effect on the ventricular mass is the same. One of the ventricles lacks its inlet component and, hence, is incomplete and rudimentary (Fig. 17.6). When there is a univentricular atrioventricular connection to a dominant left ventricle, the right

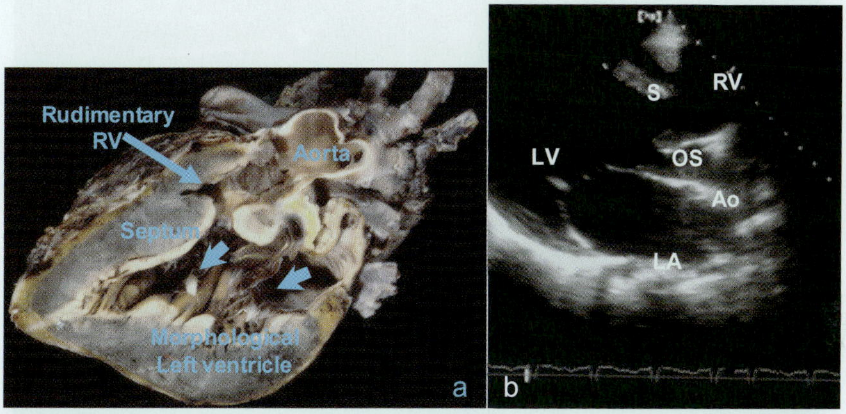

Figure 17.6 (a) This section simulating the parasternal long axis plane shows a double inlet (arrows) to a dominant left ventricle. The right ventricle situated antero-superiorly is small and rudimentary. It lacks an inlet component. (b) Parasternal long axis section showing posterior deviation of the outlet septum causing aortic stenosis in the double inlet left ventricle.

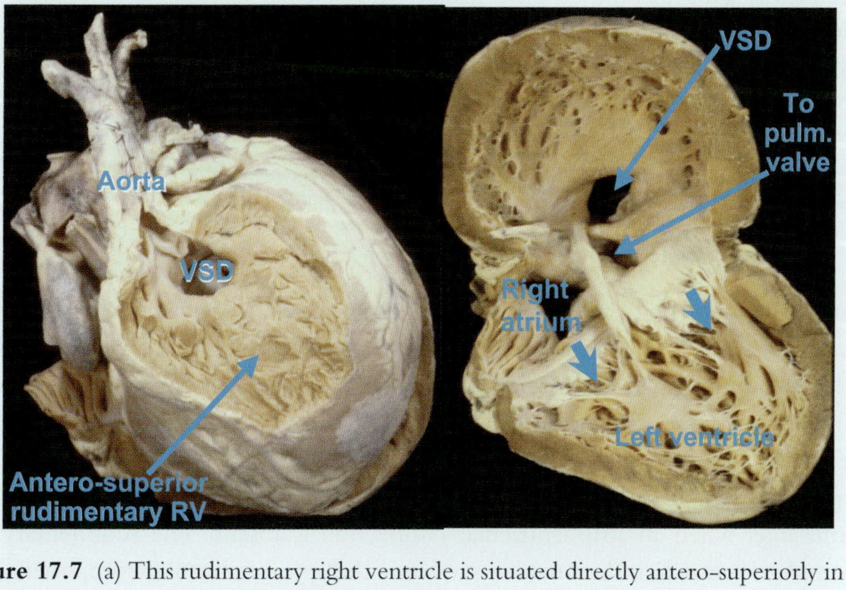

Figure 17.7 (a) This rudimentary right ventricle is situated directly antero-superiorly in the ventricular mass. (b) The dominant left ventricle receives flow from both atrial chambers via two discrete atrioventricular valves (arrows).

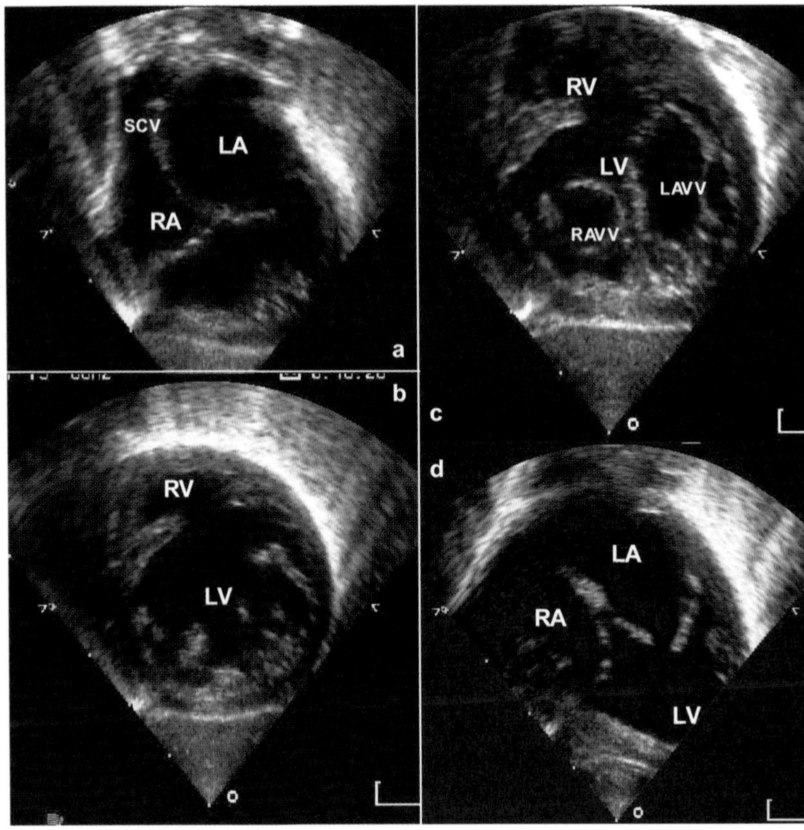

Figure 17.8 Echocardiograms showing a case of double inlet left ventricle. (a) Subcostal section showing the right and left atrial chambers. (b) Subcostal short axis section showing the rudimentary right ventricle situated antero-superiorly relative to the dominant morphologically left ventricle. (c) Subcostal short axis section showing both right and left atrioventricular valves (RAVV, LAVV) in the dominant left ventricle. (d) Parasternal four-chamber section showing both atrial chambers opening into the dominant left ventricle via two discrete valves.

ventricle is rudimentary and incomplete. Usually the right ventricle retains its outlet component, either subaortic or subpulmonary. Rarely, it may give rise to both outlets. The incomplete ventricle retains its apical trabecular component, which is found antero-superiorly within the ventricular mass, either to the right or the left side of the dominant left ventricle (Figs. 17.7 and 17.8). Also, infrequently, the dominant left ventricle may give rise to both outlets as well as receiving both inlets, or one inlet when an atrioventricular connection is absent. The rudimentary and incomplete ventricle is then made up of only the apical trabecular component.

There can also be a univentricular atrioventricular connection to a dominant right ventricle. It is then the left ventricle that is incomplete and rudimentary.

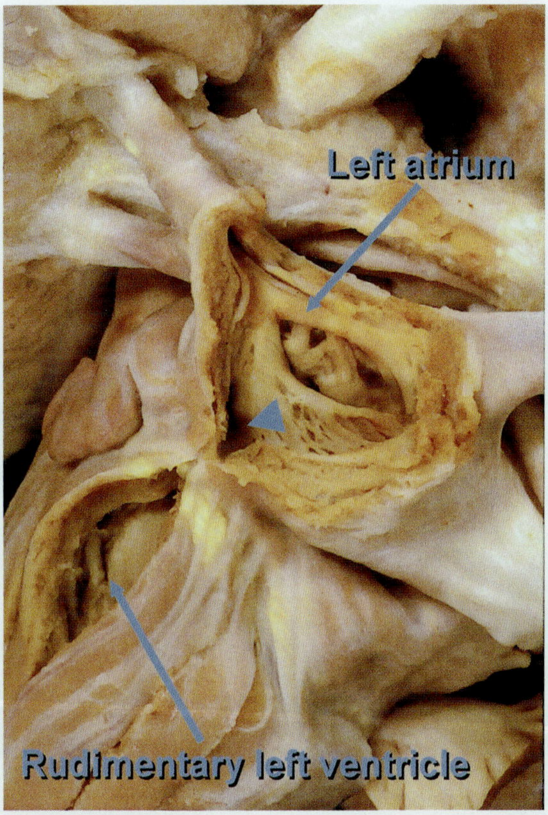

Figure 17.9 This heart is viewed from the postero-inferior aspect. It shows absence of the left atrioventricular connections with the left atrium ending in a muscular floor (Δ). The rudimentary left ventricle situated in the left and inferior position is slit-like and without a ventricular septal defect.

Rudimentary left ventricles are always positioned postero-inferiorly to the dominant right ventricle, usually to the left, but sometimes to the right (Fig. 17.9). Often, they are composed only of the apical trabecular component, both ventricular outlets arising from the dominant right ventricle.

The majority of hearts with univentricular atrioventricular connection will have either a dominant left ventricle with a rudimentary right ventricle, or else a dominant right ventricle with a rudimentary left ventricle. A rare variant is found when there is a univentricular connection to an apparently solitary ventricle. This arrangement can occur when the solitary ventricle is of right, or rarely left, morphology, and the rudimentary ventricle is so small as to be undetectable except by histological examination. Occasionally, nonetheless, the ventricular mass is made up of a truly solitary chamber of indeterminate morphology (Figs. 17.10 and 17.11). Such rare hearts are the only true anatomic examples of 'univentricular hearts' or 'single ventricles'.

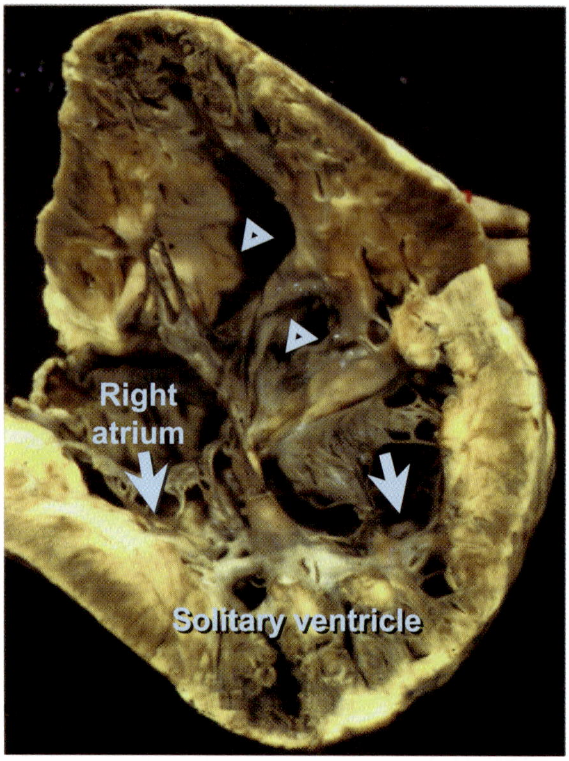

Figure 17.10 This heart has double inlet (arrows) to a solitary and indeterminate ventricle. Both great arteries arise from this chamber (ΔΔ).

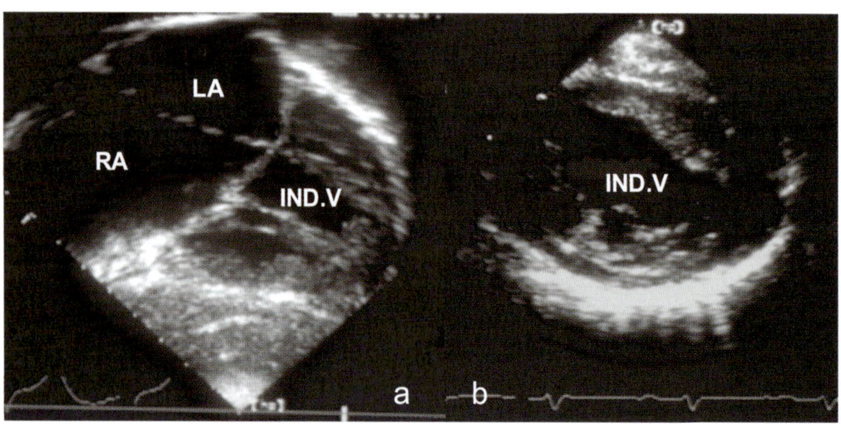

Figure 17.11 (a) Subcostal 'four-chamber' section showing a solitary ventricular chamber connecting to both atrial chambers. Note the typical extremely coarse trabeculations, proven at autopsy. (b) This subcostal short axis section confirms a solitary ventricle.

Straddling and Overriding Atrioventricular Valves

The tension apparatus of an atrioventricular valve may straddle the crest of the ventricular septum. One atrioventricular junction is then shared between both ventricles. Depending on the degree of overriding, there is a spectrum of malformations between biventricular and univentricular connections with a double inlet (Fig. 17.12). Precise description of the connection depends on the nature of the straddling valve and the topological arrangement of the ventricular mass. The overriding valve is assigned to the ventricle supporting the greater part of its circumference. The double inlet ventricle is more appropriately defined, therefore, as the arrangement with the greater part of both atrioventricular junctions connected to the same ventricle. A solitary valve can also, rarely, straddle and override when one atrioventricular connection is absent. This produces a particular arrangement in which the atrioventricular connection is uniatrial but biventricular (Figs. 17.13 and 17.14). In these circumstances, both ventricles are incomplete and rudimentary to varying degrees. Usually, one is dominant and the other rudimentary, but rarely the two incomplete ventricles may be of comparable size.

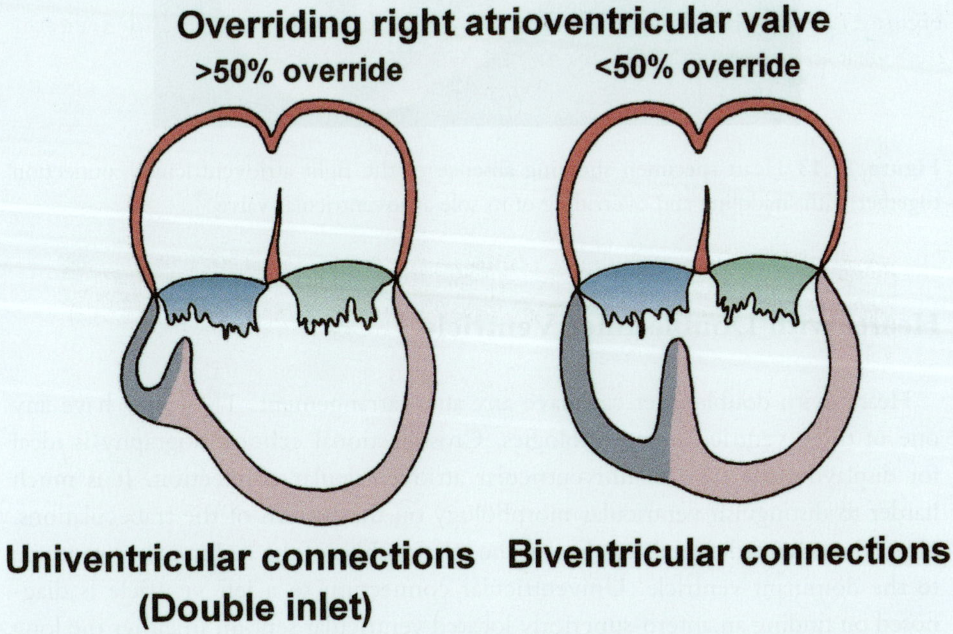

Figure 17.12 The degree of overriding of the atrioventricular valve confers the type of atrioventricular connections. The overriding valve is assigned to the ventricle supporting the greater part of its circumference (more than 50%).

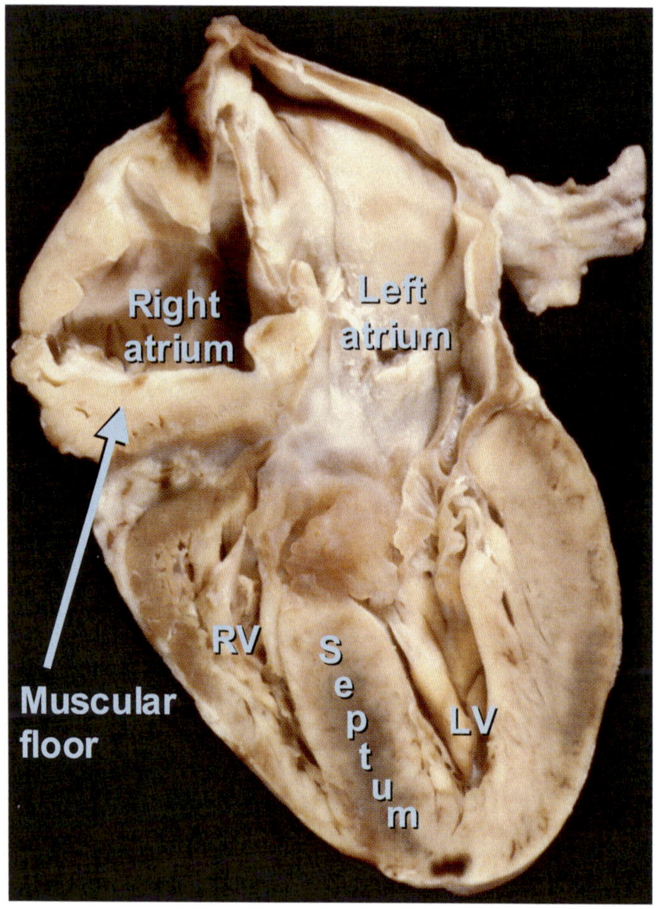

Figure 17.13 Heart specimen showing absence of the right atrioventricular connection together with straddling and overriding of its sole atrioventricular valve.

Hearts with Double Inlet Ventricle

Hearts with double inlet can have any atrial arrangement. They may have any one of three ventricular morphologies. Cross-sectional echocardiography is ideal for displaying the type of univentricular atrioventricular connection. It is much harder to distinguish ventricular morphology on the pattern of the trabeculations. Here, the echocardiographer relies on the relationships of the rudimentary ventricle to the dominant ventricle. Univentricular connection to a left ventricle is diagnosed on finding an antero-superiorly located ventricular septum in either the long axis cut parallel to the atrial septum, the parasternal plane or in the short axis cut. When the septum is found posteriorly and inferiorly, then the dominant ventricle is of right morphology. Failure to identify a rudimentary chamber is indicative of a solitary and, most probably, an indeterminate ventricle. A solitary right or left

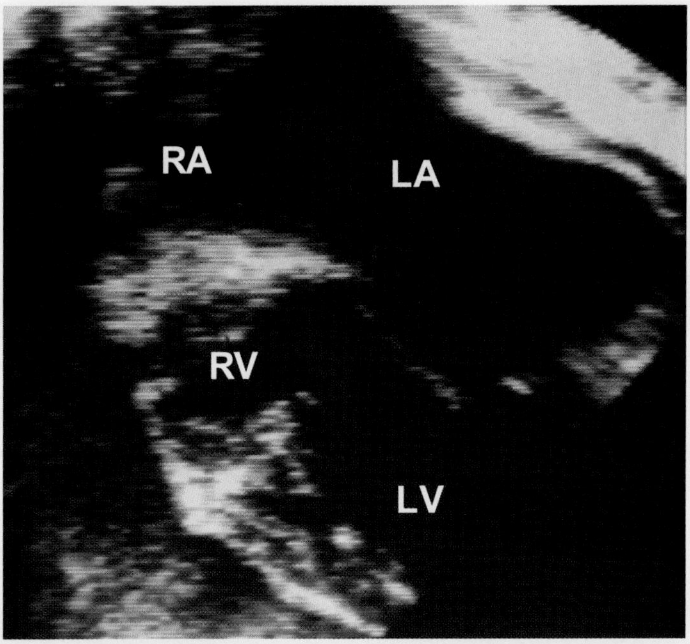

Figure 17.14 Echocardiogram of a case similar to that shown in Fig. 17.13.

ventricle, however, cannot be ruled out. Straddling and common atrioventricular valves are readily distinguished using the four-chamber long axis cuts. Imperforate valves can also be recognised, the valvar membrane being seen as an intact structure both during ventricular systole and diastole. There may be various malformations of the atrioventricular valves, any ventriculo-arterial connection, diverse relationships between dominant and rudimentary ventricles, and miscellaneous associated anomalies. Any combination may occur, but the most frequent pattern is the double inlet to a dominant left ventricle with rudimentary right ventricle on either the left or right side and discordant ventriculo-arterial connections. Another important pattern is the double inlet left ventricle with right-sided rudimentary right ventricle and concordant ventriculo-arterial connections. This is also called the Holmes heart.

Hearts with Atrioventricular Valvar Atresia

Just as much anatomical variability is possible when one atrioventricular connection is absent as when there is a double inlet ventricle. Atrioventricular valvar atresia can be produced by an imperforate valve, as well as absence of an atrioventricular connection. This must be borne in mind when using descriptions such as tricuspid or mitral atresia. Echocardiographically, the absent connection is identified by means of the thick band of the atrioventricular groove, which separates the atrial floor from the ventricular mass (Fig. 17.15). Tricuspid atresia is usually due to absence of the

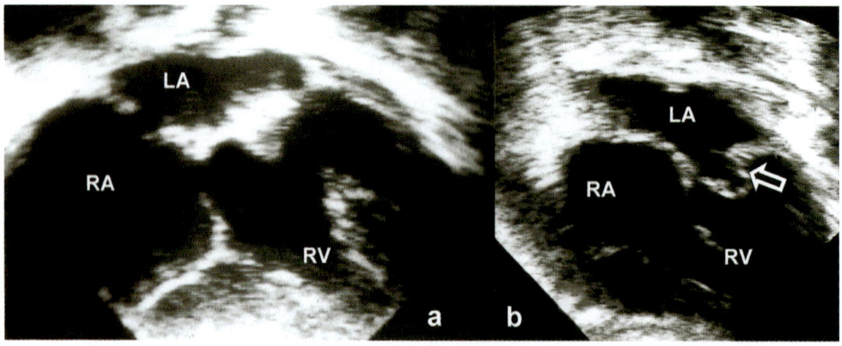

Figure 17.15 (a) Subcostal four-chamber section showing absence of the left atrioventricular connection. (b) Subcostal four-chamber section showing double inlet to dominant right ventricle associated with an imperforate left atrioventricular valve (arrow) ballooning into the right ventricle.

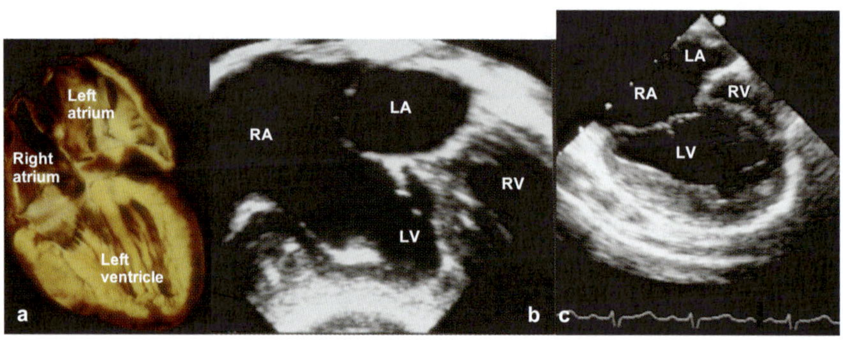

Figure 17.16 (a) This heart specimen shows absence of the left atrioventricular connections in which the right atrium is connected to the morphologically left ventricle. This case demonstrates the potential for confusion in describing it as mitral atresia. (b) Parasternal four-chamber section of a case with corresponding morphology. (c) Subcostal four-chamber section with absent left connection. The morphologically right atrium opens into the morphologically left ventricle.

right atrioventricular connection, with the left atrium connected to the dominant left ventricle with a rudimentary right ventricle. This can occur with concordant or discordant ventriculo-arterial connections, and with various degrees of pulmonary obstruction. Complete obstruction of flow from the morphologically right atrium can also be produced by an imperforate valve with either concordant or double inlet atrioventricular connections. The same haemodynamic picture can also be produced by an imperforate right valve with discordant atrioventricular connections. This last example, in morphological terms, might be described as mitral atresia, but would produce the haemodynamic picture of tricuspid atresia. This conflict between the haemodynamic and anatomical descriptions is also seen when there is absence of the left atrioventricular connection and the right atrium is connected to a dominant left ventricle, with the rudimentary right ventricle being antero-superior and left sided (Fig. 17.16). It is likely that, in this setting, if the left atrioventricular connection had formed, it would have been guarded by a morphologically tricuspid valve. Such a heart, therefore, has absence of the left atrioventricular connection, but is, morphologically, tricuspid atresia. It produces the clinical picture of mitral atresia.

18

Ebstein Malformation

First described by Wilhelm Ebstein in 1866, this valvar lesion has characteristic features, but also variations in the underlying anatomy that can make its diagnosis difficult. The illustration of the case described by Ebstein showed absence of part of the septal leaflet of the tricuspid valve, with abnormal attachments of the mural, or inferior, leaflet to the diaphragmatic wall of the right ventricle. In addition, the antero-superior leaflet, although hinged at the atrioventricular junction, was larger than usual, and its leading edge was abnormally attached. Overall, the deranged configuration of the tricuspid valve produces a valvar mechanism that coapts not close to the level of the atrioventricular junction, but well within the ventricular cavity (Fig. 18.1). Morphologically, the constant feature is the origin of some part of the valvar leaflets within the ventricular cavity rather than at the normal hingeline at the atrioventricular junction, an arrangement usually described as 'downward displacement', although the displacement is rotational rather than strictly downwards. Even within this basic definition, variations in degree of displacement are found. In the mildest form, the degree of displacement is difficult to distinguish from the normal offset arrangement at the septum between the hinges of the tricuspid and mitral valves. For a better understanding of this malformation, it is helpful first to review the structure of the normal tricuspid valve.

The Normal Tricuspid Valve

Most commonly, three leaflets can be distinguished in the tricuspid valve. All three leaflets are hinged to the atrioventricular junction, where a fibro-fatty tissue plane insulates the atrial from the ventricular myocardium. When open, the valve

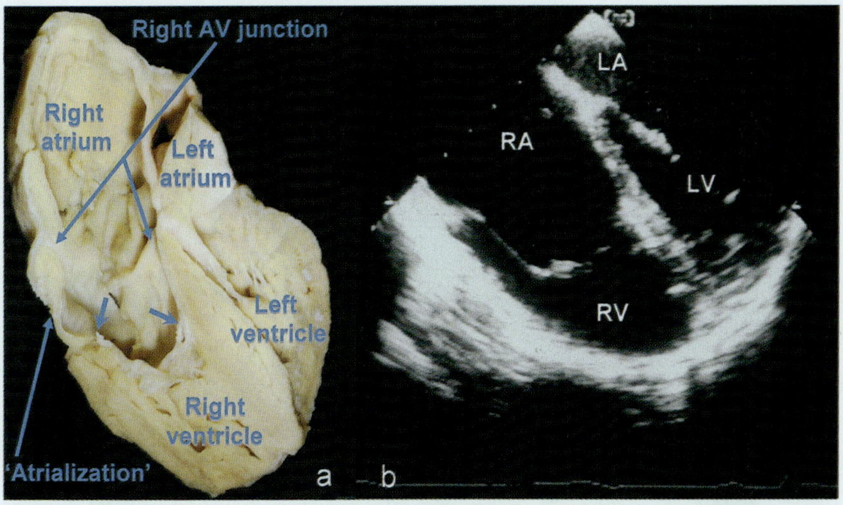

Figure 18.1 (a) This heart specimen shows gross displacement of the hingelines (arrows) of the septal and mural leaflets towards the right ventricular apex. There is thinning of the inferior wall ('atrialisation'). (b) Echocardiogram from transoesophageal window (four-chamber section) showing the apically displaced hinge of the tricuspid valve but normally attached antero-superior leaflet.

has a relatively triangular configuration, with the peripheral parts of the zones of apposition, the so-called commissures, reaching close to the level of the atrioventricular junction to resemble the points of the triangle (Fig. 1.11). The tethering of the leaflets is characteristic. The septal leaflet has direct cordal attachments to the septum (Fig. 1.12). The inferior, or mural, leaflet is supported by a variable number of small papillary muscles that arise from the diaphragmatic wall of the ventricle, usually supporting the space between septal and inferior leaflets. The remaining leaflet, the antero-superior leaflet, is usually tethered to a large anterior papillary muscle that arises from the apical extension of the septomarginal trabeculation (Fig. 1.11). The junction between the antero-superior leaflet and the septal leaflet is supported by the medial papillary muscle, which is attached to the upper portion of the septomarginal trabeculation along the ventricular septum. It is the distortion of the leading edge of the antero-superior leaflet that contributes to further variations in Ebstein's malformation.

The Tricuspid Valve in Ebstein Malformation

Ebstein malformation almost always affects the morphologically tricuspid valve, but occasionally affects the mural leaflet of the mitral valve. When affecting the tricuspid valve, the greatest point of displacement of the effective hingeline involves the adjacent parts of the inferior and septal leaflets (Fig. 18.2). Although the same

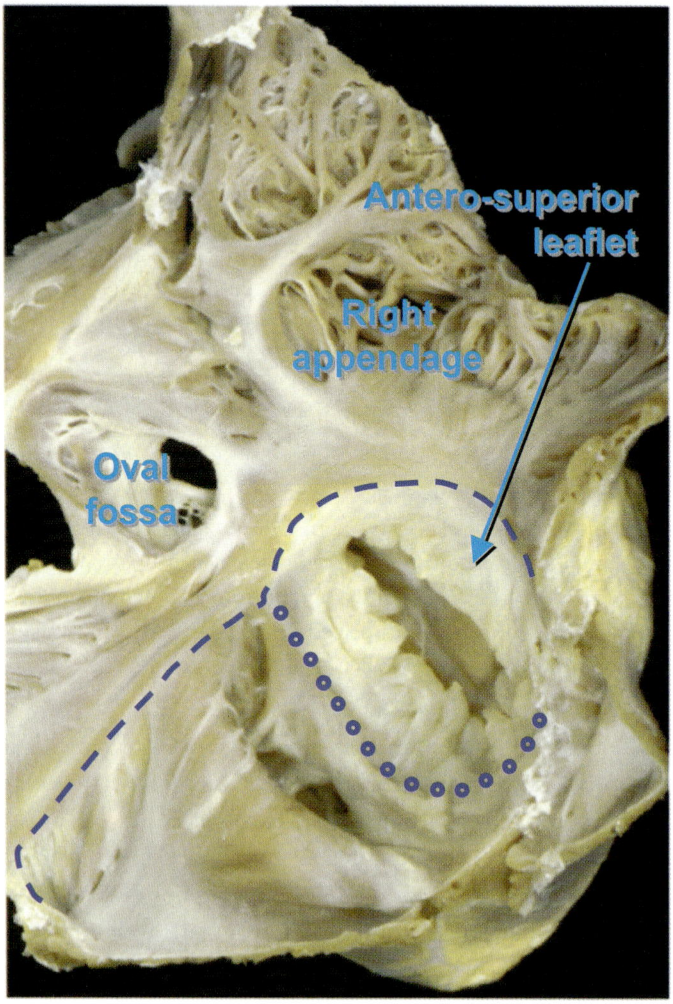

Figure 18.2 This view of the tricuspid valve from the right atrium shows the hingeline of the septal and mural leaflets (ooooo) displaced from the atrioventricular junction (- - - -). The hingeline of the antero-superior leaflet remains at its normal level.

nomenclature is used for the leaflets, the valve may be so malformed that it is not possible to clearly distinguish one leaflet from another using the analogy of the three points of a triangle, as described above. At one extreme end of the spectrum, all three leaflets may be joined and adherent to the ventricular wall, producing a 'tricuspid' sack which may even lack an orifice. More commonly two, and occasionally three, leaflets can be identified even in cases in which the triangular shape of the valvar orifice is distorted. As in the index case, part of the septal leaflet may be absent.

When displacement is minimal, it can give problems in echocardiographic diagnosis. This is because the septal leaflet of the tricuspid valve is normally offset relative to the attachment of the mitral valve (Fig. 3.4), and it is then necessary to determine how much offset is too much. The displacement of the inferior leaflet is more readily recognisable but, in practice, this region is difficult to image during life. Going along with displacement of the inferior leaflet is thinning, or atrialisation, of the ventricular wall in many cases seen at autopsy. In the more severe cases, the inferior leaflet is immobile, and lacks its division from the antero-superior leaflet.

The antero-superior leaflet is usually hinged at its normal level, but its distal attachments are often abnormal. This enlarged and sail-like leaflet is usually the most mobile of the three leaflets. In some hearts, this leaflet retains normal focal attachment to the anterior papillary muscle, and the inferior leaflet is also relatively normal. The septal leaflet in hearts of this type is virtually absent, or else represented by cauliflower-like remnants on the septal surface. In other hearts, the distal attachment is linear to a muscular shelf situated between the inlet and apical trabecular components of the ventricle, with continuity between the antero-superior and inferior leaflets. Occasionally, gaps in the linear attachment due to spaces between tendinous cords, or fenestrations, produce a hyphenated appearance (Fig. 18.3). The keyhole which normally exists between the edge of the antero-superior leaflet and the septum becomes increasingly narrowed, especially when there is fusion between the distal

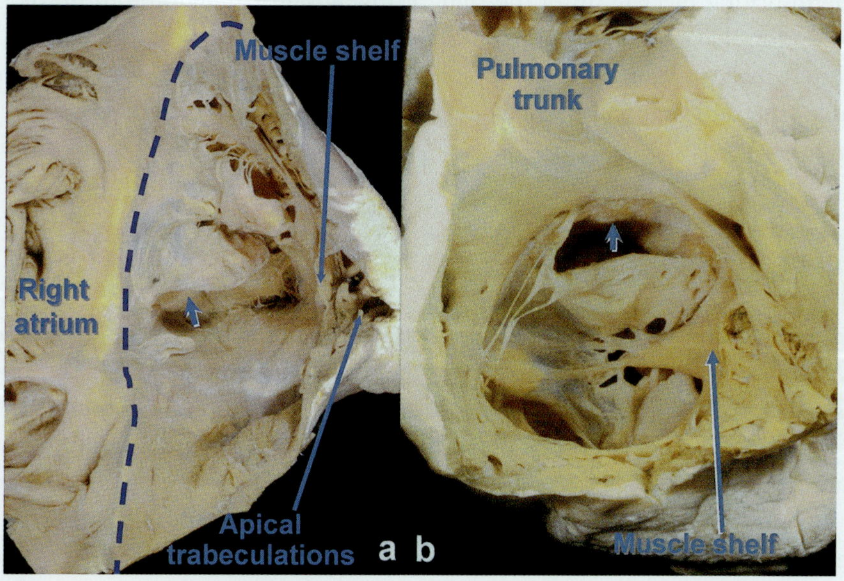

Figure 18.3 (a) The distal edge of the antero-superior leaflet is attached to a bizarre arrangement of papillary muscles and bands in this heart. These muscular structures coalesce into a shelf-like structure sequestrating the right ventricular inlet from the apical component. Outflow is through the displaced valvar orifice (arrow) between the remnant of the septal leaflet and the antero-superior leaflet as well as through the spaces at the edge of the latter leaflet. The spaces give the distal edge a 'hypenated' appearance. The broken line marks the atrioventricular junction. (b) This outlet view shows the keyhole orifice between the antero-superior leaflet and the septum.

margins of the antero-superior and inferior leaflets to form a 'hammock'. Thus, the varied combinations of proximal and distal attachments of the leaflets result in a spectrum of displacement of the effective valvar orifice, and a further spectrum concerning its size.

Associated Features

Thinning of the right ventricular wall, or atrialisation, varies from case to case. When the tricuspid valve is incompetent, the atrium and the inlet of the right ventricle also dilate. In addition to the inlet portion, thinning may also affect the apical and outlet parts, with implications for ventricular function, since these components serve as the pump. In contrast, some hearts, especially those with congenitally corrected transposition, rarely show thinning of the morphologically right ventricle situated on the left side. In adults, functional abnormalities of the ventricular septum and left ventricle have been observed.

Ventricular pre-excitation of the Wolff–Parkinson–White variant is particularly common in the setting of Ebstein malformation. It is thought to be an abnormality of the insulating mechanism of the right atrioventricular junction, but histological investigations have found the atrioventricular junctions to be well formed.

Ebstein malformation can occur in isolation, but well-recognised associated lesions include atrial and ventricular septal defects, congenitally corrected transposition and pulmonary atresia.

Conclusions

In essence, Ebstein malformation has characteristic features that are compounded by variability in the structure and arrangement of the valvar leaflets at their hingelines and distal attachments. In most autopsied examples, the valvar leaflets are also dysplastic. Dysplasia of normally attached valves is also known to produce tricuspid regurgitation, so it is the displacement of the hingelines away from the atrioventricular junction that is the diagnostic feature for Ebstein malformation. The degree and extent of atrialisation of the right ventricle will determine its function.

19

Aortic Coarctation and Interruption

Aortic coarctation is defined as a narrowing or obstruction of the aortic arch. In the past, coarctation has been divided into 'infant' and the 'adult' forms. This is an oversimplification. It is difficult to separate cases in this way on the basis of the morphological features.

Coarctation with a Closed Duct

The word 'coarctation' derives from a Latin word that means 'a drawing together'. When Morgagni performed a postmortem on a monk in 1760, he drew attention to a narrowing of the aorta a short distance from the heart. The waist-like constriction found in Morgagni's case is seen more frequently in children and adults rather than infants, in whom the morphology of the lesion is more variable. In older patients, the arterial duct is almost always closed and ligamentous (Fig. 19.1). The coarctation is usually adjacent to the site of insertion of the arterial ligament. Frequently, in the lumen of the aorta, at the level of a marked waist, there is a diaphragmatic shelf with a pin-hole orifice (Fig. 19.2). The lumen of the aorta is usually dilated distal to the coarctation. This so-called adult form is often associated with a bifoliate aortic valve, but usually is otherwise an isolated lesion. There are often well-developed collateral arteries. The intercostal arteries, the internal thoracic arteries, the scapular vessels and others form an anastomotic network and feed the descending aorta. The characteristic rib-notching seen in chest radiographs of older children with this lesion is produced by the enlarged intercostal arteries.

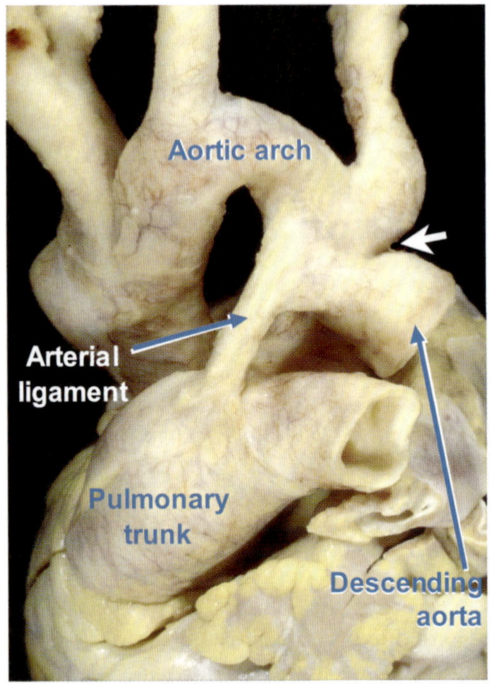

Figure 19.1 This heart specimen from an adult shows the posterior indentation (arrow) in the aorta at the site of the coarctation lesion.

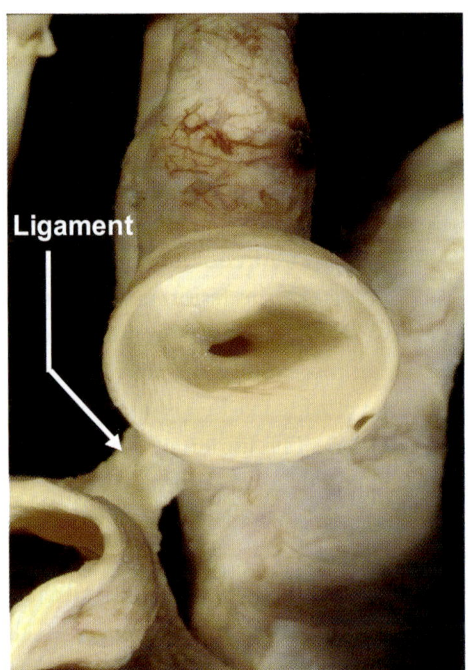

Figure 19.2 This view from the descending thoracic aorta shows the pin-hole orifice in the specimen shown in Fig. 19.1.

Coarctation and the Patent Duct

When found in infancy, coarctation usually has a different morphological pattern. The duct is patent in the majority of cases, and the obstruction tends to be at the junction of the aortic isthmus with the duct and the descending aorta. The isthmus is the part of the aortic arch between the origin of the subclavian artery and the insertion of the arterial duct. Occasionally, the obstruction is a simple waist-like constriction with infolding of the aortic wall. More often, a shelf also projects into the lumen (Fig. 19.3). The shelf forms a circle around the junction of the isthmus with the descending aorta. It is continuous with the muscular tissue of the wall of the arterial duct (Fig. 19.4). When the duct is open, the precise location of the obstruction determines the flow from the duct into the aorta in cases with aortic atresia. The obstruction can be found at preductal, paraductal and postductal locations (Fig. 19.5). The preductal position is most frequently encountered in infants and young children. The postductal position is rare, but can exist with an open duct.

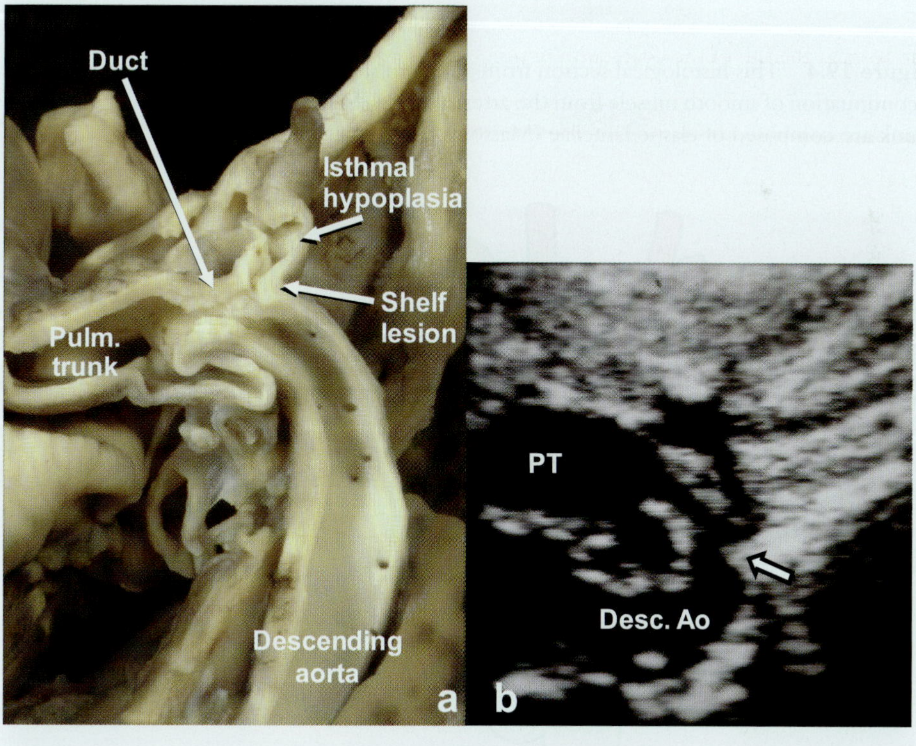

Figure 19.3 (a) This specimen from an infant shows a shelf lesion surrounding the entrance of the aortic isthmus. (b) Suprasternal parasagittal section showing a coarctation lesion (arrow) with arch hypoplasia.

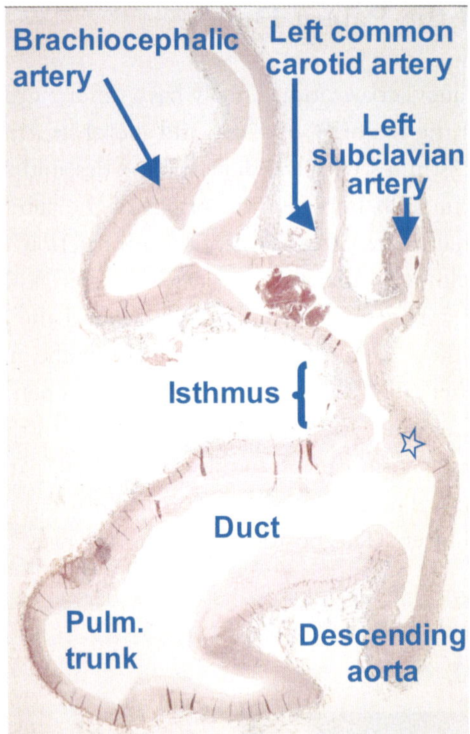

Figure 19.4 This histological section from an infant shows the coarctation shelf (☆) to be a continuation of smooth muscle from the arterial duct. The walls of the aorta and pulmonary trunk are composed of elastic lamellae (Masson's trichrome stain).

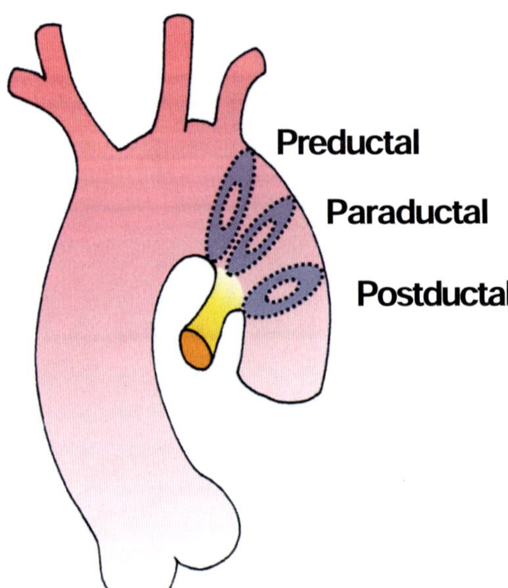

Figure 19.5 Diagram showing the location of the coarctation relative to the opening of the arterial duct or insertion of arterial ligament.

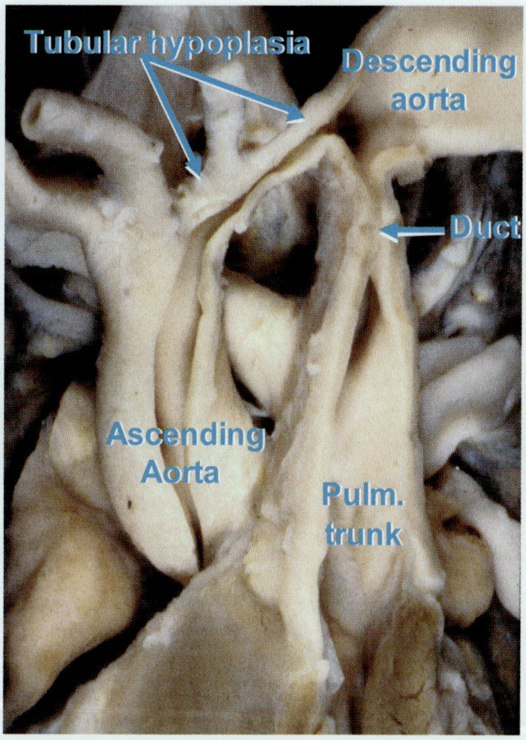

Figure 19.6 The aortic arch has a long and narrow segment from the origin of the brachiocephalic artery to the insertion of the arterial duct.

Tubular Hypoplasia

Another obstructive lesion of the aortic arch that is sometimes included under the general heading of 'coarctation' is a tubular narrowing of an entire segment of the arch. This tubular hypoplasia usually affects the aortic isthmus. It is found most often in infants. Frequently, it coexists with discrete waist and shelf lesions. Tubular hypoplasia can also exist in isolation (Fig. 19.6). Sometimes the narrow segment is longer, and affects the arch from the origin of the left common carotid artery to the insertion of the duct (Fig. 19.7). More rarely, it involves the arch between the brachiocephalic and left common carotid arteries. Varying degrees of narrowing are seen. In its most severe form, the hypoplastic segment is no more than a fibrous strand (Fig. 19.10). Interruption of the aortic arch can be considered as the most extreme form of aortic arch obstruction, and is considered separately below.

Associated Lesions

Apart from a bilfoliate aortic valve, the anomaly most often associated with coarctation is patency of the arterial duct. Abnormalities of the subclavian artery are also

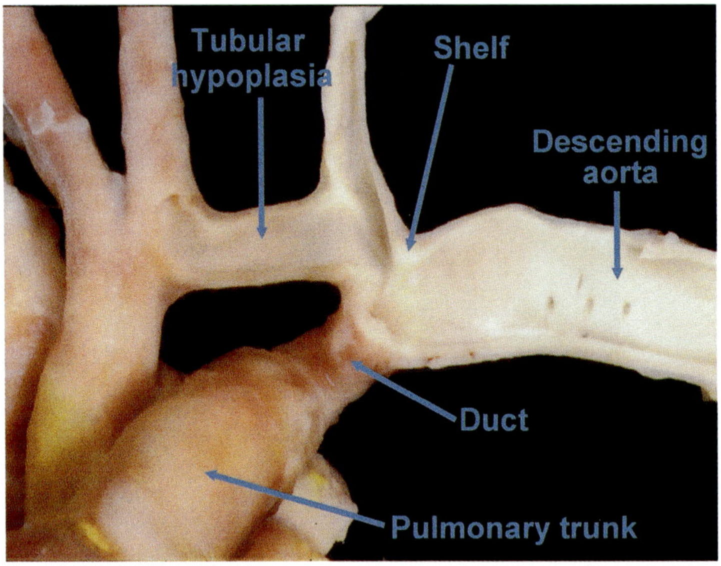

Figure 19.7 This specimen shows tubular hypoplastic of the transverse arch associated with a shelf lesion.

common, particularly a retro-oesophageal origin. The position of the origin of the subclavian artery relative to the insertion of the duct or ligament determines the length of the aortic isthmus. Usually the isthmus is long. Occasionally, it is short or non-existent, in which case the orifice of the left subclavian artery is close to, or surrounded by, ductal tissue. Retro-oesophageal origin of a subclavian artery can also be found, most frequently with interruption.

The Influence of Flow

Intracardiac anomalies that encourage flow into the pulmonary rather than the aortic pathway during foetal life are frequently associated with both coarctation and interruption. In otherwise normal hearts, an unusual type of perimembranous ventricular septal defect with overriding of the aortic valve has been found to predominate. The right ventricular margin of the defect is often restricted by tissue tags derived from the tricuspid valve. In contrast, when there is interruption rather than coarctation there is usually posterior deviation of the outlet septum, or a fibrous remnant of the septum. Congenital mitral stenosis, or a supravalvar ring within the left atrium, are also linked to obstruction within the aortic arch. Hearts with abnormal connections, for instance a univentricular atrioventricular connection to a dominant left ventricle with discordant ventriculo-arterial connections and a restrictive ventricular septal defect, are also associated with coarctation. Coarctation may also be found in double outlet right ventricle or transposition when there is a restrictive subaortic infundibulum. The majority of hearts have lesions that favour flow through the pulmonary trunk, but there are some with defects that do not. Very rarely, examples are found with defects that produce a reduction in pulmonary flow.

Interruption of the Aortic Arch

This lesion is characterised by an absence of a segment of the aortic arch. The interrupted arch is usually left sided, but a few cases of interruption have been described in right arches. The three sites of interruption (Fig. 19.8) were designated Types A, B and C by Celoria and Patton. Our preference is to use descriptive terminology. Thus, interruption can be found at the isthmus (type A), between the left common carotid and left subclavian artery (type B), or between the brachiocephalic artery and the left common carotid artery (type C). The arterial duct is usually patent, channelling flow distal to the site of interruption to the lower body. Any of the types of interruption can be found with an aberrant origin, or isolation, of a subclavian artery. Isolation, however, is exceedingly rare. Interruption between the left common carotid and left subclavian arteries is most common in autopsy series (Fig. 19.9), and this form is more frequently associated with the Di George syndrome. Interruption at the isthmus (Fig. 19.10) is less common, but is more often associated with an aortopulmonary window. The third form, interruption between the carotid arteries, is very rare.

Interruption of the aortic arch is almost always associated with other congenital cardiovascular lesions. Patency of the arterial duct and a ventricular septal defect, in the setting of concordant ventriculo-arterial connections, is most common. The ventricular septal defect is characteristically of malalignment type with the outlet

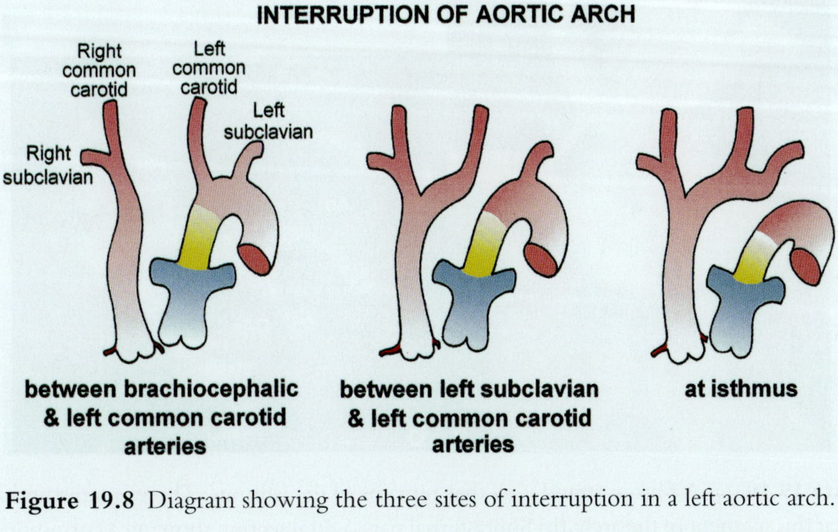

Figure 19.8 Diagram showing the three sites of interruption in a left aortic arch.

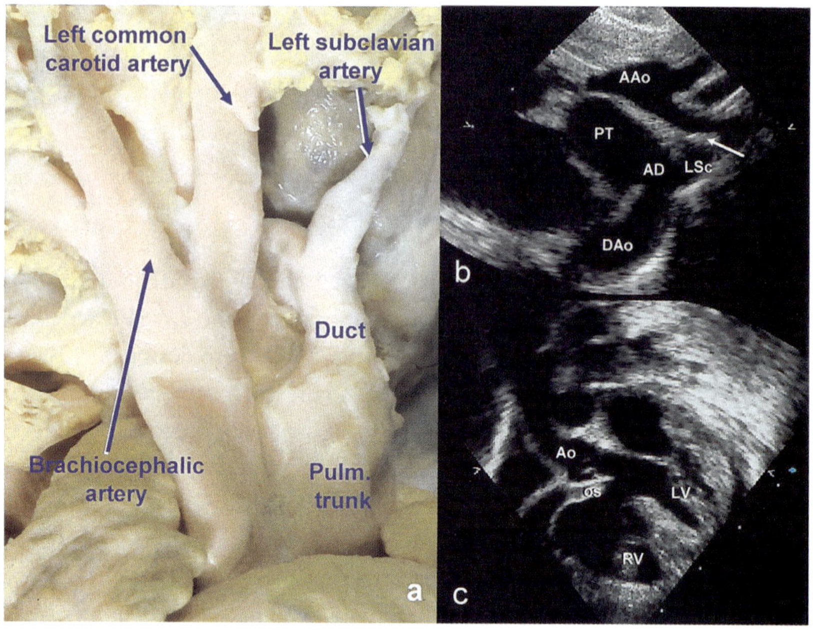

Figure 19.9 (a) The aortic arch is interrupted between the origins of the left common carotid artery and the left subclavian artery. Flow to the left subclavian artery and descending aorta is from the pulmonary trunk via the arterial duct. (b) Suprasternal parasagittal section showing interruption (arrow) of the aortic arch with the left subclavian artery (LSc) arising from the descending aorta (DAo) which is dependent on flow from the pulmonary trunk via the arterial duct (AD). (c) This subcostal section shows deviation of the outlet septum (OS) encroaching upon the left ventricular outflow tract.

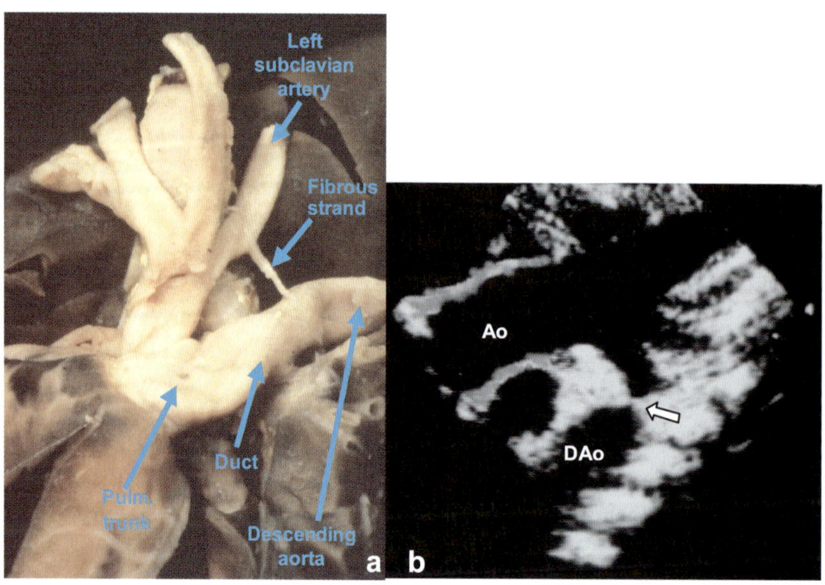

Figure 19.10 (a) A fibrous strand is all that remains of the isthmus. There is interruption of flow at this segment of the arch. (b) Suprasternal parasagittal section showing a corresponding site of interruption (arrow) probably due to a severe coarctation lesion.

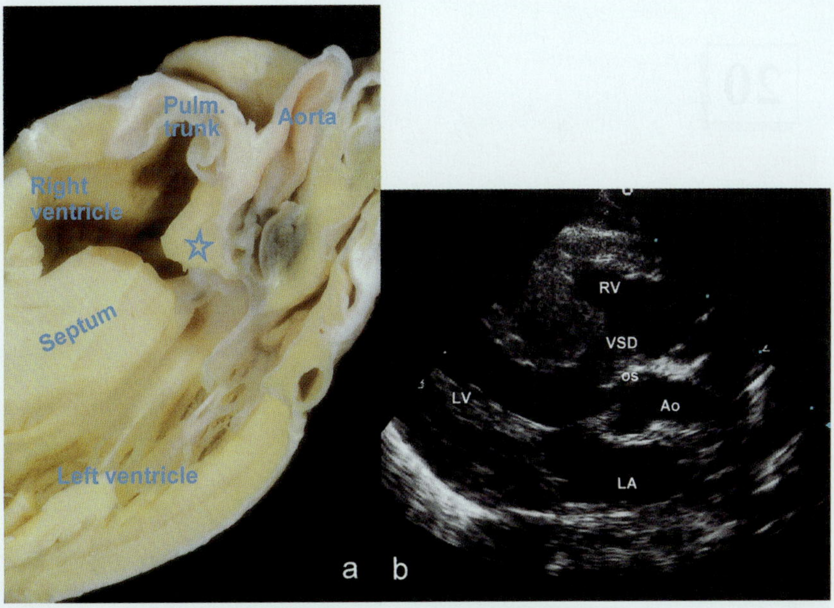

Figure 19.11 (a) Interruption of the aortic arch is frequently associated with deviation of the outlet septum (☆) into the left ventricle. (b) Echocardiogram showing malalignment of the outlet septum.

septum deviated posteriorly, narrowing the left ventricular outflow tract (Fig. 19.11). Hearts with doubly committed juxta-arterial defect, lacking an outlet septum, are also frequent. In some cases, the ventricular septum is intact, and flow to the distal arch occurs through an aorto-pulmonary window. Interruption of the arch can also exist in association with abnormal ventriculo-arterial connections, such as common arterial trunk, double outlet right ventricle with subpulmonary ventricular septal defect, and transposition and congenitally corrected transposition.

There are occasional reports of interruption of the arch as an isolated lesion. In these cases, the arterial duct is closed. Flow to the descending aorta occurs through profuse collateral arteries between the two separated segments. All three sites of interruption have been found in isolation.

20

The Arterial Duct

The arterial duct, an important channel in foetal circulation, usually closes spontaneously after birth. Patency of the arterial duct in postnatal life can occur as an isolated anomaly, in association with interruption or coarctation of the aortic arch, with aortic or pulmonary atresia, with intracardiac lesions, or as part of a vascular ring.

Normally, the duct arises from the left pulmonary artery very close to the bifurcation of the pulmonary trunk. It inserts into the aortic arch at the area of transition from the arch to the descending aorta (Fig. 20.1). The pulmonary end of the duct is covered by the reflection of the pericardium. In the newborn, the duct enters the aorta at its anterolateral aspect (Fig. 20.1), and is frequently seen bulging laterally beyond the border of the aorta. With growth, the duct or ligament joins the aorta more medially. Postero-inferiorly, the duct is related to the left main bronchus, while anteriorly it is crossed by the vagus nerve. The recurrent laryngeal nerve, arising from the vagus nerve, forms a loop under the duct near the aortic end before passing behind the aortic arch to ascend into the neck.

In the newborn, the duct is usually between 7 and 11 millimetres in length. When associated with pulmonary atresia, the duct is frequently described as long and meandering (Fig. 20.2). Rarely, the duct has no length at all. In the situation referred to as a window duct, the defect is a oval opening in the opposed walls of the aorta and pulmonary trunk (Fig. 20.3). The shape of the duct varies considerably. It may be cylindrical, take an hour-glass shape, be funnel shaped with constriction usually at the pulmonary end, or be aneurysmally dilated.

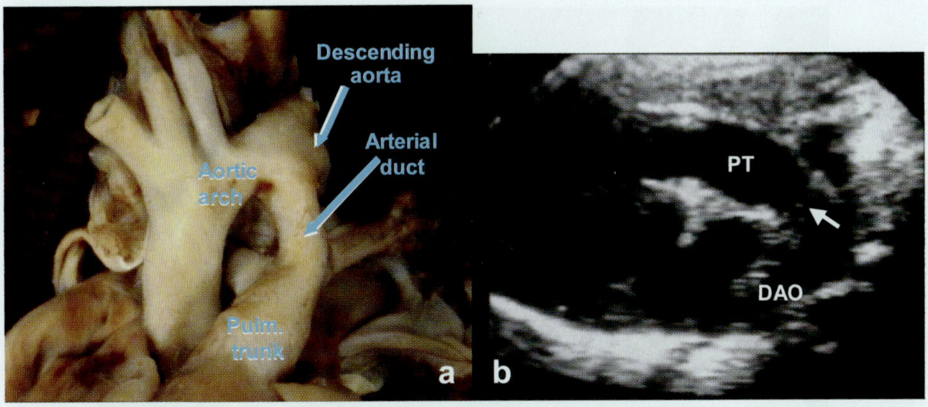

Figure 20.1 (a) The arterial duct in this newborn looks wide on the outside but intimal cushions are already well developed internally. (b) High parasternal long axis of the pulmonary trunk demonstrating a patent arterial duct (arrow) in a neonate.

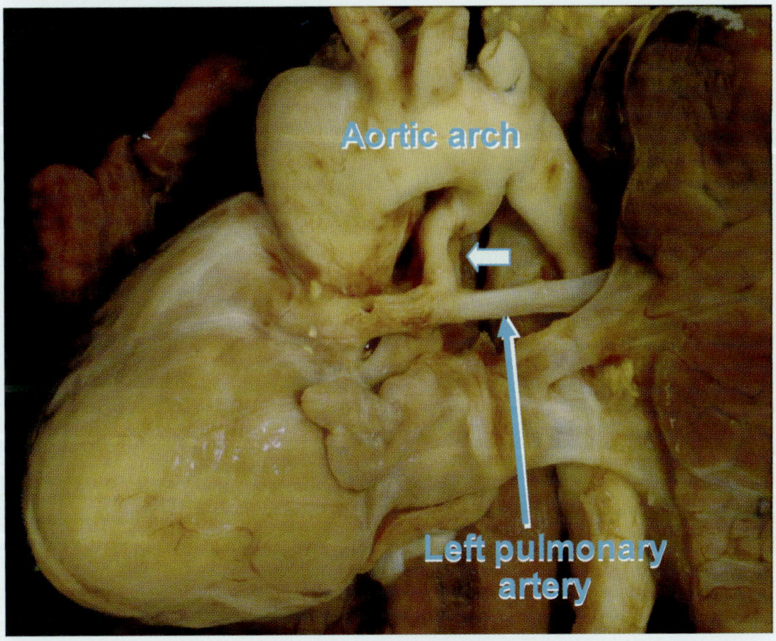

Figure 20.2 The arterial duct (arrow) is sigmoid shaped in this specimen with pulmonary atresia.

Normal Closure of the Arterial Duct

Functional closure of the arterial duct in the normal full term infant occurs within 10 to 15 hours of birth. The lumen is usually occluded by the second or third week, and the vessel ultimately becomes a fibrous ligament. The preparation for

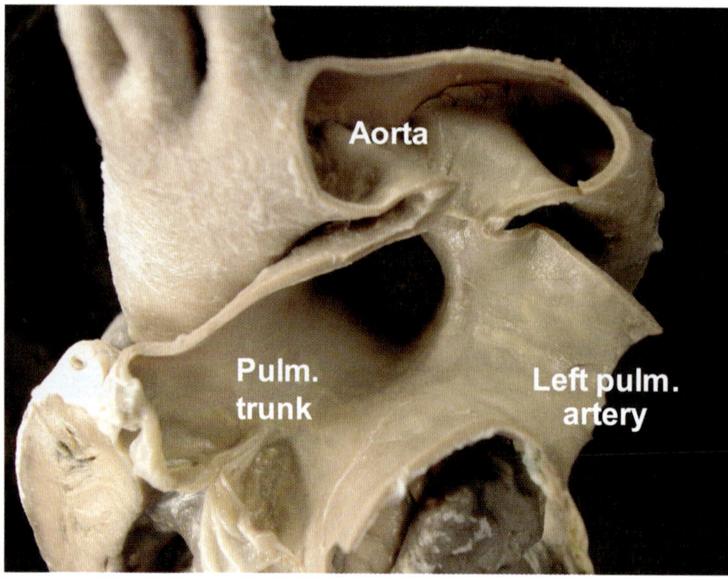

Figure 20.3 This duct in an adult specimen has hardly any length.

closure, however, begins several weeks before birth. The arterial duct is structurally different from its adjoining vessels, the aorta and the pulmonary artery. In gross dissection, the luminal surface of the newborn duct is less smooth than that of the great arteries, and has irregular ridges running lengthwise. Its wall is also thicker. Histologically, it is easily distinguished from the fibroelastic aorta and pulmonary trunk. The normal duct, near term, has an intima, a fragmented internal elastic lamina, a thick muscular media, and an adventitial layer. Intimal cushions or mounds, composed of smooth muscle and strands of elastic tissue, protrude into the lumen. The inner media has a longitudinal arrangement of muscle bundles, whereas the muscle bundles in the outer media are circularly arranged. At birth, the distal wall is constricted by coincident contracture of the muscle fibres. The lumen is closed anatomically by postnatal intimal proliferation, a progressive process taking up to three months, finally converting the duct to a fibrous strand.

Persistent Patency of the Arterial Duct

When the duct remains patent in infants older than three months, it is considered to be persistently patent. This situation applies to infants born at term, and is distinct from delayed ductal closure in preterm neonates. Delayed closure is also seen in infants that are small for dates, and infants born by caesarian section. These ducts progress to close normally. The persistent duct, in contrast, remains as an undesirable shunt. The flow is usually from the aorta to the pulmonary trunk, resulting in increased flow of blood to the lungs and overload of the left heart. On histological

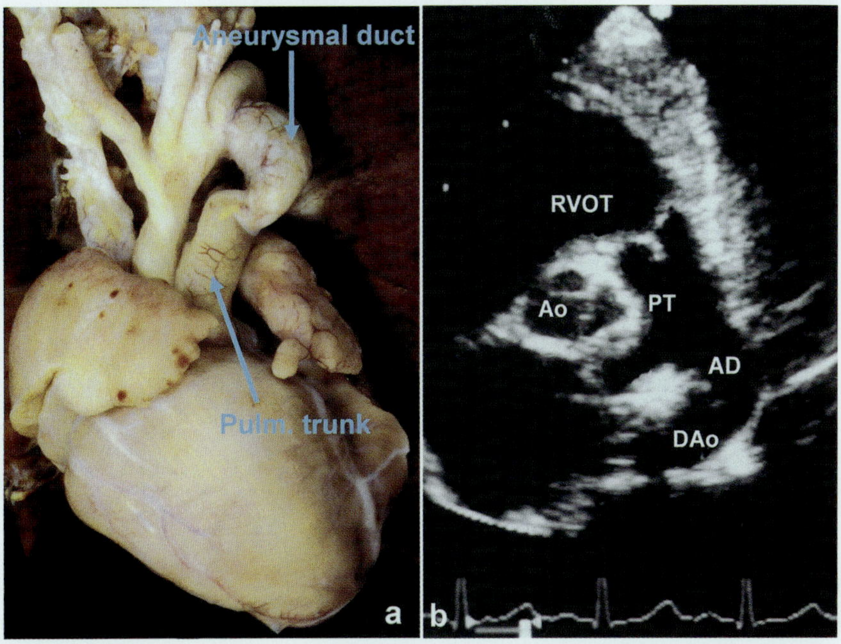

Figure 20.4 (a) This aneurysmal duct is closed at its pulmonic end. (b) Suprasternal section showing a widely patent arterial duct.

examination, the persistently patent duct is characterised by preservation of an intact elastic lamina.

Aneurysm of the Arterial Duct

True aneurysm of the duct is rare, although more than sixty cases have been reported in the literature. These are regarded as congenital, since they develop in the setting of persistently patent ducts. Ductal closure usually begins at the pulmonary arterial end of the vessel. If the aortic end fails to close, an aortic diverticulum develops, which occasionally progresses to become aneurysmal. Two types of ductal aneurysm are recognised clinically. The type found in infancy has a closed pulmonary arterial end and an open aortic end (Fig. 20.4). The other type, manifest in childhood or adulthood, is patent at both ends. The likely complications of both types are rupture, dissection, embolisation and effects of pressure on neighbouring structures.

Index

D

P

U

V

W

X

Z